OCCUPATIONAL LUNG DISEASE

CONTEMPORARY ISSUES in PULMONARY DISEASE
Volume 2

SERIES EDITORS

Neil S. Cherniack, M.D.
Professor of Medicine
Chief, Division of Pulmonary Medicine
Case Western Reserve University School of Medicine
Veterans Administration Medical Center
Cleveland, Ohio

Norman H. Edelman, M.D.
Professor of Medicine and Physiology
Chief, Pulmonary Diseases Division
Rutgers Medical School
New Brunswick, New Jersey

Volumes Already Published

Vol. 1 Chronic Obstructive Pulmonary Disease
Hugo D. Montenegro, M.D., Editor

Forthcoming Volumes in the Series

Vol. 3 Pulmonary Circulation
Edward H. Bergofsky, M.D., Editor

Vol. 4 Noninvasive Monitoring in Pulmonary Disease
Michael L. Nochomovitz, M.D., and Neil S. Cherniack, M.D., Editors

Vol. 5 Sleep and Breathing
Norman H. Edelman, M.D., Editor

OCCUPATIONAL LUNG DISEASE

Edited by

J. Bernard L. Gee, M.D.

Professor of Medicine
Department of Internal Medicine
Yale University School of Medicine
New Haven, Connecticut

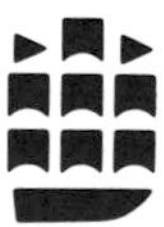

CHURCHILL LIVINGSTONE
NEW YORK, EDINBURGH, LONDON, AND MELBOURNE
1984

Acquisitions editor: William R. Schmitt
Copy editor: Peggy Brigg
Production editor: Karen Goldsmith Montanez
Production supervisor: Joe Sita
Compositor: Bi-Comp, Inc.
Printer/Binder: The Maple-Vail Book Manufacturing Group

Distributed in the United Kingdom by Churchill Livingstone, Robert Stevenson House, 1-3 Baxter's Place, Leith Walk, Edinburgh EH13AF and by associated companies, branches and representatives throughout the world.

First published 1984
Printed in U.S.A.

ISBN 0-443-08252-9
7 6 5 4 3 2 1

Library of Congress Cataloging in Publication Data
Main entry under title:

Occupational lung disease.

(Contemporary issues in pulmonary disease; v. 2)
Bibliography: p.
Includes index.
1. Lungs--Dust diseases. 2. Occupational diseases.
I. Gee, J. Bernard L. II. Series. [DNLM: 1. Lung Diseases.
2. Occupational Diseases. 3. Pneumoconiosis.
W1 C0769MRS v.2 / WF 600 0151]
RC773.028 1984 616.2'44 84-11349
ISBN 0-443-08252-9

Manufactured in the United States of America

Contributors

Mario C. Batigelli, M.D.
Professor of Medicine and Environmental Health, University of North Carolina School of Medicine, Chapel Hill, North Carolina

Gerald J. Beck, Ph.D.
Associate Professor of Biostatistics, Yale University, School of Medicine, New Haven, Connecticut

Margaret R. Becklake, M.D.
Professor of Medicine and Epidemiology and Health, McGill University, Montreal, Quebec, Canada

Jean Bignon, M.D.
Professor of Medicine, University of Paris-Val de Marne, Clinique de Pathologie Respiratoire et Environement, Creteil, France

Brian Boehlecke, M.D.
Associate Professor of Medicine, University of North Carolina School of Medicine, Chapel Hill, North Carolina

Brian T. Butcher, Ph.D.
Associate Professor of Medicine, Tulane University Medical Center, New Orleans, Louisiana

Ronald P. Daniele, M.D.
Professor of Medicine and Pathology, Cardiovascular-Pulmonary Division, University of Pennsylvania School of Medicine, Philadelphia, Pennsylvania

Guillermo A. doPico, M.D.
Professor of Medicine, University of Wisconsin Medical School, Madison, Wisconsin

Pierre Ernst, M.D.
Assistant Professor, School of Occupational Health, McGill University, Montreal, Quebec, Canada

J. Bernard L. Gee, M.D.
Director, Occupational Lung Disease Clinic, Department of Internal Medicine, Yale University School of Medicine, New Haven, Connecticut

Yehia Y. Hammad, D.Sc.
Associate Professor of Medicine, Tulane University Medical Center, New Orleans, Louisiana

David J. Hendrick, M.D.
Consultant Chest Physician, Newcastle General Hospital, Newcastle-upon-Tyne, England

Marie-Claude Jaurand, Ph.D.
Unité de Recherches sur la Biopathologie Rénale et Pulmonaire, Inserm U139, Creteil, France

James E. Lockey, M.D.
Assistant Professor of Medicine, Division of Respiratory, Critical Care, and Occupational (Pulmonary) Medicine, Rocky Mountain Center for Occupational and Environmental Health, University of Utah College of Medicine, Salt Lake City, Utah

Farhad Moatamed, M.D.
Assistant Professor of Pathology, University of Utah School of Medicine; Electron Microscopy Laboratory, Veterans Administration Medical Center, Salt Lake City, Utah

W. K. C. Morgan, M.D.
Professor of Medicine, University of Western Ontario; Director, Chest Diseases Service, University Hospital, London, Ontario, Canada

Attilio D. Renzetti, Jr., M.D.
Professor of Medicine; Chief, Division of Respiratory, Critical Care, and Occupational (Pulmonary) Medicine, Department of Internal Medicine, University of Utah School of Medicine, Salt Lake City, Utah

David J. Riley, M.D.
Associate Professor of Medicine, UMDNJ-Rutgers Medical School, New Brunswick, New Jersey

Ragnar Rylander, M.D.
Department of Environmental Medicine, University of Gothenberg, Gothenberg, Sweden

E. Neil Schachter, M.D.
Associate Professor of Medicine, Yale University School of Medicine, New Haven, Connecticut

Preface

This volume is intended to provide an in-depth coverage of currently important topics in occupational lung disease and thereby complement the more compressed information available in the standard textbooks on the subject. The topic of occupational lung disease extends from basic biologic, scientific mechanisms to public health policy and hence legislation. Between these poles, clinicians of many disciplines are essential, including those who see the disorders first, namely the chest physicians and physicians practicing with either industry or labor affiliations; industrial hygienists; public health and occupational nurses; and toxicologists. We believe this volume contains material of interest to all these professionals, even though both the editor and the international group of authors have a major focus on lung disease.

In addition to a spread of interest among professional disciplines, we have sought to consider a geographical range of interests. Thus, aside from the classic subjects of miners and minerals, we have addressed the major problem of the American South, the cotton industry, and the more geographically widespread problems of farming, animal husbandry, and the rural environment in general.

A few comments on some specific chapters are in order. The first chapter describes the biochemistry of pulmonary fibrosis, the most common form of irreversible dysfunction in the occupational setting. A later chapter deals with the use of specific immunological challenge in identifying beryllium lung disease. Two chapters describe fiber toxicology, covering asbestos and nonasbestos fibers. The extent of the asbestos-related health problems and their financial costs to society, estimated at $18.2 billion dollars, makes understanding fiber toxicology essential if the newer man-made fibers (e.g., fiberglass) are not to cause history to repeat itself. Additionally, with regard to asbestos, its relation to airway damage is carefully reviewed. This issue has been frequently raised in the course of the presently continual asbestos litigation.

Occupational asthma in its classical aspect has received much attention already, but we believe the Tulane group herein gives us a unique and practical account of how to identify the responsible agents. From this chapter, which gives much detail, it is clear that while some previously recognized agents can easily be inculpated in a particular patient setting, others require both persistence and extensive facilities.

The hazards of the rural environment are not usual features in the dreams of the city dweller. Living in the country is one thing, but Dr. doPico gives us a practical and encyclopedic account of the hazards of working in the country.

The chapters on byssinosis indicate the need for more mechanistic studies and also highlight the often heated controversy over the long-term effects of cotton dust on airway function. The readers may judge the evidence for themselves!

Finally, we include more general health considerations. There is much popular current demand for monitoring the health of the worker. Much emotion, activist vigor, and fiscal resources are already involved by industry, labor, and certain segments of society. Dr. Boehlecke's chapter brings us back to the reality of what this entails, if it is not to be an expensive, fruitless, and even anxiety provoking endeavor. Dr. W. Keith C. Morgan provides some pungent comments on how workplace health standards (for silica) should NOT be set. Dr. Renzetti extends the critique by addressing the Black Lung Act as an example of how NOT to design legislation to meet the socially and humanistically essential needs of compensating the workers suffering from occupational lung diseases.

J. Bernard L. Gee, M.D.

Acknowledgments

The editor expresses appreciation for the thoroughness and lucidity with which the authors have expressed their thoughts. Additionally, he acknowledges the support of the offices of Churchill Livingstone and thanks his secretary, Mrs. Margaret Chase, for her continued organizational and secretarial support.

Contents

1 Pulmonary Connective Tissue in Occupational Lung Disease

David J. Riley

The connective tissue network of the lung supports the airways, pulmonary vasculature, and cells lining the airspaces. This framework is normally thin and spread over a large surface area so gas exchange is not impeded. The connective tissue gives the lung its elasticity, acts as a tether to prevent overdistension, and provides a scaffold on which injured lung cells are replaced by normal cells.

Aberrations of the normal connective tissue of the lung occur in two major groups of noninfectious disease of the lungs: pulmonary emphysema and pulmonary fibrosis. Emphysema is thought to be caused by destruction of the elastin component of the connective tissue. Pulmonary fibrosis is characterized by an excess accumulation of connective tissue, particularly collagen, and destruction of the normal architecture of the lung parenchyma. The environmental lung diseases of major importance produce pulmonary fibrosis. In this review most of the emphasis will be the biochemistry of collagen and mechanisms of fibrosis. Acute toxic inhalations, however, may result in destruction of lung connective tissue. Therefore, proteolysis of connective tissue will also be considered.

The purpose of this chapter is threefold: (1) to define the connective tissue of the normal lung and discuss mechanisms controlling its presence; (2) to summarize current concepts of altered connective tissue in acute lung injury produced by exposure to exogenous toxic substances; and (3) to discuss fibrogenesis of lung produced by exogenous substances.

I do not attempt to review all aspects of pulmonary connective tissue in environmental lung diseases in this chapter. For more information, the reader is referred to reviews covering collagen,[1–3] elastin,[4] connective tissue in the normal and diseased lung,[5–9] mechanisms of fibrosis,[10] and mechanisms of fibrosis in occupational lung diseases.[11–12]

CONNECTIVE TISSUE OF THE NORMAL LUNG

Collagen

Identification of Collagen. *Collagen* is a term applied to a group of closely related structural proteins. Strictly speaking, collagen is a protein molecule consisting of three separate polypeptide chains, called α chains, which are arranged in a triple helix. *Procollagen* is a precursor of collagen and consists of three pro-α chains. Procollagen contains two nonhelical domains on terminal extensions, which are enzymatically cleaved off the procollagen molecule to yield collagen (Fig. 1-1). *Collagen fibrils* is an ordered array of crosslinked collagen molecules found in the extracellular matrix; under the electron microscope they range in size from 5 Å to several thousand angstroms in diameter. *Collagen fibers* are bundles of collagen fibrils which can be seen under the light microscope and are 0.10–15 μm in diameter.

Composition and Structure. Collagen exists as a highly crosslinked insoluble fiber and is difficult to extract from adult tissue. Detailed analysis of the collagen molecule shows that it consists of three α chains consisting of about 1000 amino acid residues each having a molecular weight of 95,000. The three α chains are twisted around each other and the helical structure is very specific so that the bend of the peptide chain has a regular pitch (Fig. 1-1). In order to accommodate the pitch of the helix, a small amino acid, glycine, is present every third amino acid in the sequence. The presence of a glycine every third amino acid results in the repeated sequence $[X\text{-}Y\text{-gly}]_n$, where X and Y are other amino acids. These other amino acids are often proline and hydroxyproline, so that collagen contains a relatively high content of glycine, proline, and hydroxyproline.

The triple helix is stabilized by hydrogen bonds between amino and carbonyl groups on adjacent chains. In addition, other covalent bonds and water molecules bound to the molecule may contribute to its stability. The helical structure of the molecule is reflected by the viscous property of collagen when in solution. This property is lost when the conformation is disrupted by heating, a process called denaturation, which yields a gel-like material called gelatin.

The physical properties of collagen are well suited to its role as a structural protein. The ropelike quality of the triple helix gives the molecule high tensile strength, yet the fiber is flexible. In the lung, collagen is thought to act like a tether in the alveolar wall to prevent overexpansion and rupture of the delicate lung parenchyma.

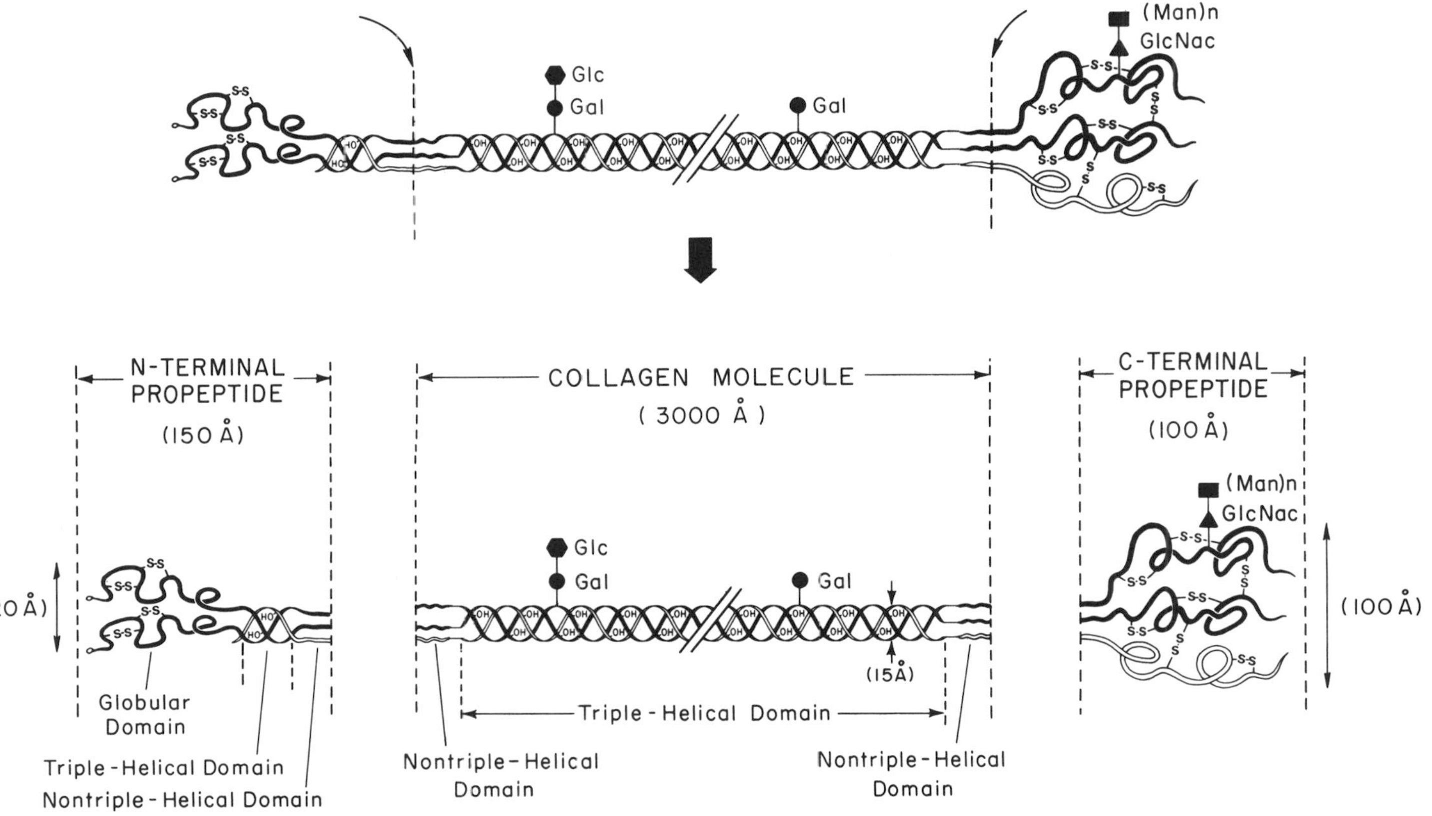

Fig. 1-1 Structure of the procollagen molecule. The procollagen molecule consists of a central helical portion and two propeptide extensions, one at the C-terminal end and the other at the N-terminal end of the molecule. The peptide chains at the propeptide extensions are linked by disulfide bonds. The procollagen molecule is linked to simple sugars. (Reprinted, by permission of the New England Journal of Medicine, from Prockop DJ, Kivirikko KI, Tuderman L, et al: The biosynthesis of collagen and its disorders. N Engl J Med 301:13, 1979.)

Types and Distribution of Collagen. In the lung, there are five types of collagen with structurally distinct properties. The distinction between types is based on the amino acid composition of the α chains. The type of collagen depends on the combination of α chains in the molecule. Roman numerals are used to designate the major types of collagen.

Type I collagen contains two different α chains; there are two $\alpha 1(I)$ chains and one $\alpha 2$ chain in each triple helix. This is designated as $[\alpha 1(I)]_2\alpha 2$. Type I collagen is the largest component of collagen in the lung, contributing about 60% of all collagen. It is found in largest amounts associated with pulmonary blood vessels and the alveolar interstitium. Type I fibers form parallel arrays and have cross-striated fibers with a regular periodicity, as seen in the electron microscope.

Type II collagen contains three α chains all of the same type, designated as $[\alpha 1(II)]_3$. In the lung, Type II collagen is found only in cartilagenous rings of the trachea and in irregular plates on the bronchial walls. This type of collagen forms a fibrillar network that supplies rigidity to the proteoglycan component of cartilage.

Type III collagen also contains three identical α chains, $[\alpha 1(III)]_3$. Type III collagen generally has the same distribution in the lung as type I collagen and is the second largest component of collagen in the lung, contributing about 30% of all collagen. It is found in the interstitium and surrounds the openings of the alveolar ducts. It appears as an irregular network of fibrils under the electron microscope and does not have the periodocity found in Type I collagen.

Type IV collagen is confined exclusively to basement membranes. Two distinct polypeptide chains, $\alpha 1(IV)$ and $\alpha 2(IV)$, have been isolated and characterized. A third component, designated 7S collagen, has been isolated and is thought to be the crosslinking region of Type IV collagen. There are two basement membranes of the lung, one found under the alveolar epithelium and one under the capillary endothelium. Basement membranes are complex structures and may contain several types of collagenous proteins.

Type V collagen is also found in basement membranes. This collagen consists of chains αA and αB and has been designated AB_2. The function of this type of collagen is presently not understood. It has been identified in bronchial basement membrane, bronchial epithelium, and basement membranes in the lung.

The basement membranes in the lung cover a large surface area and play an important role in regulating fluid flux between compartments of the lung. Basement membranes are also thought to provide a framework for the cellular constituents of the lung. In this regard, the basement membrane may play a role in directing repair of cellular constituents after tissue injury. Collagenous proteins in the basement membrane may also provide relative rigidity to basement membranes.

Biosynthesis of Collagen. Collagen synthesis occurs in a sequence of steps. These steps can be divided into two major stages: intracellular processing and modification of procollagen, and extracellular conversion of procollagen to collagen and the incorporation of collagen molecules into covalently crosslinked fibrils (Fig. 1-2).

Collagen synthesis begins with the transcription of genetic information in DNA. The production of each pro-α chain is under the control of a separate gene. Recent work has led to the isolation of a mRNA for Type I collagen and DNA fragments corresponding to sections of the genetic message for collagen.[13] The isolation of these genes is expected to be useful in determining abnormalities of certain hereditary disorders of connective tissue, such as osteogenesis imperfecta and the Ehlers-Danlos syndromes.

Like all proteins, pro-α chains are synthesized on membrane-bound ribosomes and are processed in the cisternal space of the rough endoplasmic reticulum. The initial pro-α chains synthesized have globular extensions at the amino terminal ends, which act as "signal" sequences to direct the pro-α chains into the rough endoplasmic reticulum. These signal sequences are cleaved before completion of protein synthesis.

Within the rough endoplasmic reticulum are hydroxylating enzymes that result in the conversion of prolyl residues to hydroxyprolyl residues. This reaction is mediated by the enzyme prolyl hydroxylase and requires the availability of several cofactors (Fig. 1-2). The hydroxylation reaction is critical for collagen formation, since only hydroxylated pro-α chains will fold into triple helical conformation. If fewer than a critical number of prolyl residues remain unhydroxylated, a stable triple helix does not form and the pro-α chains undergo degradation.

The presence of the enzyme prolyl hydroxylase and its increased activity during fibrogenesis have been of interest as a possible mechanism regulating collagen accumulation. However, it is currently believed that hydroxylation of prolyl residues is not rate limiting for collagen synthesis. Nevertheless, the parallel increase in prolyl hydroxylase activity and increased collagen synthesis has made measurement of the enzyme level a useful tool for detecting fibrogenesis.

A step which may be important in regulating collagen synthesis is the intracellular degradation of newly synthesized pro-α chains. In fetal cell cultures from rabbits, 20–30% of all newly synthesized collagen is degraded intracellularly.[14] It has been suggested that this mechanism selectively destroys "defective" pro-α chains,[15] but the importance of this mechanism in the overall regulation of collagen synthesis remains to be determined.

Nondegraded pro-α chains next undergo linkage to simple sugars. This occurs in two steps, and the attachment of sugar moieties to the proteins are thought to be necessary for later exocytosis of the procollagen molecule from the cell.

At this point in synthesis, the pro-α chains have to be brought together in order to intertwine to form a triple helix. This is brought about by the formation of disulfide linkages in the carboxypeptide extensions of the pro-α chains. Once the disulfide bonds bring the pro-α chains into alignment, spontaneous triple helical formation occurs. The next event after procollagen synthesis is the

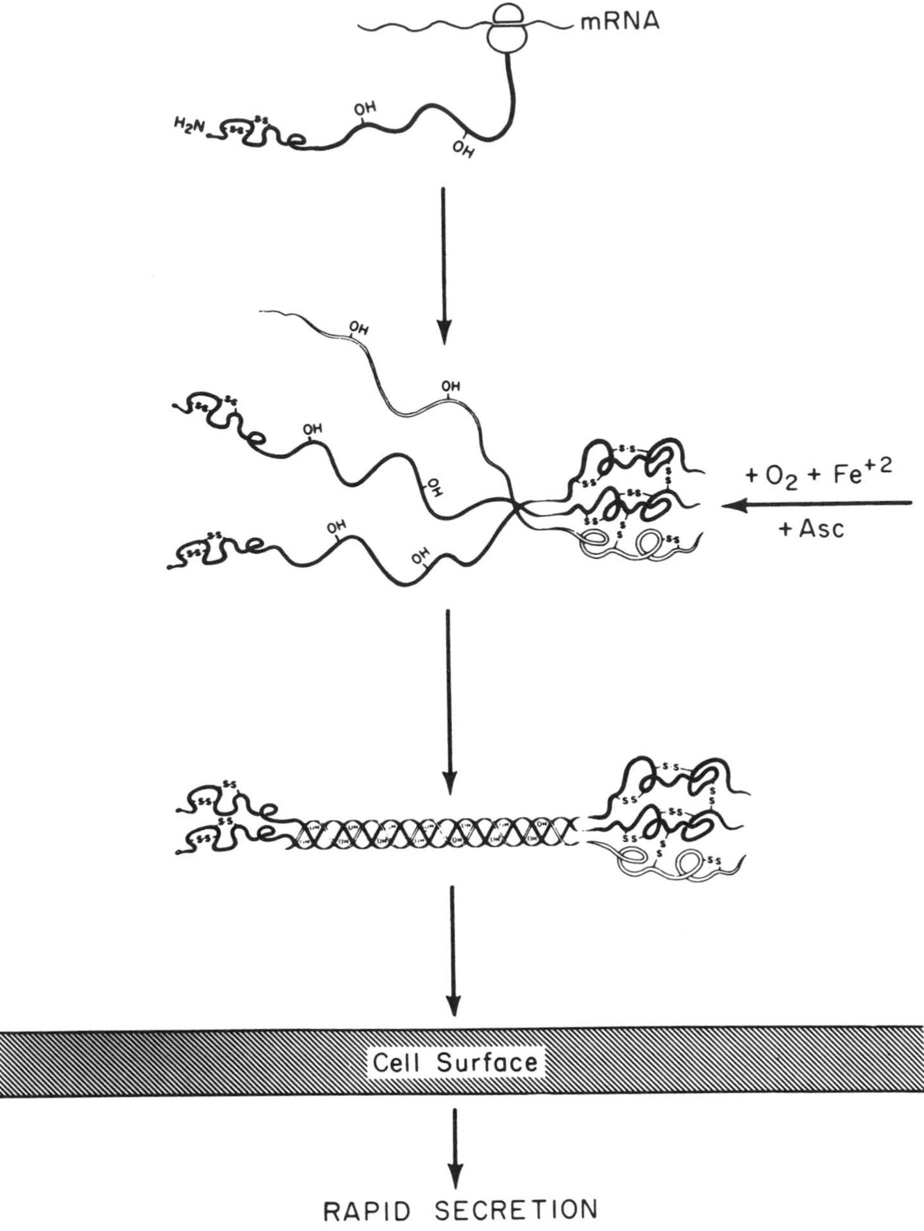

Fig. 1-2 Scheme of intracellular synthesis and processing of procollagen molecules. Pro α chains are synthesized in ribosomes in the rough endoplasmic reticulum. The prolyl and lysyl residues are hydroxylated by the enzyme lysyl oxidase (arrow) which requires the cofactors molecular oxygen, ferrous iron, and ascorbate. The molecule then undergoes triple helical formation and is secreted from the cell. (Reprinted, by permission of the New England Journal of Medicine, from Prockop DJ, Kivirikko KI, Tuderman L, et al: The biosynthesis of collagen and its disorders. N Engl J Med 301:13, 1979.)

packaging of procollagen molecules into Golgi vacuoles and the secretion from the cell into the extracellular matrix.

The series of extracellular steps is almost as complex as the intracellular steps. After secretion, the first step is the enzymatic removal of the terminal extensions, called propeptides, from both ends of the pro-α chains. These propeptides may play a role in regulating collagen synthesis, since in cultured tissue cells propeptides of Type I collagen have been found to inhibit Type I collagen production.[16] The measurement of these propeptides may be of value in detecting fibrosis, since elevated blood levels of one propeptide to Type III collagen has been found in humans with fibrosing liver diseases.[17] It might be possible to detect propeptide fragments in lung lavage fluid from patients with pulmonary fibrosis to provide an index of collagen synthesis.

After cleavage of the propeptide extensions, the product is a collagen molecule (Fig. 1-1). These newly formed collagen molecules have less tensile strength and are more soluble in salt solutions than "mature" collagen molecules. The "immature" collagen molecules undergo covalent linkage, which produces great tensile strength and causes the molecule to be much less soluble in salt solutions.

The crosslinking step involves several stages. The first step is the oxidative deamination of lysyl and hydroxylysyl residues by the enzyme lysyl oxidase. This produces reactive aldehyde groups, which participate in two major types of crosslinking reactions: condensation of two aldehyde groups and a condensation between an aldehyde group and an amino group.

The enzyme lysyl oxidase, which produces the reactive aldehyde groups needed for the crosslinking reactions, has been extensively studied. Its activity increases in tissues undergoing scar formation, and it has been used as a marker for increased rate of extracellular collagen formation. The activity of lysyl oxidase can be decreased by copper deficiency, since copper is a required cofactor. Lysyl oxidase can also be inhibited by lathyrogens such as β-aminoproprionile and DL-penicillamine. Lysyl oxidase is genetically deficient in a strain of mice called blotchy mice. Interference with crosslinking produced by copper deficiency,[18] β-aminopropionitrile,[19] and in the blotchy mouse[20] produces an emphysemalike picture, suggesting that intramolecular crosslinking is important in maintaining stability of the alveolar walls in normal lungs.

The precise mechanics that control this assembly of the fibril during growth and tissue repair remain unknown. It is probable that the initial stages of fibril formation occurs in secretory vacuoles within the cells prior to extracellular secretion.[21] There are probably a number of pathways by which lateral and longitudinal association of collagen molecules occur. It is possible that noncollagenous material surrounding the collagen fibrils, such as proteoglycans, glycoproteins, and fibronectin, affect fibril growth. Also, frictional forces may play a role in directing collagen fibril deposition.

Lung Cells Involved in Collagen Production. Several lung cells are involved in collagen production,[8] the most important of which is the fibroblast. The endothelial, epithelial, and smooth muscle cells may also contribute to collagen production in the lung. A wide variety of stimuli may be responsible for controlling the lung cells that produce collagen, but these factors are largely undefined. It is postulated that some factors may act through recruitment of cells, while others induce mitogenesis of cells committed to fibroblastic activity. Furthermore, there may be transformation of the normal population of cells of the lung to cells with enhanced potential to produce collagen.

Degradation of Collagen. The metabolic turnover of collagen in the normal adult lung is slow. The normal production of collagen is balanced by an equivalent rate of catabolism so that the net amount of collagen remains the same. The major mechanism modulating collagen degradation is tissue collagenases or enzymes that specifically degrade collagen molecules. Although collagenases are the major enzymes initiating the process of collagen breakdown, some nonspecific neutral proteases[22] and an "elastase"[23] have been recently reported to degrade collagen molecules at neutral pH. In addition, cathepsin B, an enzyme located in lysosomes, can degrade collagen at acid pH.[24] Once collagenase cleaves the native collagen molecule at a specific site, the cleaved fragment uncoils and becomes susceptible to degradation by less specific tissue proteases.

Since tissue collagenase is the key enzyme in degradation of collagen, it would seem that measuring tissue activity of this enzyme might be a way to assess degradation of collagen. However, there are a number of problems inherent in measuring the activity of this enzyme in tissue.[25,26] First, there are potent inhibitors of the enzyme in serum and tissue, the most important of which is α_2-macroglobulin. Second, there is a large pool of latent enzymes, which may be activated by a variety of factors. Third, there are several types of collagenases specific for collagen types. Finally, the several types of collagens have variable resistences to collagenases. Because of this complexity of factors, it has proven difficult to relate tissue collagenolytic activity to degradation of collagen.

The source of collagenase in the normal lung is primarily the fibroblasts, but in some species macrophages contribute a small amount.[5,26] Collagenase from the fibroblast is released in an inactive form and must be activated by a neutral proteinase. The neutrophil, which is not normally present in the lung, can release large amounts of active collagenase, and this is considered an important source of collagenolytic activity in lung injury.

Regulation of Collagen Synthesis. Relatively little is known about factors that regulate collagen biosynthesis, deposition, and degradation. In regard to collagen biosynthesis, information at the level of transcription and translation is just beginning to accumulate because of the recent application of recombinant DNA technology.[13] These techniques should shortly be applied to the study of the normal production of collagen in tissues and cells. It is now possible, for example, to measure the rate of collagen production by measuring the level of mRNA for pro-α chains.[13]

The posttranslational steps in collagen synthesis are well known, but factors that control these steps are poorly defined. Earlier studies showed that several poorly characterized factors from exudative cells and experimentally injured tissues stimulate collagen synthesis.[10] Also, factors from normal macrophages have been shown to be capable of stimulating fibroblast proliferation[27] and collagen biosynthesis by the fibroblast.[28] Factors that stimulate the intracellular levels of cyclic AMP, such as prostaglandin E_1 and β-agonists, have been found to decrease the rate of collagen synthesis.[29] In summary, it is possible that stimulatory signals from the inflammatory process stimulate fibroblast proliferation and collagen production. Once repair has been established, factors that inhibit collagen synthesis may be secreted and terminate the repair process.

Noncollagenous Connective Tissue of the Lung

The other connective tissue components of the lung are elastin, proteoglycans, and fibronectin. Elastin clearly influences the structure and function of the normal and diseased lung. The roles of proteoglycans and fibronectin in the normal and diseased lung are largely undefined. There is little need to extensively discuss the biochemistry of noncollagenous connective tissue. Several reviews of elastin,[4,30] proteoglycans,[30] and fibronectin[31] are available.

Elastin. Elastin represents about 30–35% of the connective tissue of the normal lung. Elastin is a heterogeneous material with both amorphous and fibrillar components. The fibrillar constituents, called microfibrils, are elongated structures lying within the amorphous component in a semiparallel array. The amorphous component is synthesized initially as tropoelastin chains. The chains subsequently undergo crosslinking, which requires the enzyme lysyl oxidase. This enzyme converts a lysyl residue in tropoelastin to an aldehyde, which subsequently joins three other lysyl groups in tropoelastin chains to form crosslinks. The chemical composition of this crosslinked region is thus composed of four amino acids and is called desmosine. Desmosine linkages are unique to elastin, and their presence in body fluids and tissue is a convenient "marker" for elastin. Little is known about elastin biosynthesis or the factors that control its rate of synthesis and degradation. The source of elastin in the lung is not identified, but is likely to be the fibroblast and smooth muscle cell.

The degradation of elastin occurs very slowly in adult lung tissue. The major mechanism controlling elastin breakdown is the enzyme elastase, although it is likely that a number of other enzymes are involved in elastin breakdown. There has been a great deal of interest in factors which control elastolysis in the lung because this process is central to the development of emphysema.[32]

Elastic fibers are highly compliant and possess rubberlike elastic properties. This property of the elastic fiber is presumed to be responsible for the elasticlike tissue mechanical properties of the lung. Compared to collagen, elastin has high extensibility and low tensile strength. How this feature of elastin affects the mechanical properties of the lung is uncertain because of the complex anatomic and biochemical interactions of the various components of connective tissue.

There has been little investigation of the role of elastin in lung fibrosis. In bleomycin-induced fibrosis in the hamster. there is a proportionate increase in the amount of both collagen and elastin in the lung.[32] This suggests that there is a common avenue of stimulation for increased synthetic rates of both collagen and elastin, but the factors that cause this response remain to be identified. In the bleomycin model, the number of desmosine crosslinks per elastin molecule remained the same as normal,[33] suggesting that there is no qualitative change in lung elastin in bleomycin-induced fibrosis.

Proteoglycans. Proteoglycans are composed of a core of protein with polysaccharide side chains called glycosaminoglycans. In the parenchyma of the adult lung, there are six types glycosaminoglycans with the following approximate proportions: hyaluronic acid, 10%; hyaluronate-4-sulfate, 20%; dermatin sulfate, 30%; heparin and heparin sulfate, 35%.[30] Proteoglycans form large aggregates in the interstitium of the lung, and the composition of the glycosaminoglycans varies with age. Proteoglycans are most abundant in the trachea and are less dense in the lung parenchyma. Since glycosaminoglycans have viscous properties in solution, they may play a role in lung compliance. Another postulated role of proteoglycans is that they may function as a charge-dependent filtering barrier in basement membranes, similar to their postulated role in the glomerulus. In the developing lung, proteoglycans may direct collagen fibril formation and may be important in cell attachment. In the adult lung, they may influence cell renewal during repair of lung injury.

Several experimental studies have demonstrated increases in lung glycosaminoglycan content after lung injury produced by silica exposure[34,35] and after endotracheal instillation of bleomycin,[36] N-nitroso-N-methylurethane,[37] and amosite asbestos.[38] It appears that glycosaminoglycan content increases in parallel with other connective tissue components as a general response to fibrotic lung injury. Whether the increased viscous properties of glycosaminoglycans account for the increased tissue resistance in the fibrotic lung is unknown.

Fibronectin. Fibronectin is a large glycoprotein that used to be known as "cold insoluble globulin" when measured in blood. In the lung, it is found in insoluble form in basement membranes and it forms a loose matrix that is found throughout the interstitium.[31] Fibronectin appears to play a critical role in cell–cell and cell–matrix adhesion. Fibronectin is secreted from cells and is deposited in the extracellular matrix where it binds to collagen, proteoglycons, and other matrix components. As a result of these multiple interactions, fibronectin probably functions as an adhesive glycoprotein. Moreover, it is secreted from human alveolar macrophages and may serve as an endogenous factor to promote the binding of bacterial, connective tissue degradation products, and other macromolecules to the alveolar macrophages.[39] In lung disorders, the role for fibronectin remains to be clarified. Fibronectin levels in the bronchopulmonary lavage fluid of patients with interstitial lung disease is elevated compared to normals.[40] It has been postulated that fibronectin produced by the human alveolar macrophage recruits fibroblasts to sites of tissue injury in interstitial lung diseases.[41]

ALTERATIONS IN PULMONARY CONNECTIVE TISSUE IN ACUTE LUNG INJURY PRODUCED BY EXOGENOUS TOXIC SUBSTANCES

Accidental exposure to toxic and irritant gases is an important health hazard in certain occupations. A number of inhaled gases are known to cause serious injury to the lungs: nitrogen dioxide (NO_2), ozone (O_3), high concentrations of oxygen, and cadmium (Cd) have been studied most intensively. The injury produced by these agents depends on the dose and duration of exposure. Under severe exposure conditions, some agents may produce noncardiogenic pulmonary edema. The broad subject of acute lung injury is too voluminous to describe here; this section is restricted to changes in lung connective tissue during exposure to these four toxic gases.

Much of the information about the effects of toxic gases on lung connective tissue has been derived from animal studies using NO_3, O_3, oxygen toxicity, and Cd. Certain generalizations can be made about the injury and repair sequence produced by these gases. The initial reaction in the lung is an intense inflammatory and edematous reaction of the distal lung units. The initial response is followed by a more widespread inflammatory and edematous reaction involving alveolar lining cells, the interstitium, and capillary endothelial cells. If the exposure is discontinued and the animals are allowed to recover, repair of the cellular damage occurs by replacement of damaged cells by a new population of normal cells.[42] Whether the repair process is complete depends on the extent and severity of the initial injury and individual animal's responses to the injury. If the injury is too severe, with destruction of the basal lamina of the basement membrane, permanent derangement of the tissue will be found after the cellular proliferative response has subsided. One of the features of permanent damage following recovery from exposure to toxic gases is fibrosis, which is recognized histologically as increased connective tissue and biochemically as increased synthesis and accumulation of collagen and elastin in the tissue. Increased collagen synthesis or content in the lung is found after oxygen toxicity[43] and exposure to O_3[44] and NO_2[45]; elastin content of lung is increased after oxygen toxicity[46] and O_3[47] and NO_2[45] exposure.

Animal models of lung injury produced by exposure to toxic gases allow assessment of the subsequent physiologic and morphologic consequences of the exposure attributable to alterations of connective tissue. One of the common features of the morphologic changes in rodent lungs, following exposure to toxic gases, is dilatation of parenchymal airspaces and loss of alveoli resembling emphysema. Emphysemalike changes have been described following oxygen toxicity,[48] NO_2,[49,50] O_3,[51] and Cd.[52] In addition to morphologic evidence of emphysema, there is physiologic evidence of loss of lung elastic recoil several weeks after recovery from exposure to toxic concentrations of oxygen,[48] NO_2,[50] O_3,[51] and Cd.[52]

These late emphysemalike findings suggest a common pathogenetic mechanism. Although it has been suggested that the lesions produced by Cd are due to scar emphysema,[53] another possibility is that the emphysematous lesions result from destruction of pulmonary connective tissue during acute exposure to toxic gases followed by replacement of fibers which are functionally "abnormal" either in type or arrangement of fibers.[54] This idea was suggested because there is a net decrease of hydroxyproline in the lung[55] and increased urinary excretion of hydroxyproline[54] during the acute phase of oxygen toxicity. An early decrease in collagen and elastin content of lung followed by an increase in content have also been found following exposure to NO_2.[45,56] Human studies have been limited, but collagen breakdown, indicated by increased urinary excretion of hydroxyproline, occurred in three astronauts who were accidentally exposed to toxic fumes of nitrogen dioxide.[57]

The mechanism by which these gases destroy connective tissue is unknown, but a common mechanism for lung damage for these agents is the formation of free radicals.[58,59] It has recently been shown that free-radical generating systems cause early depletion of immunofluorescent-staining material for collagen in lung[60] and in lung content of hydroxyproline.[61] Several mechanisms of this destruction of collagen are possible: activation of latent collagenases; influx of cells such as polymorphonuclear leukocytes and monocytes, which release collagenolytic active enzymes;[62] inactivation of antiproteases;[63] or direct damage to molecular collagen.[64,65] More work is needed to determine mechanisms leading to destruction of connective tissue in oxidant injury and the relation of the connective tissue alterations to the late emphysemalike changes found in the experimental models. The relevance of the animal experiments to human disease is unclear because there has been little study of connective tissue changes in humans after exposure to oxidant gases.

FIBROGENESIS OF LUNG PRODUCED BY EXOGENOUS SUBSTANCES

Silica

Intensive efforts have been made to understand the pathogenesis of silicosis for the last 50 years. Despite the extensive investigation that has been done, the events leading to the accumulation of inflammatory cells, granuloma, and connective tissue in the silicotic lung are poorly understood. Several reviews of the pathogenesis of silicosis have appeared.[66–68] The discussion here will be limited to current concepts of mechanisms by which silica induces fibrosis. It must be pointed out, however, that there are often conflicting results of different workers in this field, in part due to important differences in methods and experimental design.[68] Because of these difficulties, there is often insufficient evidence to draw firm conclusions about fibrogenesis induced by silica.

Central to the role of silica in producing fibrosis is the interaction of the silica particle with the pulmonary alveolar macrophage. Silica particles reaching the lower respiratory tract are ingested by macrophages and lie within phagosomes. The phagosomes interact with lysosomes, which release enzymes into the phagosomal vacuoles. This process eventually leads to the destruction of the cell due to the release of lysosomal enzymes. The silica particle, thereby released from the cell, is ingested by another macrophage, and so in turn perpetuates cell autolysis. Although immune factors are important in the pathogenesis of silicosis, immune mechanisms probably do not participate directly in the killing of macrophages by silica. Immune factors may, however, be involved in the recruitment of macrophages to the area of injury, and this may contribute to the perpetuation of the process and formation of granuloma.

The significance of the effects of silica on macrophages in producing fibrosis is not clear, but there appears to be a good correlation between cytotoxicity for macrophages and fibrogenicity of a silica particle.[69–71] The steps by which macrophages mediate fibrosis is believed to involve the release of a soluble mediator, which stimulates fibroblasts to increase collagen synthesis.[72] In these experiments, the effect of an unstimulated macrophage alone or silica particles alone was excluded. However, other investigators, using similar methods, presented evidence that the "macrophage fibrogenic factor" is not soluble,[73] and work from other species could not confirm the presence of a factor from macrophages which stimulates fibroblasts to synthesize collagen.[74] As pointed out by Reiser and Last,[68] these studies have methodologic difficulties, which may account for some of the conflicting results. There are too few critical studies to evaluate the manner in which silica-exposed macrophages affect collagen biosynthesis by fibroblasts in vitro. The theory of macrophage mediation of fibroblast to produce collagen may be correct, but critical evidence that this punitive mediator is the mechanism by which silica induces fibrosis in humans has not been found. Furthermore, the relevance to the activation of macrophages in human silicosis is not clear, since macrophages obtained by lung lavage from silicotic patients are normal in number and function.[75]

Other factors may also influence the fibrogenic response to silica. There is an apparent synergistic role of infection in the induction of pulmonary fibrosis in silica-exposed rats.[76] Also, lipids may have an important role in mediating the silicotic response by controlling macrophage accumulation or interacting with the surface of the silica particle.[77] The role of other lung cells capable of synthesizing collagen is largely unknown, and the direct effect of silica on fibroblasts is unclear.[68]

In summary, experiments using tissue culture to study the interaction of silica and macrophage and of macrophage and fibroblast have led to a better understanding of the pathogenesis of fibrosing silicosis. The central role of the macrophage in silica ingestion seems clear. It appears that this cytotoxic process leads to release of a factor that stimulates fibroblasts to replicate and/or increase collagen synthesis. There are many unanswered questions about the molecular mechanism involved and the relevance of these observations to silicosis in humans.

It is clear, however, that silica instillation in lungs increases collagen synthesis and content.[78–81] Total content of hydroxyproline in the lung is increased above control levels within six days of exposure of rats to silica,[81] most likely due to an enhanced rate of collagen synthesis.[79] An increased rate of degradation of collagen may occur at a later time.[81] It is somewhat surprising that, despite marked increases of collagen content in the lung, lung mechanics remain relatively unaffected in humans with simple silicosis[82] and in animal models.[83] This is most likely explained by a high concentration of connective tissue located in focal silicotic nodules, which may not be sufficiently extensive to produce measurable effects on lung mechanics, even though they contribute to the greater than normal increase in collagen content of the lungs.

Asbestos

There has been considerable interest in the mechanism by which asbestos induces disease because of the well-known hazards and widespread use of this fibrous mineral. Among the diseases caused by asbestos exposure, asbestosis of the lung is among the most important. This disease has many features in common with the other chronic interstitial lung diseases[6] and is distinguished by a history of exposure to asbestos and the presence of asbestos fibers in the lung. There are many factors that influence the extent of parenchymal lung disease which develops after exposure to asbestos. These factors are the type and size of the fiber, the duration and intensity of exposure, and individual susceptibility.[84–86] This discussion will be focused on current concepts of the fibrogenesis of asbestos fibers in the lung.

It is currently asserted that asbestos fibers may injure the lung parenchyma by direct action of the fiber on cells[87] or through the mediation of factors released from activated macrophages.[88] There is good evidence that when resident macrophages attempt to ingest asbestos fibers they become activated.[89,90] Furthermore, macrophages that have ingested asbestos produce a factor that stimulates fibroblasts to produce increased amounts of connective tissue.[91] The mechanism for this increase in collagen in the lung could be either an increase in the number of fibroblasts producing collagen or an increase in the rate of collagen synthesis per fibroblast. Recent evidence suggests the former mechanism, namely secretion of a factor causing replication of fibroblasts.[92]

The physicochemical properties of types of asbestos fibers and their fibrogenic effects has been a subject of investigation for many years and has been reviewed by Harington and associates.[91] Several general principles emerge from this experience. Most types of asbestos tested are fibrogenic in vivo. Of the various types of asbestos, however, only chrysotile shows marked activity. The physical nature of the asbestos fiber rather than its chemical composition is more important in fibrogenesis, since glass fibers and other nonasbestos fibers stimulate collagen synthesis.[93] Most authors agree that longer fibers are more fibrogenic than shorter ones.[94] This might be explained by the aggregation of several macrophages around a long fiber and the release of stimulating factors from the combined cells. Macrophages are not destroyed by ingestion of asbestos as readily as by silica, and lysosomal enzymes may be released from cells into the culture medium in the absence of cell death.[88]

There are several lung cells, other than the macrophage, which may mediate the fibrogenic response to asbestos. The uptake of chrysotile by fibroblasts causes their proliferation and stimulates collagen synthesis. It is possible that interstitial fibroblasts may directly initiate the fibrogenic process. Although blood lymphocytes from patients with asbestosis have abnormalities that suggest impaired cellular and humoral immunity,[95] the role of the lung lymphocytes in the fibrogenic response to asbestos has not been evaluated. An immunologic stimulus mediated by complement may render asbestos fibers more cytotoxic,[96] possibly by potentiating the release of factors that stimulate macrophages to attract neutrophils.[97] The neutrophil may act as another cell that can degrade lung tissue in the early stages of asbestos exposure, since this cell is attracted to asbestos-activated macrophages[97] and neutrophils are found in bronchoalveolar lavage fluid from patients with asbestosis.[90,97]

It is postulated that, where progression of the fibrosis continues after the exposure to the offending dust has terminated, self-perpetuating host responses are involved. The mechanism involved is not clear, but it has been shown that antibodies to lung connective tissue can stimulate macrophages to release a collagen-stimulating factor.[98] It is not known whether this observation explains the postexposure progression of fibrosis in man. However, nonspecific autoantibodies to connective tissue have been found in humans exposed to fibrogenic dusts.[99–100]

There has been relatively little work in experimental asbestosis in animals. The studies of a Canadian group on asbestosis in sheep have been recently reported.[101] Although a variety of animals develop fibrosis after exposure to asbestos,[102–106] there is considerable variability in animal response to asbestos exposure.[105] Which factor or factors stimulate and modulate the production of connective tissue in these models has yet to be determined.

Agents Other Than Silica and Asbestos

Many environmental agents other than silica and asbestos are known to cause interstitial lung disease.[6] These agents vary greatly in their fibrogenicity to lung tissue. Most of the information about the fibrogenicity of dusts is provided by human epidemiologic studies and examination of human pathology specimens. Animal studies are also useful in predicting the fibrogenicity of dusts. Several recent reviews have appeared on this subject;[107–110] this section will focus on what is known about connective tissue changes in the lung due to environmental agents other than silica and asbestos.

Coal and Carbon. Coal and carbon are not cytotoxic, and they behave as inert dusts, causing only mild reticulin proliferation in the lungs of experimental animals.[109] Experimental studies in animals show fibrosis due to coal dust is related to the quartz content of the dust. After inhalation by rats of a mixture of coal dust containing 2% quartz, no fibrosis was observed,[111] but fibrosis was present when rats inhaled a mixture containing 20% quartz[112] and after 18 months when rats inhaled a 5% mixture.[113] The implication of these studies is that coal dust itself is nonfibrogenic, but even a small quantity of quartz may cause fibrosis. The quartz content in human lungs with "simple" coal workers' pneumoconiosis is 2–4%,[109] an amount sufficient to cause a minimal fibrotic response if the animal studies can be applied to humans.

Simple coal workers' pneumoconiosis is characterized pathologically by the coal macule, which is initially characterized by a focal collection of dust-laden phagocytes situated near the terminal bronchiole. Later in the evolution of this lesion, reticulin can be found on light microscopic examination.[109] No studies have appeared on the biochemistry of simple coal workers' pneumoconiosis.

The appearance of progressive massive fibrosis, in contrast, shows conglomerate masses of dense collagenous fibrous tissue as well as deposits of coal and a few scattered lymphocytes.[114] The biochemical composition of the tissue from the lesions of progressive massive fibrosis were shown to contain coal, calcium, phosphate, and protein, and that collagen comprised 25–30% of the protein.[115] In addition, there were also elevated levels of glycosaminoglycans. The collagen was present primarily at the periphery of the lesion; the centers contained noncollagenous protein. Also, the turnover of collagen in tissues of patients with simple and complicated coal workers' pneumoconiosis appears to be slow as indicated by normal values of urinary hydroxyproline.[116,117]

Nonasbestos Fibrous Minerals. Over 150 minerals other than asbestos occur in fibrous form, and many of these have biologic activity.[107] Whether pure talc causes a pneumoconiosis is uncertain;[109] the diffuse interstitial fibrosis found in humans exposed to talc may be due to associated tremolite or anthophyllite asbestos. Animal experiments using talc of known high purity showed no fibrosis of the lung.[118,119] Most reports suggest that kaolin, fuller's earth, bentonite, and mica are nonfibrogenic in rodents, although local macrophage accumulations or foreign body response may occur in the lungs after exposure of animals to these substances. Man-made fibers, such as slug wools, rock wool, and glass wool, cause no fibrosis after inhalation by rats or hamsters, nor is there evidence from epidemiologic surveys or human postmortum studies that man-made fibers cause disease.[110]

Metals. In general, inorganic mineral dusts are nonfibrogenic provided they are free of toxic impurities and contain <1% quartz. Siderosis, or inhalation of metallic iron or iron compounds, is the most common pneumoconiosis due to inert dusts, and there is no evidence of fibrosis in this disorder.[109] Hematite, the material from pulverized rock containing both iron and free silica, causes fibrosis because of its silica content.[120] Whether aluminum is fibrogenic is unsettled; although metallic aluminum in high doses can cause fibrosis in animals,[121] there is little evidence of fibrosis in humans exposed to aluminum.[108] However, in cases of fibrosis reported in humans, it has been attributed to mineral oil which was used to coat the flaked aluminum metal;[122] however, the mineral oil-coated aluminum flake did not enhance fibrosis in rats.[123] The apparent fibrogenicity of aluminum in rodents but not man may represent species differences in reaction to the dust. Tin oxide exposure in man causes aggregation of dust-laden macrophages but no fibrosis, even after 50 years of exposure.[124] Tin oxide does not cause fibrosis in the lungs of experimental animals.[125] Similarly, barium, antimony, zirconium, chromate, titanium, rare earths, vanadium, and silver appear to be harmless to man and experimental animals.[108,109]

Cobalt, on the other hand, is potentially allergenic and cytotoxic. Inhalation of high concentrations of cobalt fumes has caused a fibrosing alveolitis.[108,109] In chronic exposure in humans, a diffused interstitial pulmonary fibrosis is found with collagen and elastin prominent in the alveolar walls.[109] Cobalt metal instilled in the lungs of animals produces acute diffuse lung injury;[126,127] longer term studies using cobalt oxide in swine showed electron microscopic evidence of collagen in alveolar septae.[128] Cobalt is bound with tungsten to produce tungsten-carbide, which is used as a hard metal for cutting tools. Tungsten-carbide alone and particulate tungsten metal do not produce fibrosis.[108,109]

Inert dusts of low radiodensity, such as limestone, marble, Portland cement, gypsum, and silicon carbide, are nonfibrogenic provided the silica content is less than 1–2%.[109]

Some researchers believe that chronic inhalation of cadmium oxide fumes causes emphysema in humans,[129,130] but there is considerable debate as to whether the association of cadmium exposure and emphysema are cause and effect. Emphysema can be produced by cadmium exposure in animals by some investigators[131] but not by others.[52] If cadmium does produce emphysema, its mechanism is entirely unclear. There is general agreement that cadmium is not fibrogenic in humans.

Accidental exposure to mercury vapors can cause serious lung injury similar to a chemical peumonitis. In humans surviving the acute insult, diffuse interstitial pulmonary fibrosis can be found weeks to months after exposure.[132,133] Similarly, nickel carbonyl vapor may cause an acute pneumonitis and interstitial fibrosis.[134] Experimental animals exposed to the same compound develop pulmonary fibrosis.[135]

Beryllium. Chronic berylliosis is a granulomatous disorder resulting from exposure to beryllium. Fibrosis can be found around the granuloma in almost all cases, and in some the granuloma may be wholly fibrotic. In these cases the fibrosis may be associated with honeycombing and causes severe respiratory impairment.[109] No biochemical analyses of the connective tissue changes in the lungs in berylliosis have been performed.

Radiation. Although lung cancer is the major risk of workers exposed to ionizing radiation, there is some evidence to suggest that chronic irradiation may be synergistic with silica in uranium miners to produce pulmonary fibrosis.[136] Pickrell[137] has shown that exposure of animal lung tissue to clays containing ionizing radiation directly stimulates collagen synthesis.

ACKNOWLEDGMENTS

This work was supported in part by U.S. Public Health Service grant HL 24264. The author is the recipient of a Pulmonary Academic Award HL 00443 from the National Heart, Lung and Blood Institute, National Institutes of Health.

REFERENCES

1. Prockop DJ, Kivirikko KI, Tuderman L, Guzman NA: The biosynthesis of collagen and its disorders. N Engl J Med 301:13,77, 1979.
2. Bornstein P, Beyers PH: Disorders of collagen metabolism. In: Metabolic Control and Disease, 8th ed, eds. Bondy PK, Rosenberg LE. Philadelphia, Saunders, 1980, p 1089.
3. Minor RR: Collagen metabolism. A comparison of diseases of collagen and diseases affecting collagen. Am J Pathol 98:227, 1980.
4. Sandberg LB, Soskel NT, Leslie JG: Elastin structure, biosynthesis, and relation to disease states. N Engl J Med 304:566, 1981.
5. Hance AJ, Crystal RG: The connective tissue of the lung. Am Rev Respir Dis 112:657, 1975.
6. Keogh BA, Crystal RG: Chronic interstitial lung disease. In: Current Pulmonology, vol 3, ed. Simmons DH. New York, Wiley, 1981, p 237.
7. Crystal RG, Gadek JE, Ferrans VJ, et al: Interstitial lung disease: Current concepts of pathogenesis, staging, and therapy. Am J Med 70:542, 1981.
8. Crystal RG: The biochemical basis of pulmonary function. In: Lung Biology in Health and Disease, vol 2, ed. Lenfant C. New York, Marcel Dekker, 1976.
9. Pickrell JA: Lung Connective Tissue: Location, Metabolism, and Response to Injury. Boca Raton, Fla., CRC Press, 1981.
10. Fuller GC, Mann SW: Mechanisms of fibrosis. Rev Biochem Toxicol 3:193, 1981.
11. Bateman ED, Emerson RJ, Cole P: Mechanisms of fibrogenesis. In: Occupational Lung Diseases: Research Approaches and Methods, eds. Weill H, Turner-Warwick M. New York, Marcel Dekker, 1981, p 237.
12. Crystal RG, Rennard SI: Pulmonary connective tissue and environmental lung disease. Chest 80(Suppl):33S, 1981.
13. Prockop DJ: Present and future research on collagen and genes for collagen. Med Biol 58:289, 1980.
14. Bienkowski RS, Cowan MJ, McDonald JA, Crystal RG: Degradation of newly synthesized collagen. J Biol Chem 253:4356, 1978.
15. Berg RA, Schwartz ML, Crystal RG: Regulation of the production of secretory proteins: Intracellular degradation of newly synthesized "defective" collagen. Proc Natl Acad Sci USA 77:4746, 1980.
16. Wiestner M, Krieg T, Hörlein D, et al: Inhibiting effect of procollagen peptides on collagen biosynthesis in fibroblast culture. J Biol Chem 254:7016, 1979.
17. Rohde J, Vargas L, Hahn E, et al: RIA for type III procollagen peptide and its application to human liver disease. Eur J Clin Invest 9:451, 1979.
18. O'Dell BL, Kilburn KH, McKenzie WN, Thurston RJ: The lung of the copper-deficient rat: A model for developmental pulmonary emphysema. Am J Pathol 91:413, 1978.
19. Kida K. Thurlbeck WM: The effect of β-aminoproprionitrile on the growing rat lung. Am J Pathol 101:693, 1980.
20. Fisk DE, Kuhn C: Emphysema-like changes in the lungs of the blotchy mouse. Am Rev Respir Dis 113:787, 1976.
21. Trelsted RL: Multistep assembly of type I collagen fibrils. Cell 28:197, 1982.
22. Sellers A, Murphy G: Collagenolytic enzymes and their naturally occurring inhibitors. Int Rev Connect Tissue Res 9:151, 1981.
23. Gadek JE, Fells GA, Wright DG, Crystal RG: Human neutrophil elastase functions as a type III collagen "collagenase." Biochem Biophys Res Commun 95:1815, 1980.

24. Otto K: Cathepsin B1 and B2. In: Tissue Proteinases, eds. Barret AJ, Dingle JT. Amsterdam, North-Holland Publishing, 1971, p 1.
25. Cawston TE, Murphy G: Mammalian collagenases. Meth Enzymol 80:711, 1981.
26. Harper, E: Collagenases. Ann Rev Biochem 49:1063, 1980.
27. Tchòrzewski H, Denys A, Lipiǹski S: The influence of polymorphonuclear leucocytes and macrophages on the growth of lymphocytes and fibroblasts in vitro. Exp Pathol Bacteriol 10S:289, 1975.
28. Jalkanen M, Peltonen J, Kulonen E: Isoelectric focusing of macrophage culture media and the effects of the fractions on the synthesis of DNA and collagen by fibroblasts. Acta Pathol Microbiol Scand Sect C 87:347, 1979.
29. Baum BJ, Moss J, Breul SD, Crystal RG: Association in normal human fibroblasts of elevated levels of 3′:5′-monophosphate with a selective decrease in collagen production. J Biol Chem 253:3391, 1978.
30. Horwitz AL, Elson NA, Crystal RG: Proteoglycans and elastic fibers. In: The Biochemical Basis of Pulmonary Function, ed. Crystal RG. New York, Marcel Dekker, 1976, p 273.
31. Mosher DF, Proctor RA, Grossman JE: Fibronectin: Role in inflammation. In: Advances in Inflammation Research, vol 2, ed. Weissman G. New York, Raven Press, 1981, p 187.
32. Karlinsky JB, Snider GL: Animal models of emphysema. Am Rev Respir Dis 117:1109, 1978.
33. Starcher BC, Kuhn C, Overton JE: Increased elastin and collagen content in the lungs of hamsters receiving an intratracheal injection of bleomycin. Am Rev Respir Dis 117:299, 1978.
34. Schnaidman IM, Dzhangozina DM: Lesion of mucopolysaccharide metabolism in rat lungs in experimental silicosis. Vopr Med Khim 13:157, 1969.
35. Vasilieva GN: Content of soluble collagen and protein-carbohydrate components in lungs of rats in experimental silicosis. Vopr Med Khim 17:277, 1971.
36. Karlinsky JB: Glycosaminoglycans in emphysematous and fibrotic hamster lungs. Am Rev Respir Dis 125:85, 1982.
37. Cantor JO, Bray BA, Ryan SF, et al: Glycosaminoglycan and collagen synthesis in N-nitroso-N-methylurethane-induced pulmonary fibrosis. Proc Soc Exp Biol Med 164:1, 1980.
38. Misra V, Rahman Q, Viswanathan PN: Biochemical changes in guinea pig lungs due to amosite asbestos. Environ Res 16:55, 1978.
39. Villiger B, Kelley DG, Engleman W, et al: Human alveolar macrophage fibronectin: Synthesis, secretion, and ultrastructural localization during gelatin-coated latex particle binding. J Cell Biol 90:711, 1981.
40. Rennard SI, Crystal RG: Fibronectin in human bronchopulmonary lavage fluid-elevation in patients with interstitial lung disease. J Clin Invest 69:113, 1982.
41. Rennard SI, Hunninghake GW, Bitterman PB, Crystal RG: Production of fibronectin by the human alveolar macrophage-mechanism for the recruitment of fibroblasts to sites of tissue injury in interstitial lung disease. Proc Natl Acad Sci USA 78:7147, 1981.
42. Bowden DH: Alveolar response to injury. Thorax 36:801, 1981.
43. Välimäki M, Juva K, Rantanen J, et al: Collagen metabolism in rat lungs during chronic intermittent exposure to oxygen. Aviat Space Environ Med 46:684, 1975.
44. Last JA, Greenberg DB, Castleman WL: Ozone-induced alterations in collagen metabolism of rat lungs. Toxicol Appl Pharmacol 51:247, 1979.
45. Kleinerman J, Ip MPC: Effects of nitrogen dioxide on elastin and collagen contents of lungs. Arch Environ Health 34:228, 1979.

46. Richmond V, D'Aoust BG: Effects of intermittent hyperbaric oxygen on guinea pig elastin and collagen. J Appl Physiol 41:295, 1976.
47. Dubick MA, Rucker RB, Last JA, Cross CE: Does ozone exposure alter lung elastin metabolism? Fed Proc 39, 1030, 1980.
48. Riley DJ, Berg RA, Edelman NH, Prockop DJ: Prevention of collagen deposition following pulmonary oxygen toxicity in the rat by cis-4-hydroxy-L-proline. J Clin Invest 65:643, 1980.
49. Freeman G, Juhos LT, Furiosi NJ, et al: Pathology of pulmonary disease from exposure to interdependent ambient gases (nitrogen dioxide and ozone). Arch Environ Health 29:203, 1974.
50. Niewoehner DE, Kleinerman J: Effects of experimental emphysema and bronchiolitis on lung mechanics and morphometry. J Appl Physiol 35:25, 1973.
51. Bartlett D Jr, Faulkner CS II, Cook K: Effect of chronic ozone exposure on lung elasticity in young rats. J Appl Physiol 37:92, 1974.
52. Snider GL, Karlinsky JB: Relation between the elastic behavior and connective tissues of the lungs. Pathobiol Annu 7: 115, 1977.
53. Thurlbeck WM, Foley FD: Experimental pulmonary emphysema. The effect of intratracheal injection of cadmium chloride solution in the guinea pig. Am J Pathol 42:431, 1963.
54. Riley DJ, Kerr JS, Yu SY, et al: Pulmonary oxygen toxicity. Connective tissue changes during injury and repair. Chest 83(Suppl): 98S, 1983.
55. Riley DJ, Kerr JS, Yu SY, et al: Degradation of lung connective tissue following oxygen exposure in rats. Fed Proc 41:488, 1982.
56. Droždž M, Kucharz E, Szyja J: Effect of chronic exposure to nitrogen dioxide on collagen content in lung and skin of guinea pigs. Environ Res 13:369, 1977.
57. Hatton DV, Leach CS, Nicogossian AE, DiFerrante N: Collagen breakdown and nitrogen dioxide inhalation. Arch Environ Health 32:33, 1977.
58. Mustafa MG, Tierney DF: Biochemical and metabolic changes in the lung with oxygen, ozone, and nitrogen dioxide toxicity. Am Rev Respir Dis 118:1061, 1978.
59. Amoruso MA, Witz G, Goldstein BD: Enhancement of rat and human phagocyte superoxide anion radical production by cadmium in vitro. Toxicol Lett 10:133, 1982.
60. Sandblom R, Johnson K, Killen P, et al: Lung injury due to oxygen metabolites alters the composition of extracellular matrix. Fed Proc 41:941, 1982.
61. Phan SH, Armstrong G, Sulavik MC, et al: A comparative study of pulmonary fibrosis by bleomycin and an O_2 metabolite-producing enzyme system. Chest 83(Suppl): 44S, 1983.
62. Fox RB, Hoidal JR, Brown DM, Repine JE. Pulmonary inflammation due to oxygen toxicity: Involvement of chemotactic factors and polymorphonuclear leukocytes. Am Rev Respir Dis 123:521, 1981.
63. Bruce MC, Boat TF, Martin RJ, et al: Inactivation of $alpha_1$ proteinase inhibitor in infants exposed to high concentrations of oxygen. Am Rev Respir Dis 123:166, 1981.
64. Greenwald RA, Moy WW: Inhibition of collagen gelation by action of the superoxide radical. Arthritis Rheum 22:251, 1979.
65. Venkatasubramanian K, Joseph KT: Action of singlet oxygen on collagen. Indian J Biochem Biophys 14:217, 1977.
66. Heppleston AG: The biological response to silica. In: Biology of Fibroblast, eds. Kulonen E, Pikkarinen J. New York, Academic Press, 1973, p 529.
67. Chvapil M, Hurych J, Cmuchalova B, et al: Conflicting hypotheses on experimental silicotic fibrogenesis: New experimental data. Environ Res 1:89, 1967.

68. Reiser KM, Last JA: Silicosis and fibrogenesis: Fact and artifact. Toxicology 13:51, 1979.
69. Harington JS: Investigative techniques in the laboratory study of coal workers' pneumoconiosis: Recent advances at the cellular level. Ann NY Acad Sci 200:816, 1972.
70. Zaidi SH: Experimental Pneumoconiosis. Baltimore, Johns Hopkins Press, 1969.
71. Harington JS: Fibrogenesis. Environ Health Perspect 9:271, 1974.
72. Heppleston AG, Styles JA: Activity of a macrophage factor in collagen formation by silica. Nature 214:521, 1967.
73. Kilroe-Smith TA, Webster I, Van Drimmelen M, Marasas L: An insoluble fibrogenic factor in macrophages from guinea pigs exposed to silica. Environ Res 6:298, 1973.
74. Harington JS, Ritchie M, King PC, Miller K: The in vitro effects of silica-treated hamster macrophages on collagen production by hamster fibroblasts. J Pathol 109:21, 1973.
75. Schuyler MR, Gaumer HR, Stankus RP, et al: Bronchoalveolar lavage in silicosis. Lung 152:95, 1980.
76. Heppleston AG, Wright NA, Stewart JA: Experimental alveolar lipoproteinosis following the inhalation of silica. J Pathol 101:293, 1970.
77. Gross P, deTreville RTP: Experimental "acute" silicosis. Arch Environ Health 17:720, 1968.
78. Dale K: A method for inducing unilateral silicosis in rabbits by an injection technique with some observations on lung clearance and quantitative evaluation of experimental silicosis. Scand J Respir Dis 54:157, 1973.
79. Halme J, Uitto J, Kahanpää K, et al: Protocollagen proline hydroxylase activity in experimental pulmonary fibrosis of rats. J Lab Clin Med 75:535, 1970.
80. Dauber JH, Rossman MD, Pietra GG, et al: Experimental silicosis. Morphologic and biochemical abnormalities produced by intratracheal instillation of quartz into guinea pig lungs. Am J Pathol 101:595, 1980.
81. Chvapil M, Eskelson CD, Stiffel V, Owen JA: Early changes in the chemical composition of rat lung after silica administration. Arch Environ Health 34:402, 1979.
82. Teculescu DB, Stanescu DC, Pilat L: Pulmonary mechanics in silicosis. Arch Environ Health 14:461, 1967.
83. Davis GS, Hemenway DR, Evans JN, et al: Alveolar macrophage stimulation and population changes in silica-exposed rats. Chest 80(Suppl):8S, 1981.
84. Selikoff IJ, Hammond EC: Health hazards of asbestos exposure. Ann NY Acad Sci 330:1, 1979.
85. Selikoff IJ, Lee DHK: Asbestos and Disease. New York, Academic Press, 1978.
86. Becklake MR: Asbestos-related diseases of the lung and other organs: Their epidemiology and implications for clinical practice. Am Rev Respir Dis 114:187, 1976.
87. Richards RJ, Wusteman FS, Dodgson KS: The direct effects of dusts on lung fibroblasts grown in vitro. Life Sci 10:1149, 1971.
88. Davies P, Allison AC, Ackerman J, et al: Asbestos induces selective release of lysosomal enzymes from mononuclear phagocytes. Nature 251:423, 1974.
89. Miller K, Kagan E: The in vitro effects of asbestos on macrophage membrane structure and population characteristics of macrophages: A scanning electron microscopic study. J Reticuloendothel Soc 20:159, 1976.
90. Jaurand MC, Gaudichet A, Atassi K, et al: Relationship between the number of asbestos fibres and the cellular and enzymatic content of bronchoalveolar fluid in asbestos exposed subjects. Bull Eur Physiopathol Respir 16:595, 1980.

91. Harington JS, Allison AC, Badami DV: Mineral fibers: Chemical, physiochemical, and biological properties. Adv Pharmacol Chemother 12:291, 1975.
92. Bitterman P, Rennard S, Schoenberger C, Crystal R: Asbestos stimulates alveolar macrophages to release a factor causing human lung fibroblasts to replicate. Chest 80(Suppl):38S, 1981.
93. Davis JMG: The fibrogenic effects of mineral dusts injected into the pleural cavity of mice. Br J Exp Pathol 53:190, 1972.
94. Davis JMG, Coniam SW: Experimental studies on the effects of heated chrysotile asbestos and automobile brake lining dust injected into the body cavities of mice. Exp Mol Pathol 19:339, 1973.
95. Kagan E, Solomon A, Cochrane JC, et al: Immunological studies of patients with asbestosis. II. Studies of circulating lymphoid cell numbers and humoral immunity. Clin Exp Immunol 28:268, 1977.
96. Miller K, Weintraub Z, Kagan E: Manifestations of cellular immunity in the rat after prolonged asbestos inhalation. I. Physical interactions between alveolar macrophages and splenic lymphocytes. J Immunol 123:1029, 1979.
97. Gadek J, Hunninghake G, Schoenberger C, et al: Pulmonary asbestosis and idiopathic pulmonary fibrosis: Pathogenetic parallels. Chest 80(Suppl):63S, 1981.
98. Lewis DM, Burrell R: Induction of fibrogenesis by lung antibody-treated macrophages. Br J Ind Med 33:25, 1976.
99. Turner-Warwick M, Haslam P: Antibodies in some chronic fibrosing lung diseases. I. Non-organic specific autoantibodies. Clin Allergy 1:83, 1971.
100. Turner-Warwick M, Haslam P, Weeks J: Antibodies in some chronic fibrosing lung diseases. II. Immunofluorescent studies. Clin Allergy 1:209, 1971.
101. Lemaire I, Rola-Pleszczynski M, Begin R: Asbestos exposure enhances the release of fibroblast growth factor by sheep alveolar macrophages. J Reticuloendothel Soc 33:275–86, 1983.
102. Sahu AP, Dogra RKS, Shanker R, Zaidis H: Fibrogenic response in murine lungs to asbestos. Exp Pathol 115:21, 1975.
103. Holt PF, Mills J, Young DK: Experimental asbestosis in the guinea pig. J Pathol Bacteriol 92:185, 1966.
104. Wagner JC: Asbestosis in experimental animals. Br J Ind Med 20:1, 1963.
105. Vorwald AJ, Durkan TM, Pratt PC: Experimental studies of asbestosis. Arch Int Hyg Occup Med 3:1, 1951.
106. Davis HV, Reeves AL: Collagen biosynthesis in rat lungs during exposure to asbestos. Am Ind Hyg Assoc J 32:599, 1971.
107. Lockey JE: Nonasbestos fibrous minerals. Clin Chest Med 2:203, 1981.
108. Brooks SM: Lung disorders resulting from the inhalation of metals. Clin Chest Med 2:235, 1981.
109. Parkes WR: Occupational Lung Disorders. London, Butterworth, 1982.
110. Hill JW: Health aspects of man-made mineral fibers. A review. Ann Occup Hyg 20:161, 1977.
111. King EJ, Zaidi S, Harrison CV, Nagelschmidt G: The tissue reaction in the lungs of rats after the inhalation of coal dust containing 2% of quartz. Br J Ind Med 15:172, 1958.
112. Ross HF, King EJ, Yoganathan M, Nagelschmidt G: Inhalation experiments with coal dust containing 5 percent, 10 percent, 20 percent and 40 percent quartz: Tissue reactions in the lungs of rats. Ann Occup Hyg 5:149, 1962.
113. Martin JC, Daniel-Moussard H, Le Bouffant L, Policard A: The role of quartz in the development of coal workers' pneumoconiosis. Ann NY Acad Sci 200:127, 1972.

114. Wagner JC: Immunologic factors in coal workers' pneumoconiosis. In: Inhaled Particles III, vol 2, ed. Walton WH. London, Unwin, 1971, p 573.
115. Wagner JC: Etiologic factors in complicated coal workers' pneumoconiosis. Ann NY Acad Sci 200:401, 1972.
116. Resnick H, Lapp NL, Morgan WKC: Urinary hydroxyproline excretion in coal workers' pneumoconiosis. Br J Ind Med 26:135, 1969.
117. Resnick H, Morgan WKC: Hydroxyproline excretion in complicated pneumoconiosis. Am Rev Respir Dis 103:849, 1971.
118. Wehner AP, Zwicker GM, Cannon WC, et al: Inhalation of talc baby powders by hamsters. Food Cosmet Toxicol 15:121, 1977.
119. Wagner JC, Berry G, Cooke TJ, et al: Animal experiments with talc. In: Inhaled Particles IV, eds. Walton WH, McGovern B. Oxford, Pergamon Press, 1977, p 647.
120. Faulds JS, Nagelschmidt GS: The duct in the lungs of haematite miners from Cumberland. Ann Occup Hyg 4:255, 1962.
121. Gross P, Harley RA Jr, DeTreville RTP: Pulmonary reaction to metallic aluminum powders. Arch Environ Health 26:227, 1973.
122. Mitchell J, Manning GB, Molyneaux M, Lane RE: Pulmonary fibrosis in workers exposed to finely powdered aluminum. Br J Ind Med 18:10, 1961.
123. Roche AD, Picard D, Vernhes A: Silicosis of ocher workers. A clinical and anatomo-pathologic study. Am Rev Tuberc 77:839, 1958.
124. Robertson AJ, Rivers D, Nagelschmidt G, Duncumb P: Stannosis. Pneumoconiosis due to tin dioxide. Lancet 1:1089, 1961.
125. Fischer HW, Zimmerman GR: Long retention of stannic oxide. Lack of tissue reaction in laboratory animals. Arch Pathol 88:259, 1969.
126. Harding HE: Notes on the toxicology of cobalt metal. Br J Ind Med 7:76, 1950.
127. Schepers GWH: The biological action of particulate cobalt metal. Arch Ind Health 12:127, 1955.
128. Kerfoot EJ, Frederick WG, Domeier E: Cobalt metal inhalation studies on miniature swine. Am Ind Hyg Assoc J 36:17, 1975.
129. Bonnell JA, Kazantzis G, King E: A follow-up study of man exposed to cadmiun oxide fumes. Br J Ind Med 16:135, 1959.
130. Lane RE, Campbell ACP: Fatal emphysema in two men making a copper cadmium alloy. Br J Ind Med 11:118, 1954.
131. Snider GL, Hayes JA, Korthy AL, Lewis GP: Centrilobular emphysema experimentally induced by cadmium chloride aerosol. Am Rev Respir Dis 108:40, 1973.
132. Liebow AA: Definition and classification of interstitial pneumonias in human pathology. Prog Respir Res 8:1, 1975.
133. Hallee TJ: Diffuse lung disease caused by inhalation of mercury vapor. Am Rev Respir Dis 99:430, 1969.
134. Jones Williams W: The pathology of the lungs in five nickel workers. Br J Ind Med 15:235, 1958.
135. Barnes JM, Denz FA: The effect of 2,3-dimercapto-propanol (BAL) on experimental nickel carbonyl poisoning. Br J Ind Med 8:117, 1951.
136. Trapp E, Renzetti AD, Kobayashi T, et al: Cardiopulmonary function in uranium miners. Am Rev Respir Dis 101:27, 1970.
137. Pickrell JA, Schnizlein CT, Hahn FF, et al: Radiation-induced pulmonary fibrosis: Study of changes in collagen constituents in different lung regions of beagle dogs after inhalation of beta-emitting radionuclides. Radiat Res 74:363, 1978.

2 Asbestos Exposure and Airway Responses

Margaret R. Becklake
Pierre Ernst

A recent review of the pathogenesis of asbestos-related respiratory disease[1] lists the following entities: parenchymal fibrosis (asbestosis), pleural lesions both benign and malignant, bronchogenic cancer, and cancer of the digestive system and other organs. A similar list was given nine years earlier in a much-quoted review[2] published in the United Kingdom. No mention was made in either paper of the possibility that airway dysfunction might also be related to asbestos exposure, although the issue had been raised elsewhere[3] and the conclusion reached on the basis of a review of the literature to date (1976) that because "the character of the function impairment may be obstructive in a certain number of cases, until further evidence is available an open mind should be kept in this regard."[4] This chapter reviews the subsequent evidence (since 1976) as well as some of the earlier evidence in an attempt to throw light on the question: does exposure to asbestos cause airway dysfunction? The question remains a current clinical issue.[5]

AIRWAY RESPONSES

Alteration in airway function may give rise to symptoms described by the patient, physical signs detected by the physician, and lung function abnormality measured by physiologic tests. In general the chest radiograph lacks sensitivity in the detection of airway dysfunction, particularly in subjects exposed to asbestos in whom parenchymal fibrosis may also be present.

The clinical indicators of airway dysfunction are not specific. For instance, symptoms such as cough and shortness of breath may be the consequence of airway dysfunction, but in asbestos-exposed workers may also be associated with the early stages of radiographic pulmonary fibrosis.[4] Sputum production, often used as the diagnostic criterion for bronchitis[6] because it probably reflects mucus gland hyperplasia, is perhaps more suggestive of airway dysfunction; also, both wheezing and rhonchi may be manifestations of airflow limitation and possibly airway lability.

Compared to the other clinical indicators lung function tests provide the best quantitative and qualitative measurements of airway dysfunction. However, here again lack of specificity is a problem because of the interdependence of airway and parenchymal function[7] such that measurements of the former are inevitably affected by changes in the latter.

Problems also arise in the interpretation of results of lung function tests, particularly those that appear to reflect small airway function[8] (such as measurements derived from the single breath nitrogen test and forced expiratory flow rates at low lung volumes). Thus there are few studies correlating small airway structure and function,[9–12] and most measurements were adopted on the basis of their capacity to discriminate between smokers and nonsmokers,[13] in line with the hypothesis that small airway abnormality precedes large airway disease in those smokers who will eventually develop chronic disabling airflow limitation.[14] It is not surprising to find that in occupational surveys abnormalities are found most often in smokers. An additional problem in the interpretation of their association with asbestos exposure arises from the fact that functional abnormalities of the small airways have been described in other interstitial pulmonary diseases such as sarcoidosis[15] and cryptogenic fibrosing alveolitis.[16]

HUMAN EXPOSURE TO ASBESTOS

Human exposure to asbestos may occur under a wide variety of circumstances.[4,17,18] These include exposure (1) in mining asbestos-bearing rock and milling the fiber; (2) in manufacturing the very large number and variety of products that incorporate this material, as well as in the use and application of such products; (3) in the use of this material in the home for improvements and hobbies, by contamination of the home environment with material transported on work clothes; and (4) environmental pollution due to the proximity of the home to a workplace where asbestos is produced or used.

Nonmalignant (chronic inflammatory or fibrotic) as well as malignant pulmonary disease may follow exposure, and these have been the subject of several recent reviews.[5,18–20] In general the risk of developing disease has been shown to be related to exposure.[18,19] Human risk may also be influenced by circumstances under which exposure occurs, as well as by fiber type.[18,19] In assessing the evidence for a relationship between asbestos exposure and airway responses, these factors should not be ignored, nor should we fail to recognize the potential contribution of other environmental contaminants in the workplaces where the exposure to the asbestos occurred. In practice it is usually not possible to separate the consequences of an occupational exposure to an environment that includes pollution by asbestos particles from the consequences of direct exposure to asbestos particles per se, except where the latter are the only environmental contaminants.

ASSOCIATION AND CAUSALITY

Certain criteria have been proposed to determine whether the association between a disease that is common in the general population is causally related to a particular environmental exposure. These criteria include the strength and consistency of the association, time and dose–response relationships, and the biologic plausibility and coherence of the evidence.[21] One application would be to assess the relationship between asbestos exposure and lung cancer.[22]

Dose–response relationships used to assess causality should ideally reflect the dose of the agent in question (in this case, asbestos particles) delivered to the target organ (in this case, the airways) and retained in contact with the target organ for sufficient time to evoke a biologic response. In practice, it is necessary to use exposure measurements as a substitute for measurement of biologic dose. Certain factors, such as particle size, that affect aerodynamic properties of particles can often be taken into account in the assessment of exposure, but other factors cannot be quantified with precision, for example, the very effective pulmonary clearance mechanisms and personal characteristics that may influence penetration, deposition, and clearance of inhaled materials.

REVIEW OF THE EVIDENCE: APPROACH AND CLASSIFICATION

This review is based on a search of the medical literature using (1) the National Library of Medicine "medline" to identify publications dealing with asbestos and lung function or disease from January 1979 to April 1982, (2) the Sourcebook on Asbestos Diseases[23] to identify articles dealing with lung function or pathology for the years 1971–1979, and (3) a selection of material published prior to 1971 culled from an earlier comprehensive review of the literature on the topic.[24]

All material was classified into one of four categories for the purpose of abstracting:

1. Experimental studies: in which exposure (or not) was controlled by the researcher and subjects (in this case, only animals) were randomly assigned to either group.[25–29]

Table 2-1. Asbestos Exposure and Airway Responses: Clinical Studies

First Author	Ref.	Subjects	Exposure	Response Measurements			Findings
				Clinical	PFTs	x-ray	
Williams (1960)	30	21 certified cases of asbestosis, 19 exposed workers	Not given	+	+	+	Rhonchi in 9/21 workers with certified asbestosis, and an increase in FEV_1/FVC following a bronchodilator in 8/10 without radiologic disease; no information on smoking
Bader (1970)	31	598 members of a union of insulators	Years worked	+	+	+	FEV_1/FVC less than 70% in 29 men; rhonchi heard in 24; no information on smoking
Muldoon (1972)	32	60 cases referred for a pneumoconiosis panel	Years worked	+	+	+	10/13 subjects with "obstruction" (TLC normal or increased, SG_{aw} reduced) had normal chest radiographs
Zedda (1973)	33	368 chrysotile miners and 356 men in mills or manufacturing	Years worked	+	+	+	Of 398 subjects with chest radiographs 0/0 or 0/1, 11% with less than 10 years exposure and 24% with over 10 years exposure had "COPD"

Harless (1978)	34	23/79 construction workers who cut asbestos floor boards	Short (5 months); heavy (over 2 f/ml)	+	+	+	12 (3 nonsmokers) had some function abnormality; 8 months later CV/VC% had increased in 7
Rodriguez-Roisin (1980)	35	40 workers referred to a pneumoconiosis panel	Years since first exposure		−	+	34/40 subjects had reduced flows on MEFV curve; of these 22 (7 nonsmokers) had otherwise normal function, 6 a restrictive and 6 an obstructive profile; weak relationship to smoking, none to exposure
Sulotto (1980)	36	200 workers referred to a compensation panel	Years worked; chrysotile and crocidolite		+	+	67 smokers, 67 nonsmokers showed abnormal small airway function; FVC, FEV_1, $\dot{V}_{max\,50}$ and $\dot{V}_{max\,25}$ lower in those with crocidolite exposure
Pearle (1981)	37	88 male shipyard workers referred for assessment	Years worked	+	+	+	18 workers had FEV_1/FVC less than 70%, of whom 17 were smokers (over 10 pk. yrs)
Pearle (1982)	38	131 male shipyard workers referred for assessment	Years worked	+	+	+	26 men with FEV_1/FVC less than 70%; related to smoking but not exposure; pleural abnormality also related to exposure but not parenchymal abnormality

Table 2-2. Asbestos Exposure and Airway Responses: Pathologic Studies

First Author	Ref.	Subjects	Source	Exposure	Findings
Hourihane (1966)	40	69 cases of asbestosis	Autopsy	Not stated	Conclude "the basic lesion is a peribronchiolar fibrosis which obliterates surrounding alveoli as it extends outwards"
Turner-Warwick (1974)	41	1 case	Not stated	Not stated	An example in the author's experience of the "occasional case of asbestosis where the fibrosis is almost exclusively peribronchiolar"
DiMenza (1976)	42	1 case	Not stated	Not stated	Pneumonectomy specimen showing gramlonatous changes in the distal bronchiole with narrowing
Becklake (1982)	43	1 case	Pleural biopsy		Pleural effusion in a 28-year-old man 10 years following last exposure; subpleural areas showed peribronchiolar fibrosis
Churg (1982)	44	15 exposed 15 nonexposed (age, sex, smoking matched)	Autopsy material	Not stated	More fibrosis in the membranous bronchioles and alveolar ducts of the exposed workers than in those of the nonexposed workers

2. Clinical studies: essentially descriptive studies of workers and other exposed individuals without information on how representative they were of the workforce or exposed population to which they belong(ed)[30–39] (see also Table 2-1).

3. Pathologic studies: for the most part in the same category as clinical reports[17,40–44] (see also Table 2-2).

4. Epidemiologic studies: conducted so that the subjects studied could in some way be related to the source population[45–63] (see also Table 2-3).

Each category of study has strengths and weaknesses[64] and their relative weight in assessing the case for or against a causal association between asbestos exposure and airway dysfunction varies. The evidence will be discussed by category.

Table 2-3. Asbestos Exposure and Airway Responses

First Author	Ref.	Subjects	Exposure	Response Measurements			Findings
				Clinical	PFTs	x-ray	
A Epidemiologic Studies of Workforces Exposed in Mining and Milling							
McDonald (1972)	45	1015 Quebec chrysotile miners and millers	Cumulative exposure index for each subject	+			Phlegm and wheeze related to smoking, and in men over 50 to cumulative exposure; 11% had radiologic fibrosis
Becklake (1972)	46	1015 Quebec chrysotile miners and millers	Cumulative exposure index for each subject		+		In nonsmokers MMEF, and in smokers MMEF and FEV_1/FVC decreased with exposure: 11% had radiologic fibrosis
Fournier-Massey (1978)	47	1015 Quebec chrysotile miners and millers	Cumulative exposure index for each subject	+	+	+	Comparable prevalence of obstructive and restrictive profiles; neither related to exposure; obstructive group had more smokers and higher exposures
Becklake (1982)	48	1015 Quebec chrysotile miners and millers; follow-up on 722 men	Cumulative exposure index for each subject (not updated)	+	+	+	Attack and progression rates for MMEF abnormality related to age and smoking rather than exposure
Jodoin (1971)	49	1015 Quebec chrysotile miners and millers; subsample of 24 men with normal chest x-rays	Cumulative exposure index for each subject	+	+		CL, DL_{CO} were related to the exposure index; however, $\dot{V}_{max}$ at low lung volumes was also decreased
Peress (1975)	50	1015 Quebec chrysotile miners and millers; subsample of 129 men with normal chest x-rays	Cumulative exposure index for each subject		+		Closing vol% VC, slope phase III distinguished low and high exposure groups in nonsmokers and smokers

(*continued*)

Table 2-3 (*continued*)

First Author	Ref.	Subjects	Exposure	Response Measurements			Findings
				Clinical	PFTs	x-ray	
Meurman (1974)	51	787 anthophylite miners	Years worked	+		+	Cough twice as frequent in nonexposed subjects, and 4 times as frequent in subjects with over 10 yrs exposure
Grzybrowski[a]	—	126 B.C. chrysotile miners	Years worked	+	+	+	Prevalence of cough and breathlessness was 14% and 11% in those with less than 10 yrs exposure, and 49 and 53% in those with over 10 years exposure
B. Epidemiologic Studies of Workforces Exposed in Production, Manufacturing, and Utilization.							
Langlands (1971)	52	252 insulation workers	Years worked	+	+	+	In men over 40 yrs, 49% had sputum, 50% wheezed but 69% were smokers
Wallace (1971)	53	50 insulators, 50 others		+	+	+	FEV_1/FVC comparable in both groups; 14 insulators had radiologic evidence of fibrosis
Ferris (1971)	54	63 pipecoverers, 61 others	Ship repair; often over 5 mppcf	+	+	+	No differences in FEV_1, FVC, PF; 28 pipecoverers had radiologic evidence of fibrosis
Murphy (1971, 1972)	55 56	101 pipecoverers, 94 others with follow-up	Shipyard (new construction); amosite, some chrysotile; in general under 5 mppcf	+	+	+	FEV_1/FVC, Raw comparable in both groups: phlegm, wheezing more common in pipecoverers

Murphy (1978)	57	Follow-up: 77 pipecoverers, 70 others	See above	+	+	+	Wheezing recorded in 39% and 13%, respectively; "COPD" in 13% and 7%, respectively
Weill (1975)	58	859 asbestos cement workers	Cumulative exposure index for each man: chrysotile, some crocidolite	+	+	+	FEV_1, FVC, and MMEF decreased in relation to exposure; reduction slightly more marked in men exposed to crocidolite; 30% had radiologic evidence of fibrosis
Lebowitz (1977)	59	1195 men in a population based study	60% had occupational exposure to various materials including asbestos	+			Wheezing and wheezing with dyspnea significantly increased in asbestos-exposed compared to nonexposed subjects
Woitowitz (1978)	60	499 workers in 2 processing plants		+	+		Symptoms and signs increased in relation to exposure in heavy smokers: FEV_1 reduced, R_{aw} increased in exposed nonsmokers
Becklake (1980)	61	272 workers in a factory, 118 in a textile plant	Mixed fiber	+	+		Wheezing in 36% of factory workers and 40% of textile workers, compared to 11% in miners previously studied (46)
			Chrysotile only	+	+		
Hedenstierna (1981)	62	101 construction workers (55 with plaques) 56 nonexposed		+	+	+	$\dot{V}_{max\ 50}$, $\dot{V}_{max\ 25}$ were decreased and CV/VC% increased in subjects with pleural disease compared to nonexposed subjects matched for smoking
Rodriguez-Roisin (1981)	63	71 chrysotile textile workers	High exposure for an average of 4.1 years		+		FEV_1, FVC, FEV_1/FVC, MMEF, $\dot{V}_{max\ 50}$, $\dot{V}_{max\ 25}$, DLco correlated with exposure

[a] Unpublished report on miners in Cassiar, B. C.

EXPERIMENTAL STUDIES IN ANIMALS

Several elegant animal models have been devised to study the earliest pulmonary reactions to inhaled asbestos particles and the fate of such particles[25,26] as well as to correlate early pathologic lesions with abnormalities measured by pulmonary function tests.[27,28] Inhaled particles tend to collect at the origins of the respiratory bronchioles; a cellular response can also be demonstrated. For example, in a guinea pig model[26] where animals were exposed to more than 1000 fibers/ml for 9 or 18 days, the initial reaction was granulomatous and was mainly peribronchiolar in location with severe structural disruption of terminal and respiratory bronchioles. These changes were followed by peribronchiolar fibrosis, which appeared to progress into surrounding alveoli. Lung function measurements revealed an increase in resistance and a decrease in dynamic compliance corresponding to the time of maximal bronchiolar disruption. In a similar study in a sheep model[27] in which weekly intratracheal injections of chrysotile were given for six months, transbronchial biopsies revealed an alveolitis with peribronchial inflammation in over half the airways, which were at times compressed. These abnormalities were coincident with a decrease in compliance (CL), a reduced vital capacity (VC), a reduced forced expiratory flowrate at 50% lung volume ($\dot{V}_{max\ 50}$), an increase in upstream resistance and an increase in the volume of isoflow breathing helium. It remains to be shown whether these abnormalities in small airways are an early manifestation of diffuse parenchymal fibrosis, that is, asbestosis, as seems likely. Less likely, though possible, is that the lesions will in some instances remain localized to the airways, eventually leading to chronic airflow limitation. In summary, the pathologic evidence from recent animal studies, in agreement with earlier work,[29] demonstrates that the fibrotic process consequent on exposure to inhaled asbestos particles starts at the level of the small airways, and that these lesions are associated with abnormality in function tests generally believed to reflect small airway status.

CLINICAL STUDIES (See Table 2-1)

Starting at the beginning of the century, there have been a large number of case reports and clinical studies of lung function in asbestos workers;[24] of those prior to 1971, a few have been selected for comment. A study of 40 workers from a British factory led to the conclusion that asbestosis was characterized by a reduced diffusing capacity for carbon monoxide (DLco) and a reduced VC in keeping with a restrictive defect.[30] Not commented upon was the fact that rhonchi were found on auscultation of 9 out of 21 workers certified as having asbestosis and a bronchodilator response to sympathomimetics in 8 out of 10 cases with heavy exposure but not certified disease. Both findings are suggestive of obstructive airways disease. In this study, as in much of the earlier work, no data regarding smoking habits were presented. Indeed, the role of smoking in the causation of airway abnormality had not yet been fully recognized, and it is therefore difficult in such studies to assess the relative roles of smoking and asbestos exposure in the production of detected airway abnormality.

Clinical studies also fail to provide any standard of comparison for the frequency of abnormality or, in a diseased population, for the frequency of exposure. For instance, in a study of 598 currently employed workers belonging to an asbestos workers union, including men over 70 years of age, decrease in forced vital capacity (FVC) was found in 35% of subjects, while a decrease in forced expiratory volume in one second as a percent of forced vital capacity (FEV_1/FVC%) was noted in only 29 subjects, and "moderate or severe rhonchi" were heard in only 4%.[31] No nonexposed population was studied for comparison. There may also have been a selection bias toward healthy workers reflected in the fact that no significant difference in lung function was found between smokers and nonsmokers. In another study of 724 mill and factory workers, a restrictive pulmonary function pattern was found in workers with x-ray abnormalities suggestive of asbestosis.[33] In addition, in subjects with a normal chest x-ray and less than 10 years of asbestos exposure, 11% were reported as having chronic obstructive pulmonary disease (criteria not specified) as compared to 24% with more than 10 years exposure. This difference may have been due to age and/or smoking, since the group with longer exposure was on average 5 years older and no information on smoking habits was provided. The pulmonary function data reported also showed similar proportionate decreases in FEV_1 and FVC as well as similar values for residual volume as a percent of total lung capacity (RV/TLC%) in both groups, findings which do not suggest an exposure-related obstructive abnormality.

Several studies have reported detailed lung function in subjects referred to a pneumoconiois panel or compensation board for certification of asbestos-related illness. In one such report based on 60 workers, an "obstructive group" of 13 subjects was identified on the basis of a normal or increased TLC and a reduced specific airways conductance (SG_{aw}), 10 of whom had interstitial disease on chest x-ray.[32] There was no difference in mean age, duration of asbestos exposure, or smoking habits between the restrictive and obstructive groups, although there were no nonsmokers in the latter and only 4 in the group as a whole. The authors are rightly cautious in their conclusions and state only that obstructive airways disease is not uncommon in asbestos workers even with radiographic abnormalities compatible with asbestosis and that "the possibility that asbestos dust can induce bronchial damage needs further critical study." In another study of 40 workers referred to a pneumoconiosis panel, 34 of 40 subjects, including 15 with otherwise normal lung function, had reduced flowrates at low lung volumes.[35] No association with years since first exposure could be demonstrated. Although the authors state that these lung function changes could not be completely accounted for by smoking, only one of their subjects was a lifetime nonsmoker. Nevertheless, considering the many possible causes of reduced flow at low lung volumes, it seems difficult to ascribe these changes to asbestos exposure with any certainty.

The major shortcomings in reports based on subjects referred for compensation assessment is that such individuals came to medical attention because of symptoms and signs of lung disease in association with a history of asbestos exposure. The lack of reference populations matched for past experience, excluding asbestos exposure, makes any link between this exposure and their lung disease entirely conjectural. While this type of study remains important as a pointer to the presence of relationships between an environmental agent and a biologic effect, further investigations, including epidemiologic and, if possible, experimental studies, are required to determine if the association can be considered causal.

Similar reservations must be borne in mind in interpreting the results of other referral populations. For instance, two such reports[37,38] deal with 131 male shipyard workers, 97 of whom had normal chest x-rays; 21% were found to have a reduced $FEV_1/FVC\%$, which correlated with smoking but not with exposure. The author concludes that his "data strongly suggests that smoking is the primary cause of airway obstruction in asbestos exposed workers." This conclusion seems somewhat overstated when one considers that no sensitive indicators of airway obstruction, not even a maximal midexpiratory flow (MMEF) were reported. The very crude exposure grouping into three categories based on years of exposure without any consideration of job classification should make one cautious in rejecting a dose relationship to exposure. There is also a bias toward finding a better correlation with smoking, since the quantification of tobacco use was more precise. Another report[34] deals with 23 volunteers from 79 workers who had had heavy exposure for five months to asbestos dust; 12 subjects showed at least one abnormal test of small airways function with an increase in closing volume (CV) being the most frequent. Again, only one subject was a lifetime nonsmoker, there were no nonexposed subjects studied for reference, the exposure index was retrospective, and technical factors may have influenced some of the results; for instance, one subject showed a 7-fold increase in closing volume as a percent of vital capacity (CV/VC%) over eight months.

PATHOLOGIC STUDIES (See Table 2-2)

Autopsy material not surprisingly tends to reflect endstage disease; like clinical referral material, it is biased toward the more severe degrees of abnormality. Nevertheless, careful review has permitted the pathologist to develop an impression of the pathologic evolution of nonmalignant asbestos-related pulmonary disease. One of the earlier reviews,[40] based on an experience with 69 autopsies of cases of asbestosis, concluded that "the basic lesion (of asbestosis) is a peribronchiolar fibrosis which obliterates surrounding alveoli as it extends outwards from the bronchiole." Basically the same conclusions were reached recently by an expert panel assembled to prepare diagnostic criteria and a grading scheme for asbestos-associated diseases of the lungs and pleural cavities.[17] There are also a few other case reports in man[41–43] describing a predominantly peribronchiolar fibrosis. Recently, using a morphometric method,[9] Churg and Wright[44] have reported in preliminary form a comparison of autopsy findings in the lungs of 15 asbestos workers with those in 15 nonexposed persons matched for age, sex, and smoking. No details were given of exposure nor of the provenance of the nonexposed subjects nor of the method of selection. A significant increase in fibrous tissue in respiratory bronchioles and alveolar ducts was found in the asbestos-exposed group, while no difference between groups could be shown for abnormalities of small bronchioles. How these differences might be reflected clinically is unknown, and there has so far been no attempt to correlate these pathologic findings with pulmonary function results in humans. However, it is not unreasonable to suppose that they would be associated with abnormality in tests of small airway function, similar to the findings in smokers in whom the pathologic function correlation has been examined.

EPIDEMIOLOGIC STUDIES (See Table 2-3)

Studies in this category allow one to estimate the prevalence of an abnormality. This is achieved either by defining the population at risk and determining the frequency of dysfunction in the population as a whole or in a representative sample, or by a case referent approach that allows one to estimate the relative risk of exposure in affected subjects as compared to nonaffected referent subjects. The first approach or typical occupational survey avoids selecting subjects because of illness as happens in clinical studies. Such prevalence studies can be strengthened by studying an appropriate reference population which has not been exposed, using the same methods, and ensuring that the studies are conducted simultaneously or as closely in time as possible to avoid differences due to technical or temporal factors. However, studies on current workforces are studies of survivor populations and are likely to underestimate prevalence of abnormality unless past workers are included and/or turnover rates taken into account. The case referent method aims to eliminate selection bias by applying the selection process to both cases and controls. The problem here is in the selection of appropriate referents.[64] Cohort or longitudinal studies are necessary to provide estimates of incidence.

For the present review, material pertaining to mining exposures is listed in Table 2-3A, and that to exposures in production, manufacturing, and utilization in Table 2-3B. These exposures are considered separately because of the differences in the character of the environmental pollution; thus in mining there is usually a considerable amount of nonfibrous particulate airborne matter, including rockdust,[65,66] believed to be relevant in the development of industrial bronchitis,[67] while in the other industrial processes the airborne material tends to contain more, or even exclusively, asbestos fibers[61] and/or particles, with or without other contaminants.

In the mining sector, one series of reports[45–50] deals with Quebec chrysotile asbestos miners and millers; the main study population[45–48] comprised an age-stratified random sample of current workers approximately 11% of whom had radiographic changes suggestive of asbestosis. Past exposures had been extremely heavy,[65] both in terms of particle and fiber pollution.[65,66] Respiratory health was examined in relation to a cumulative exposure index based on careful job histories, length of exposure, and dust measurements. Breathlessness correlated with increasing cumulative exposure, while phlegm and wheeze were predominantly related to cigarette smoking, and only in men over 50 years of age to cumulative exposure.[45] Lung volumes were found to decrease with exposure as might be expected with developing lung fibrosis. However, there was also a progressive dose-related decrease in MMEF in nonsmokers, while smokers had both a decrease in MMEF as well as a lower $FEV_1/FVC\%$ with increasing exposure.[46] In a follow-up study of the same workers 7 years later[48] over 50% of those with a normal MMEF at the time of the initial survey had developed abnormality (defined as an MMEF less than 80% predicted), and more than 40% of subjects with an initially abnormal MMEF had worsened significantly. This rate of progression is two to three times greater than that seen when considering abnormalities in VC. Though the rates for attack and progression of abnormality could not be related to the cumulative exposure once age and smoking had been taken into account, this may in part be due to the interrelations between smoking, age, and exposure. It is possible that part of the effect attributed to age reflects residence time of dust in the lung, which, because of improving environmental conditions,[65] became progressively more strongly linked to age than to the calculated cumulative exposure. Approximately half the subjects developed new radiologic abnormality or showed progression of previous abnormality. The abnormality of function that ensued may have been the consequence of interstitial fibrotic changes or of independent airway disease or of both.

To overcome the lack of specificity of any one test of lung function, the material gathered in the cross-sectional study of Quebec miners and millers[46] was reexamined using lung function profiles based on abnormalities in lung volumes and spirometry.[47] In this way the sample was divided into groups with normal, undifferentiated, restrictive, and obstructive patterns of function. Almost equal prevalence of definite obstructive and restrictive profiles were found, 12.2% and 12.8%, respectively. Both the restrictive and obstructive profiles were more common in smokers, and neither showed a relationship to cumulative exposure. The obstructive group had both a higher proportion of heavy smokers and of higher dust indices, suggesting a possible synergistic effect.

In a study designed to look for the earliest responses to exposure,[49] i.e., before abnormalities were evident on the chest radiograph or in the usual surveillance function measurements such as FVC, a subsample of 24 subjects with normal radiographs underwent detailed studies of lung mechanics. Pulmonary compliance was related to exposure, consistent with fibrotic changes having already started to develop; however, though $FEV_1/FVC\%$ and MMEF were increased in the higher exposure group compared to the lower exposure group, flowrates at low lung volumes were decreased not increased, suggesting that the changes must have caused small airway narrowing. A larger study in the same workforce, also confined to subjects without radiologic abnormality, in which smoking history was taken into account, gave similar results.[50] This combination of findings suggestive of small airways disease does not appear to be the same airway abnormality as that found in the population as a whole (which includes those with radiologic abnormality) where young nonsmokers with high dust exposure were found to have a decreased mean MMEF with a normal $FEV_1/FVC\%$.[46] This latter combination has also been interpreted as evidence of small airways disease.[68] The natural history of neither abnormality is known. The classical restrictive findings in patients in the earlier study[49] suggest that their airway dysfunction might be due to peribronchial fibrosis, recognized as the early lesion of asbestosis. (As already indicated, similar results have also been described in patients with cryptogenic fibrosing alveolitis[16] and sarcoidosis.[15]) The decrease in MMEF in the latter study[46] is more likely to represent early obstructive airways abnormality, since it is a common abnormality in young smokers.[68]

In summary, data on Quebec asbestos miners and millers are consistent with there being a hypersecretory airway response (reflected in the complaint of sputum) to heavy exposures in older workers, as well as of acute airway reactions (reflected in the complaint of wheezing), the prevalence of which increased with increasing exposure. In addition, there was evidence that small airway abnormality may develop either as a manifestation of the peribronchiolar fibrotic reactions that precede the more diffuse interstitial fibrosis of asbestosis, or possibly as the manifestation of a primarily intraluminal small airway reaction as seen in response to other inhaled agents such as cigarette smoke. Chronic airflow limitation was a common finding, though its relationship to exposure has not been clarified.

A number of the studies in secondary industry deal with insulation workers. In a study of 252 insulation workers in Belfast, Northern Ireland,[52] a decreasing $FEV_1/FVC\%$ could be related to increasing smoking in those with a normal chest radiograph but not in those with evidence of pleural or parenchymal disease. Possible interpretations include the presence of both obstructive and restrictive abnormality affecting different parts of the lung in the same individual, resulting in a near-normal $FEV_1/FVC\%$. Another possibility is the presence of individuals in the population with both types of abnormality, obstructive and restrictive, with the result that the mean $FEV_1/FVC\%$ may be close to a normal value. In a second study based on the same workforce,[53] 50 insulation workers were selected by a random procedure and matched to 50 nonexposed subjects working in the city of Belfast, so as to control for the possible effects of a generally polluted industrial environment and to attempt to account for the usual confounders such as age, height, and smoking. The exposed group had smaller mean lung volumes and more x-ray abnormalities, including 14 cases with definite x-ray evidence of fibrosis. Questionnaires indicated they also had significantly greater frequency of cough and sputum. On the basis of similar values for $FEV_1/FVC\%$ in the exposed and nonexposed subjects, respectively, the authors conclude that there was no evidence of airways obstruction secondary to asbestos exposure. Since 28% of the insulators had frank asbestosis by chest x-ray and, as a group, had lower mean lung volumes, one would have expected a higher $FEV_1/FVC\%$ consistent with the restrictive ventilatory disorder, particularly in view of the fact that the smoking habits of both groups were comparable. The findings are thus not inconsistent with the presence of exposure-related airflow limitation in this workforce, although the authors' own interpretation of their findings is also reasonable.

Several other studies have dealt with insulation workers in shipyard industries.[54–57] One study[54] compared symptoms, simple spirometry, and chest x-ray findings in 101 pipecoverers in new ship construction with those in a group of 94 other workers from the same shipyards. Most of the same subjects were retested a year later,[55] and their results for measurements of airway resistance were published in a subsequent paper.[56] Lower lung volumes and a greater frequency of x-ray abnormality were found among exposed subjects of whom only 27.8% had a normal chest radiograph. No differences were found for FEV_1/FVC% or airways resistance. The authors concluded that there was no evidence of an excess of chronic nonspecific lung disease, either airways obstruction or chronic bronchitis, among workers with the heavier asbestos exposure. The exposed and nonexposed subjects were well matched, the studies well done, and therefore these two papers are often quoted as evidence against airways dysfunction secondary to asbestos exposure.

There are, however, objections that can be raised to the broad conclusions that have been based on this work. Although there was no excess of chronic bronchitis by clinical criteria, pipecoverers reported more cough, phlegm, and wheezing apart from colds, suggesting that clinical criteria used were too rigid for determining abnormality in a working population. Furthermore, on reevaluation of 77 of the exposed subjects and 70 of the reference subjects almost seven years later,[57] wheezing was reported in 39% and 12.9% of the two groups, while 13.1% of the pipecoverers satisfied clinical criteria for the diagnosis of chronic obstructive disease as opposed to 7.1% of others matched for age, height, and, more importantly, smoking status. Again, no difference between groups could be shown on the only test of airways obstruction reported, FEV_1/FVC%. The failure to demonstrate a difference on simple spirometry may in part be methodologic. There is certainly likely to have been some error due to misclassification, since the referent group showed radiologic evidence of asbestos exposure; for instance, 11.4% had definite parenchymal abnormality (1/0 or more on UICC classification). In addition, this population was composed of survivors at follow-up, and severe abnormality of any type had been excluded.

As part of a large nationwide study of chronic bronchitis in Germany,[60] a random sample of 499 workers from two raw asbestos processing plants were examined. Subjects were divided into high, medium, and low exposure groups on the basis of job classification, length of employment, and serial dust measurements. Using a graded profile of symptoms and physical signs, including cough, phlegm, wheeze, and auscultatory rhonchi, the authors found a greater prevalence of chronic nonspecific lung disease with increasing asbestos exposure in heavy smokers. This is similar to the findings of a Tuscon, Arizona study, the only community-based study encountered.[59] In a group of 1195 men grouped according to reported occupational exposures, more symptoms were reported in all dusty occupations. The excess was most marked in heavy smokers over the age of 45, suggesting a synergistic effect of cigarette smoke and dust exposure on symptoms. In addition, those with asbestos exposure showed a higher prevalence of wheezing. The German study also found an 8% greater incidence of an obstructive pulmonary profile among young male nonsmokers with the heaviest asbestos exposure, but could not demonstrate any difference among smokers.

In another study,[58] 859 asbestos cement workers were the subjects, 68% of whom had a normal chest x-ray and another 15% had only pleural changes. Exposure was calculated from total respirable dust measurements and detailed job histories. An exposure-related reduction in FEV_1, FVC, and MMEF was found independent of smoking or any x-ray changes. Because of proportionate decreases in FEV_1 and FVC, the FEV_1/FVC% was unchanged, again indicating that a normal FEV_1/FVC% cannot necessarily be construed as evidence against an obstructive ventilatory defect in an asbestos-exposed group. The decrease in MMEF is very similar to the results reported in Quebec chrysotile miners.[46] However, part of this obstructive pattern in the asbestos cement workers could be secondary to cement dust, also reported as causing a decrease in maximal flows at low lung volumes.[69] An analogous problem occurs in relation to many occupational exposures, since inert dust has been shown to have at least a temporary effect on FEV_1[70] and on airways resistance.[71] It is conceivable that part of the airway dysfunction associated with asbestos exposure is due to a nonspecific dust effect related to larger particles that tend to deposit in major airways. If this were the case, a lack of correlation between indices of exposure based on fiber counts and airways dysfunction would hardly be surprising.[67]

Another study examined two Quebec plants,[61] one making asbestos textiles where the exposure was to chrysotile only and another making asbestos cement products using mainly chrysotile with some amosite and in the past crocidolite. In both groups the prevalence of radiologic and function abnormality was greater than in Quebec chrysotile miners (studied some years previously by the same methods) despite their longer exposures to apparently higher dust levels compared to the plant workers. In addition, the prevalence of the complaint of wheezing was considerable higher in the two plants as was the occurrence of a low MMEF.

Textile workers were also the subjects of study in a recent report from Spain;[63] 71 of a workforce of 104 with high exposure to chrysotile (mean duration 4.1 years) were studied. Of these cases, 46 were nonsmokers and showed decreased lung volumes and maximal flows. Differences between exposed and nonexposed were less marked in subjects who smoked. The following lung functions showed a significant correlation with exposure: FVC, FEV_1, TLC, FEV_1/FVC%, MMEF, $V_{max\ 50}$, $V_{max\ 25}$, and DLco. No correlation was found between exposure and specific conductance, a test of large airways. The authors conclude that in addition to the well-recognized restrictive impairment, asbestos exposure is associated with airflow limitation occurring predominantly in small airways. This study provides evidence in favor of an asbestos effect on airways, evidence not likely to be forthcoming again, considering the very high dust levels.

Finally, a case-control study of construction workers[62] exposed to asbestos deserves comment; 55 of 423 asbestos workers were selected for the presence of isolated pleural plaques on chest x-ray and matched with 55 nonexposed workers. Cases showed an excess of cough (62% as compared to 22%), as well as an increase in CV/VC% and decreased maximal flows at low lung volumes, but no decrease in compliance. This is in contrast to the reduction in compliance reported in exposed chrysotile miners without radiologic abnormality.[49] However, the results must be considered with circumspection because of poor matching of cases and controls for socioeconomic status and even for smoking. Furthermore, cases and controls also differed in respect of other occupational exposures besides asbestos.

CONCLUSIONS

From the preceding review it is evident that there is a considerable amount of information on the nature and mechanisms (from clinical and animal studies) of airway dysfunction seen in asbestos workers. It is also clear that airway dysfunction is by no means infrequent in workers with occupational exposures primarily to asbestos fibers and/or particles as well as those in which these constitute only one component of the environmental pollution. However, in general, the epidemiologic evidence does not meet the criteria for establishing a causal association with asbestos exposure for any of the clinical syndromes of airway dysfunction. On the one hand, there is a rather surprising consistency in the evidence with epidemiologic as well as clinical studies of the exposed workforces, pointing to increased prevalences for one or more of the indicators of airway dysfunction. Since most of the epidemiologic evidence comes from prevalence studies of current workers, it is likely that the occurrence of chronic airflow limitation, a potentially disabling abnormality, has been underestimated. On the other hand, exposure–response relationships are frequently not seen; however, this may be due to imprecision or inappropriateness of the exposure measurements used.[72] These have focused on elements in the exposure believed to be important in the development of parenchymal reactions, in particular, fibers, whereas airway responses may well be the consequence of exposure to particles of other dimensions usually present in much greater numbers in the environmental dust clouds. Without pathologic material it is difficult to distinguish airway dysfunction that is the consequence of peribronchiolar fibrosis (and therefore likely to be the early stages of asbestosis) from that which is the consequence of bronchiolar wall damage, as seen in relation to other inhaled agents such as cigarette smoke and the oxides of nitrogen, and which may also be related to damage by asbestos.

While the indicators of airway dysfunction may be sensitive, they are certainly not specific (see above). Time relationships are also difficult to assess when the response is a chronic one whose onset is difficult to pinpoint. Nevertheless, because of biologic plausibility (it seems probable that breathing dust loads will affect the channels through which the dust passes), as well as a certain coherence in the evidence, it would be unreasonable to reject the idea of causal association between exposure and any of the clinical syndromes listed. Moreover, the evidence since 1976 has strengthened this conclusion considerably. However, clarification of the question is unlikely without studies specifically designed to address the issue; unfocused prevalence studies are no more likely to clarify the question than the studies to date have done.

Finally, it must be pointed out that this review has addressed the question of asbestos exposure and airway dysfunction. Whether or not the indicators of airways dysfunction considered here, separately or together, are necessarily associated with impairment and/or will lead to disability,[73] is a separate question, requiring a separate review.

The following sections discuss various clinical syndromes separately.

Small Airway Abnormality

Experimental studies in animals as well as review of human material indicates that the earliest fibrotic changes in response to asbestos exposure occur in the area around small airways. In animal studies these changes lead to dysfunction detected in tests reflecting the status of the small airways, and there is evidence that the same is true in man from both clinical and epidemiologic studies. However, the natural history of such changes remains to be clarified; for instance, it is not known whether they inevitably lead to generalized fibrosis with or without disablement, or whether they will remain essentially inflammatory reactions in the bronchiolar wall[27] with or without implications for the subsequent development of chronic airflow limitation. Both types of outcome are plausible.

Mucus Hypersecretion (Chronic Bronchitis)

Certain asbestos-exposed populations show an increase in cough and phlegm consistent with industrial bronchitis, e.g., Boston pipecoverers, Belfast insulators, and German workers in raw asbestos processing plants. In other populations, e.g., Quebec miners and millers, bronchitic symptoms appear to be related to exposure only in older subjects despite the very high dust levels. In general, there seems to be no reason to doubt the existence of an industrial bronchitis in relation to some, though apparently not all, occupational exposures involving asbestos. The emphasis should probably be placed on the occupational exposure (including all its components) rather than on asbestos as the necessary agent.

Acute Airway Reactions

Wheezing is a common symptom in a number of asbestos-exposed workforces and suggests that exposure to asbestos particles may evoke acute, presumably reversible, airflow limitation. As indicated in the section on mucus hypersecretion, emphasis should probably be placed on the occupational exposure itself (including all its components), and more information is required before asbestos can be incriminated as the agent responsible, although the Tucson study[59] based on a general population sample is suggestive. There is no evidence on the relationship of acute airway reactions to chronic airflow limitation.

Chronic Airflow Limitation

There can be little doubt that chronic airflow limitation is also common in asbestos workers. However, the nature of its relationship to occupational exposures is much less clear. Using pulmonary function profiles to avoid the lack of specificity of any one lung function test, an almost equal prevalence of obstructive and restrictive impairments has been shown in Quebec chrysotile miners.[47] However, smoking was also common in this group and its effect on airway function well documented. Both restrictive and obstructive profiles were seen more commonly in smokers, and neither could be related to exposure. This has not led to a rejection of the association between asbestos and parenchymal fibrosis because of strong evidence from numerous other studies in this and other populations. By the same token, it may be unwise to reject the association between asbestos and airways disease for several reasons. First, the effect of asbestos on airways may be similar to that of cigarettes, and if they are not simply additive, an individual's airway abnormality could be due to cigarettes and asbestos in differing proportions, depending on the dose of each delivered to the airways as well as to differing susceptibilities to each agent. Therefore, when adjusting for an effect of cigarettes, one might also remove part of the asbestos effect. Second, while an obstructive defect in tests of small airways has been related to cigarette smoking, there is no reason to assume it is specific to that exposure; indeed, the evidence is to the contrary, suggesting that other exposures may also produce this type of abnormality. Third, given that most of the studies reviewed as well as numerous clinical reports found no difference in $FEV_1/FVC\%$ with asbestos exposure, a reasonable conclusion is that this is not a sensitive test of abnormality in asbestos workers; one cannot necessarily conclude that asbestos exposure does not cause airway obstruction for the preceding reasons, of which the most important is the opposing effects of restrictive and obstructive abnormalities on this test. Indeed, the search for relationships in population studies is hampered by the fact that asbestos also results in parenchymal effects, which may obscure any possible airway effects.

The Relationship Between the Syndromes of Acute Airway Dysfunction and Chronic Airflow Limitation

The clinical syndromes of acute airway dysfunction and chronic airflow limitation are clearly not agent-specific. Each may be the response to more than one if not many environmental exposures, while a number of environmental exposures may evoke more than one response and these may or may not be interrelated. For example, cigarette exposure is associated with mucus hypersecretion as well as with chronic airflow limitation; one view is that they are independently related to this exposure (the British hypothesis);[74] in another view, chronic airflow limitation occurs only in those smokers in whom there is an asthmatic tendency (the Dutch hypothesis).[75] In the case of cotton dust exposure, acute airway reactions are well documented, but their relationship to chronic airflow limitation remains an important but unanswered question.[76] In the case of asbestos exposure (or more precisely, exposure to occupational environments that include asbestos), not only is the evidence linking acute and chronic airway dysfunction with exposure less strong, but so is the evidence on their interrelationships. However, even the present evidence cannot be ignored. Given the hypothesis that abnormalities in tests of small airways function found in cigarette smokers[14] are a precursor of disabling chronic airflow limitation, it would be reasonable to postulate a similar relationship between small airway abnormality and disabling chronic airflow limitation due to other inhaled agents, such as asbestos particles. If this were shown to be so, then it may also be necessary to accept that in an individual exposed in the past to a heavy dust load and presenting today with chronic airflow limitation, asbestos may be in part responsible even if the subject has smoked. Clearly, only further directed research will clarify this issue.

SUMMARY

Airway responses to inhaled materials include mucus hypersecretion and airflow limitation in large and/or small airways; this may be acute and reversible or chronic and at best partly reversible. In the present review the evidence linking airway responses with asbestos exposure is evaluated in order to answer the question: Does asbestos exposure cause airways dysfunction in man? Four categories of evidence were considered: experimental (in animals), clinical, pathologic, and epidemiologic. The following conclusions were reached:

1. The early pathologic charges of asbestosis occur at the level of the small airway where inhaled fibers tend to accumulate. Features include thickening of the wall of the membranous and respiratory bronchioles. These changes may manifest themselves in asbestos-exposed workers as impaired small airway function.
2. Industrial bronchitis is recognized as occurring in association with a number of occupational exposures, including some in which the inhaled materials include asbestos particles. This type of airway response probably relates to total particle load rather than specifically to the asbestos content, and is likely to be seen in relation to exposures in which dust burden is high, for instance, in mining.
3. There is some evidence that acute (and probably reversible) airflow limitation may occur in response to certain industrial exposures to asbestos fiber in some workers. The relative importance of personal factors and/or other environmental contaminants remains to be clarified.

4. Chronic airflow limitation involving, in particular, large airways is a common finding in asbestos exposed workers, whether or not they have radiologic evidence of fibrosis. In the absence of a smoking history, the evidence suggests that an obstructive functional abnormality may be the consequence of asbestos exposure. In the presence of a smoking history the relative importance of the two environmental contaminants in an individual case cannot be determined.

5. The present conclusions are based on a review study of workers exposed under a variety of different conditions to occupational environments containing usually a number of environmental pollutants of which asbestos particles were often only ore. The extent to which the industrial process, fiber type, and other contaminants may have influenced the biologic activity of the asbestos material is not known, but should always be borne in mind in assessing the individual subject.

ACKNOWLEDGMENTS

Margaret R. Becklake is a Career Investigator, Medical Research Council of Canada. Pierre Ernest is Boursier, Institut de Recherche en Sante et Securite au Travail de Quebec.

REFERENCES

1. Craighead JE, Mossman BT: The pathogenesis of asbestos-associated diseases. N Engl J Med 306:1446, 1982.
2. Parkes WR: Asbestos-related disorders. Br J Dis Chest 67:261, 1973.
3. Thomson ML, Pelzer AM, Smither WJ: The discriminant value of pulmonary function tests in asbestosis. Ann NY Acad Sci 132:421, 1965.
4. Becklake MR: Asbestos-related diseases of the lungs and other organs: Their epidemiology and implications for clinical practice. Am Rev Respir Dis 114:187, 1976.
5. Becklake MR: Asbestos-related diseases of the lungs and pleura: Current clinical issues. Am Rev Respir Dis 126:187, 1982.
6. MRC: Definition and classification of chronic bronchitis for clinical and epidemiological purposes. Lancet 1:775, 1965.
7. Mead J: Interet respectif de differentes investigations chez le malade. Bull Physiopathol Respir 7:491, 1971.
8. Dosman J, Macklem PT: Disease of small airways. Adv Intern Med 22:355, 1977.
9. Cosio M, Ghezzo H, Hogg JC, et al: The relationship between structural changes in small airways and pulmonary function tests. N Engl J Med 298:1277, 1978.
10. Niewoehner DE, Knoke JD, Kleinerman J: Peripheral airways as a determinant of ventilatory function in the human lung. J Clin Invest 60:139, 1977.
11. Berend N, Woolcock AJ, Marlin GE: Correlation between the function and the structure of the lung in smokers. Am Rev Respir Dis 119:695, 1979.
12. Petty TL, Silvers GW, Stanford RE, et al: Small airway abnormality is related to increased closing capacity and abnormal slope of Phase III in excised human lungs. Am Rev Respir Dis 121:449, 1980.

13. Bake B: Is maximum mid-expiratory flow rate sensitive to small airways obstruction? Eur J Respir Dis 62:187, 1981.
14. Macklem PT: Obstruction in small airways—A challenge to medicine. Am J Med 52:721, 1972.
15. Powell E, Renzi G, Macklem PT: Severity and site of airflow obstruction in sarcoidosis (abstract). Am Rev Respir Dis 121:(4, pt 2)178, 1980.
16. Ostrow D, Cherniak RM: Resistance to airflow in patients with diffuse interstitial lung disease. Am Rev Respir Dis 108:205, 1973.
17. Craighead JE, Abraham JL, Churg A, et al: The pathology of asbestos-associated diseases of the lungs and pleural cavities: Diagnostic criteria and proposed grading scheme. Arch Pathol Lab Med 106:541, 1982.
18. Acheson ED, Gardner MJ: The ill effects of asbestos on health. In: Asbestos, Final Report of the Advisory Committee, vol 2. Health and Safety Commission, London, Her Majesty's Stationery Office, 1979.
19. McDonald JC: Asbestos-related disease: An epidemiologic review. IARC Sci Publ 30:615, 1980.
20. Becklake MR: Exposure to asbestos and human disease. N Engl J Med 306:1480, 1982.
21. Hill AB: A Short Textbook of Medical Statistics. London, Hodder and Stoughton, 1980, p 285.
22. McDonald JC: Asbestos and lung cancer: Has the case been proven? Chest 78(suppl 2):374, 1980.
23. Peters GA, Peters BJ: Sourcebook on Asbestos Diseases. New York, Garland STPM Press, 1980.
24. Becklake MR: Lung function. IARC Sci Publ 8:40, 1973.
25. Brody AR, Hill LH, Adkins B, O'Connor RW: Chrysotile asbestos inhalation in rats: Deposition pattern and reaction of alveolar epithelium to macrophages. Am Rev Respir Dis 123:679, 1981.
26. Hiett DM: Experimental asbestosis: An investigation of functional and pathological disturbances. I. Methods, control animals and exposure conditions. II. Results for chrysotile and amosite exposure. Br J Ind Med 35:129, 1978.
27. Begin R, Masse S, Bureau MA: Morphology and function of the airways in early asbestosis of the sheep model. Am Rev Respir Dis 128:870, 1982.
28. Goldstein B, Webster I, Rendell REF, Skikne MI: The effects of asbestos-cement dust inhalation on baboons. Environ Res 16:216, 1978.
29. Wagner JC, Berry G, Skidmore JW, Timbrell V: The effects of the inhalation of asbestos in rats. Br J Cancer 29:262, 1974.
30. Williams R, Hugh-Jones P: The significance of lung function changes in asbestosis. Thorax 15:109, 1960.
31. Bader ME, Bader RA, Tierstein AS, et al: Pulmonary function and radiographic changes in 598 workers with varying duration of exposure to asbestos. Mt Sinai J Med 37:492, 1970.
32. Muldoon BC, Turner-Warwick M: Lung function studies in asbestos workers. Br J Dis Chest 66:121, 1972.
33. Zedda S, Aresini G, Ghezzi I, Sartorelli E: Lung function in relation to radiographic changes in asbestos workers. Respiration 30:132, 1973.
34. Harless KW, Watanabe S, Renzetti AD: Acute effects of chrysotile asbestos exposure on lung function. Environ Res 16:360, 1978.
35. Rodriguez-Roisin R, Merchant JEM, Cochrane GM, et al: Maximal expiratory flow-volume curves in workers exposed to asbestos. Respiration 39:158, 1980.

36. Sulotto F, Romano C, Berra A, et al: Radiographic and functional changes following exposure to different types of asbestos. IARC Sci Publ 30:565, 1980.
37. Pearle J: Exercise performance and functional impairment in asbestos exposed workers. Chest 80:701, 1981.
38. Pearle J: Smoking and duration of asbestos exposure in the production of functional and roentgenographic abnormalities in shipyard workers. J Occup Med 24:37, 1982.
39. Becklake MR: Asbestos miners and millers: Morbidity studies. In: Health Issues Related to Metallic and Nonmetallic Mining. eds. Wagner WL, Rom WN, Merchant JA. Boston, Butterworths, 1983, 263.
40. Hourihane DO'B, McCaughey WTE: Pathological aspects of asbestosis. Postgrad Med J 42:613, 1966.
41. Turner-Warwick M: A perspective view on widespread pulmonary fibrosis. Br Med J 2:371, 1974.
42. DiMenza L, Ruff F, Bignon J, et al: Obstruction des voies aeriennes perpheriques au cours de l'exposition professionelle a l'amiante. Ann Anat Pathol (Paris) 21:261, 1976.
43. Becklake MR: Asbestos-related fibrosis of the lungs (asbestosis) and pleura. In: Pulmonary Diseases and Disorders: Update 1, ed. Fishman AP. Philadelphia, McGraw-Hill, 1982.
44. Churg A, Wright JL: Airway lesions with asbestos exposure: Do specific lesions exist? Am Rev Respir Dis 125:4(pt 2)154, 1982.
45. McDonald JC, Becklake MR, Fournier-Massey G, Rossiter CE: Respiratory symptoms in chrysotile asbestos mine and mill workers of Quebec. Arch Environ Health 24:358, 1972.
46. Becklake MR, Fournier-Massey G, Rossiter CE, McDonald JC: Lung function in chrysotile asbestos mine and mill workers of Quebec. Arch Environ Health 24:401, 1972.
47. Fournier-Massey GF, Becklake MR: Pulmonary function profiles in Quebec asbestos workers. Bull Physiopathol Respir 11:429, 1978.
48. Becklake MR, Thomas D, Liddell FDK, McDonald JC: Follow-up respiratory measurements in Quebec chrysotile asbestos miners and millers. Scand J Work Environ Health 8(Suppl):105, 1982.
49. Jodoin G, Gibbs GW, Macklem PT, Becklake MR: Early effects of asbestos exposure on lung function. Am Rev Resir Dis 104:525, 1971.
50. Peress L, Hoag H, White F, Becklake MR: The relationship between closing volume, smoking and asbestos dust exposure. Clin Res 23:647A, 1975.
51. Meurman LO, Kiviluoto R, Hakama M: Mortality and morbidity among the working population of anthophyllite asbestos miners in Finland. Br J Ind Med 31:105, 1974.
52. Langlands JHM, Wallace WFM, Simpson MJC: Insulation workers in Belfast. II. Morbidity in men still at work. Br J Ind Med 28:217, 1971.
53. Wallace WFM, Langlands JHM: Insulation workers in Belfast. I. Comparison of a random sample with a control population. Br J Ind Med 28:211, 1971.
54. Ferris BG Jr, Ranadive MV, Peters JM, et al: Prevalence of chronic respiratory disease and asbestosis in ship repair workers. Arch Environ Health 23:220, 1971.
55. Murphy RHL, Ferris BG Jr, Burgess WA, et al: Effects of low concentrations of asbestos: Clinical, environmental, radiological and epidemiologic observations in shipyard pipecoverers and controls. N Engl J Med 285:1271, 1971.
56. Murphy RHL, Gaensler EA, Redding RA, et al: Low level exposure to asbestos: Gas exchange in ship pipecoverers and controls. Arch Environ Health 25:253, 1972.

57. Murphy RHL Gaensler EA, Ferris BG, et al: Diagnosis of "asbestosis": Observations from a longitudinal study of shipyard pipecoverers. Am J Med 65:488, 1978.
58. Weill H, Ziskind MM, Waggenspack C, Rossiter CE: Lung function consequences of dust exposure in asbestos cement manufacturing plants. Arch Environ Health 30:88, 1975.
59. Lebowitz MD: Occupational exposure in relation to symptomatology and lung functions in a community population. Environ Res 14:59, 1977.
60. Woitowitz HJ, Valentin H: The asbestos industry. In: DFG Research Report: Chronic Bronchitis and Occupational Dust Exposure. Bonn-Badgodesburg, Harold Boldt & Verlag KG, 1978, p 186.
61. Becklake MR, Gibbs GW, Arhirii MH: Exposure to asbestos and respiratory abnormality: The influence of fibre type and nature of exposure. IARC Sci Publ 30:763, 1980.
62. Hedenstierna G, Alexandersson R, Kolmodin-Hedman B, et al: Pleural plaques and lung function in construction workers exposed to asbestos. Eur J Respir Dis 62:111, 1981.
63. Rodriguez-Roisin R, Picado C, Ananos F, et al: Airflow obstruction in chrysotile asbestos workers. Am Rev Respir Dis 123 (4, pt2):148, 1981.
64. McDonald JC: Epidemiology. In: Occupational Lung Diseases: Research Approaches and Methods, eds. Weill H, Turner-Warwick M. New York, Marcel Dekker, 1981, p 373.
65. Gibbs GW, Lachance M: Dust exposure in chrysotile asbestos mines and mills of Quebec. Arch Environ Health 24:358, 1972.
66. Gibbs GW, Lachance M: Dust-fibre relationships in the Quebec chrysotile industry. Arch Environ Health 28:69, 1974.
67. Morgan WKC: Industrial bronchitis. Br J Ind Med 35:285, 1978.
68. McFadden ER, Linden DA: A reduction in maximum mid-expiratory flow rate. A spirographic manifestation of small airways disease. Am J Med 52:725, 1972.
69. Kalacic I: Early detection of airflow obstruction in cement workers. Arch Environ Health 29:147, 1974.
70. Andersen IB, Lundqvist GR, Proctor DF, Swift DL: Human response to controlled levels of inert dust. Am Rev Respir Dis 119:619, 1979.
71. Widdicombe JG, Kent DC, Nadel JA: Mechanism of bronchoconstriction during inhalation of dust. J Appl Physiol 17:613, 1962.
72. Acheson ED, Gardner MJ: Exposure limits—The scientific criteria. In: Recent Advances in Occupational Health, ed. McDonald JC. Edinburgh, Churchill Livingstone, 1981, p 257.
73. Epler GR, Saber FA, Gaensler EA: Determination of severe impairment (disability) in interstitial lung disease. Am Rev Respir Dis 121:647, 1980.
74. Fletcher CF, Peto R: The natural history of chronic airflow obstruction. Br Med J 1:1645, 1977.
75. Van der Lende R: Epidemiology of chronic nonspecific lung disease (chronic bronchitis). Assen, Van Gorcum and Coy NV, 1969.
76. McDonald JC: Conference summary: International conference on byssinosis. Chest 79(4)(Suppl):134S, 1981.

3 Asbestos Fiber Toxicity and Lung Disease

Jean Bignon
Marie-Claude Jaurand

Asbestos is a generic term for a variety of hydroxylated silicates that can separate into thin and flexible fibers.[1] Many minerals with asbestos characteristics and without commercial importance are encountered as natural components of the earth crust (Table 3-1).[2] It is, however, the commercially important types of asbestos that have received the most attention in terms of lung disease.

There are two main commercial varieties of asbestos, chrysotile and the amphiboles.[3] Chrysotile is a hydrated, magnesium-layered silicate from the serpentine group. Its fibrils have a hollow, cylindrical form with an outer diameter of about 30 nm. In the workplace, chrysotile fibers are formed by the association of numerous discrete fibrils in bundles of different sizes and curvilinear shapes. Chrysotile currently accounts for over 95% of the total asbestos marketed in the world. Amphibole varieties of asbestos include crocidolite, amosite, anthophyllite, and tremolite. The first two were the most frequently used in the industry. Individual amphibole fibers are generally straight with a diameter of 0.13 μm for crocidolite and 0.5 μm for other amphiboles.

AN OVERVIEW

The inhalation of asbestos dusts causes pleural and pulmonary fibrosis and also lung cancer and mesothelioma. Over the last 20 years, epidemiologic and experimental work has established the relationship between these diseases and asbestos exposure.[4,5]

At present, several areas need further studies: the biologic sequences that lead to parenchymal and pleural fibrosis; the relationship between fiber-related

Table 3-1. Asbestos, Asbestiforms, and Acicular Fragments

1. *Asbestos:*	with commercial importance
Serpentine:	chrysotile $[Mg_6(OH)_8Si_4O_{10}]$
Amphiboles:	crocidolite or riebeckite $[Na_2Fe_5(OH)_2Si_8O_{22}]$
	amosite or cummingtonite-grunerite $[Mg,Fe_7(OH)_2Si_8O_{22}]$
	anthophyllite (commercially exploited in the past)
	actinolite-tremolite $[Ca_2(Mg,Fe)_5(OH)_2Si_8O_{22}]$
2. *Asbestiforms*	
Sheet or Tubular Silicates (as chrysotile)	
halloysite, fibrous talc (beaconite or agilite), fibrous attapulgite (palygorskite), micas (muscovite, lepidolite, glauconite)	
Chain Silicates (as amphiboles)	
wollastonite, sillimanite	
Erionite-Zeolites	
Jade	

From Zoltai T: Asbestiform and acicular mineral fragments. Ann NY Acad Sci 330:621, 1979.

inflammatory diseases and cancer; the shape of the dose–response curve (particularly for low-level exposure) specifically to ascertain if a threshold value for the development of cancer exists; the documentation and explanation of the pathogenicity gradient between different fiber types for lung fibrosis as well as for lung cancer and mesothelioma. Indeed, epidemiologic and experimental evidence shows that pathologic responses are related not only to the dose of fibers (the number of fibers inhaled during a lifetime exposure) but also to the fiber types. This gradient in the pathogenicity of different types of fibers, particularly chrysotile and amphiboles, is presently a major concern for scientists and hygienists, who must make recommendations concerning the banishment of specific types of asbestos fibers.

Two areas of scientific investigation are particularly important in making these recommendations: (1) the quantitative and qualitative assessment of the asbestos fibers actually retained in the respiratory tissues will help provide better insight into the actual dose to which cells are exposed; (2) the in vivo and in vitro cellular responses to treatment with fibrous dusts will bring a better understanding of the specific toxicity of fibers in relation to their durability, their physical state (i.e., shape and size), their physicochemical properties (i.e., charge and surface reactivity), and chemistry (composition and stability in biologic fluids). Advances in the area have been reported in recent meetings.[6–8]

CONDITIONS OF ASBESTOS EXPOSURE

Because of its unique physical properties—elasticity, flexibility, and heat resistance—asbestos is used in many products.[3] Two different situations exist for occupational exposure. First, the large asbestos industries—mines, mills, and plants—process raw asbestos to make various products, such as asbestos cement pipes, friction materials, and insulation boards and sheets. Currently, these industries must comply with standards that require dust concentrations to be lower than 2 fibers of 5 μm length per cubic centimeter of air. Second, there are diverse industries using asbestos occasionally, for example, the construction industry, and shipyards. In these situations, levels of exposure may be high because the use of asbestos is usually not controlled. In considering occupational exposure, we must remember that asbestos has been employed liberally in building and ship construction during and since the second world war. Because the latency period for the diseases associated with asbestos exposure is more than 20 years, the cases we are now observing correspond to exposures that took place between 1940 and 1960. Because of the new regulations limiting exposure to 2 fibers/cm^3, occupational exposure to asbestos is decreasing. We do not, however, know to what extent these regulations will cause a diminution in the number of diseases related to occupational exposure.

Investigators are also questioning the possibility of disease caused by nonoccupational exposure to asbestos and other mineral fibers. Exposures in the home and those occurring from leisure time activities have been proven to induce asbestos-related diseases.[3] Another recently discovered source of asbestos exposure is the indoor airborne asbestos pollution coming from ceilings sprayed with asbestos fibers or from asbestos flooring.[9] Asbestiforms, such as tremolite or erionite-zeolite, have brought occupational hazards in mines[10] and in agricultural areas.[11,12]

NONMALIGNANT ASBESTOS-RELATED RESPIRATORY DISEASES

Asbestosis

Advanced Lung Fibrosis. Asbestosis, a pneumoconiosis described at the beginning of the century, is an interstitial lung fibrosis caused by the inhalation of asbestos dusts.[4,5] Clinically, radiologically, functionally, biologically, and pathologically, advanced asbestosis is not different from idiopathic pulmonary fibrosis.[13,14,15] The etiology of this pulmonary fibrosis is based on finding a history of heavy asbestos exposure and/or the discovery of asbestos fibers in lung tissue and in sputum or bronchoalveolar lavage fluid.

Bronchoalveolar lavage is an effective tool for diagnosing asbestosis. It allows the physician to identify and quantify asbestos fibers in alveolar spaces. In asbestosis, numerous coated and uncoated asbestos fibers are usually recovered in the bronchoalveolar lavage fluid.[16,17] Moreover, bronchoalveolar lavage gives a representative sample of the alveolar cell population during asbestosis, that is, an increased percentage of leukocytes, mostly polymorphonuclear neutrophils, and also eosinophils.[16] This cell proportion is similar to findings described in idiophathic pulmonary fibrosis (Figs. 3-1 and 3-2).[15] The percentage of lymphocytes may be normal in asbestosis and increased in persons with pleural fibrosis and with mesothelioma and lung carcinoma (Fig. 3-3). In a series of patients with severe asbestosis, the concentration (mg/100 ml) of albumin, IgG, IgA, alpha-1-antitrypsin, transferrin, C3, and haptoglobulin in bronchoalveolar lavage fluid was increased but usually to a lesser extent than in idiopathic

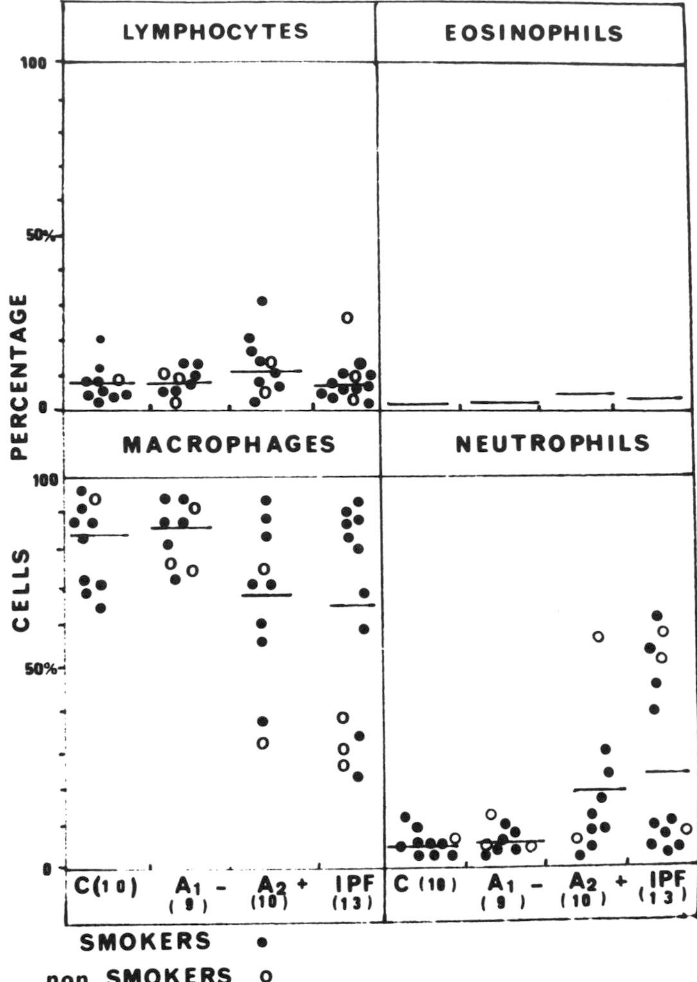

Fig. 3-1 Cells percentage (lymphocytes, eosinophils, neutrophils, and macrophages) according to disease. C: normal volunteers, A_1 = definite past asbestos exposure without lung fibrosis, A_2 = asbestosis, IPF = idiopathic pulmonary fibrosis. Number of cases are indicated in brackets.

pulmonary fibrosis (Table 3-2). These findings indicate that the alveolar reaction in asbestosis is mostly of the exudative inflammatory type. However, in our series when the different proteins were related to albumin concentrations, there was a striking relative increase in alveolar IgA (Table 3-3). The alveolar production of IgA in asbestosis is usually associated with an increase in the serum immunoglobulin levels.[18] The reason for this increase remains unknown. The high frequency of autoantibodies in patients with asbestos-related disease pro-

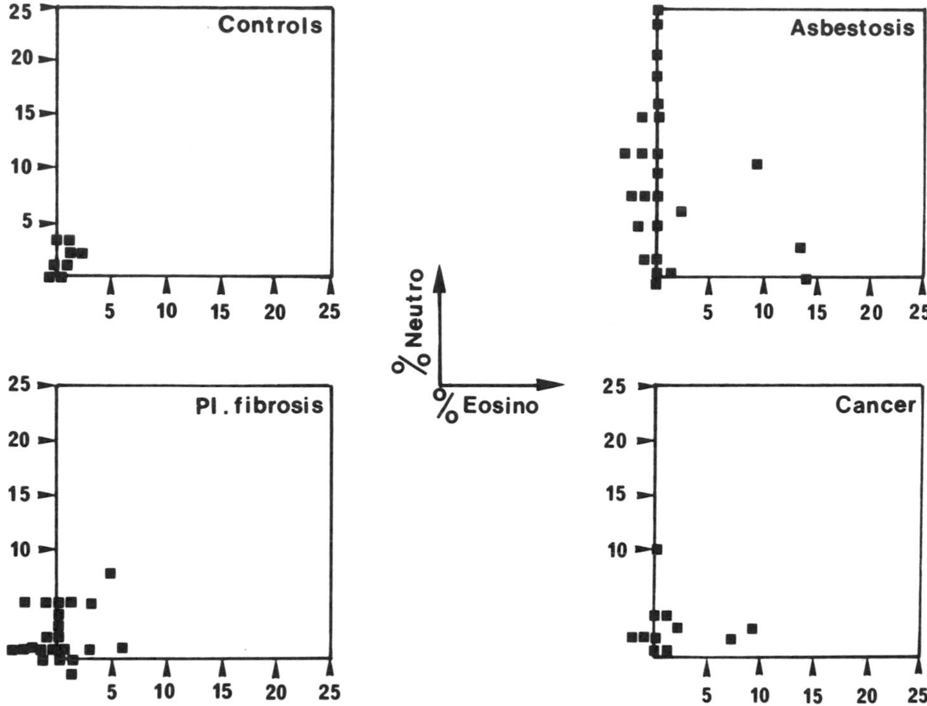

Fig. 3-2 Percentage of neutrophils (neutro) and eosinophils (eosino) in bronchoalveolar lavage fluid according to different asbestos related diseases (cases are different from Fig. 3-1). Pl. fibrosis: pleural fibrosis; cancer = lung carcinoma and pleural mesothelioma; controls = unexposed young volunteers.

vides further evidence of disturbed humoral immunity in association with asbestosis.[18,19] Disturbances in cell-mediated immunity in asbestos have been suggested by studies in patients[20,21] and in animals.[22] Recently it has been shown that the in vitro responses of normal human blood lymphoid cells to

Table 3-2. Serum Proteins in Bronchoalveolar Lavage Fluid (BALF) Measured by Immunochemical Methods[a]

Serum proteins (mg/100 ml BALF)	Controls (10 cases)	A_1 (9 cases)	A_2 (10 cases)	IPF (13 cases)
Albumin	4.9	6.4	8.2	8.7
IgG	2.93	3.34	3.7	5.1
IgA	0.2	0.38	0.96	1.3
alpha-1-Antitrypsin	0.17	0.17	0.39	0.90
Transferrin	0.57	0.97	0.90	0.85
C3	ND	ND	0.15	0.11
Haptoglobin	0.17	9.16	0.22	0.15
alpha-2-Macroglobulin	0.24	ND	0.30	0.34
IgM	ND	ND	ND	ND

[a] ND: not detectable. For symbols A_1, A_2, and IPF, see legend to Fig. 3-1.

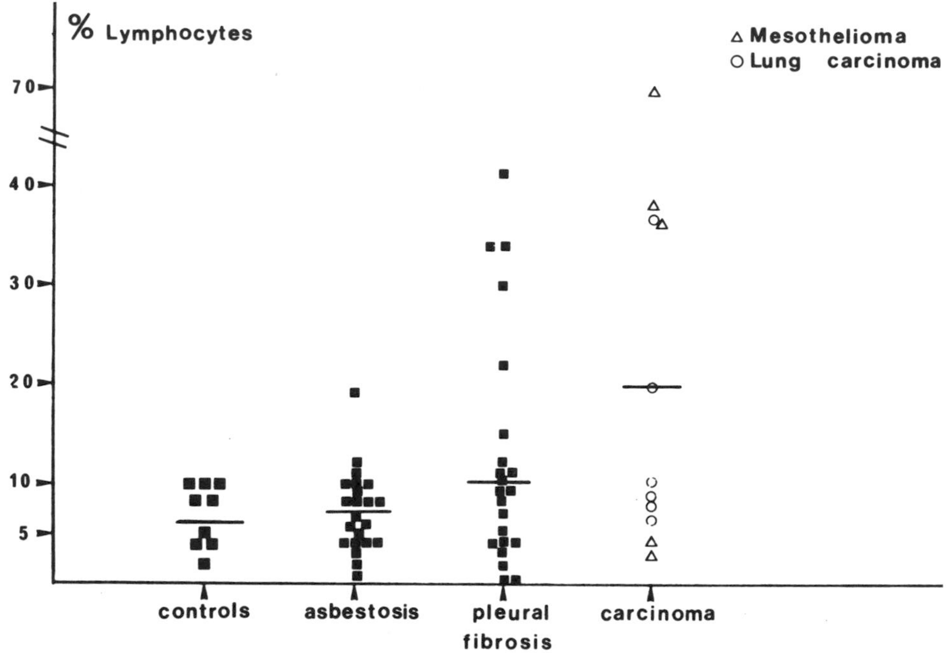

Fig. 3-3 Percentage of lymphocytes in bronchoalveolar lavage fluid according to different asbestos-related diseases. Controls were unexposed young volunteers.

phytohemagglutinin are depressed when the cells are in contact with low doses of fibrous dusts. This depression was most significant with chrysotile and least significant with glass fibers. Such a response that requires cell contact with fibers is not related to cytotoxicity.[23]

Early Asbestosis. In subjects exposed to asbestos dusts, airflow limitation in small airways, as assessed by pulmonary function tests, is often the first

Table 3-3. Ratio of IgG, IgA, and alpha-1-Antitrypsin (a1-AT) to Albumin (ALB) in Bronchoalveolar Lavage Fluid Recovered from Different Diseases[a]

Ratios	Controls (10)	A_1 (9)	A_2 (10)	IPF (13)
IgG / ALB	0.59	0.36	0.45	0.58
IgA / ALB	0.04	0.05	0.11	0.14
a1 AT / ALB	0.03	0.03	0.05	0.1

[a] For symbols A_1, A_2, and IPF, see legend to Fig. 3-1. The number of cases is in parentheses.

functional abnormality, even before radiographic changes suggest asbestosis. Observations of lung pathology from humans and rats exposed to inhalable asbestos dusts revealed that inflammation and sclerosis began mainly within the wall of terminal and respiratory bronchioles with a noticeable reduction of the airway lumen.[24,25] These data have some implication for the early detection of asbestos-related parenchymal diseases.

Dose–Response Relationship. Several studies have attempted to establish a dose–response relationship between asbestosis-related morbidity and cumulative exposure to asbestos dusts.[26,27] However, Berry et al.[28] recently surveyed workers in an asbestos textile factory and showed that it is not possible to draw any definite conclusions on the effects of the present 2 fiber/cm^3 standard. Indeed, this standard does not take into account the cumulative dose and the rate of dust elimination from the lungs. For this reason, it is possible that asbestosis could occur after 40 years of exposure to 1 or even to 0.3 fiber/cm^3. Until data are available on groups exposed to lower levels, it is not possible to assess adequately the effects of the current standards. Begin et al.,[29] studying a sheep model, have shown that the functional and biologic changes, which suggest the development of lung fibrosis, appeared only after a cumulative intratracheal dose of about 2000 mg of chrysotile. In contrast, exposure to low doses of chrysotile (up to 128 mg) produced no overall significant change in total cell yield or in the number of macrophages, lymphocytes, and neutrophils within the bronchoalveolar lavage fluid of these animals.[30] These data from animal models as well as those from humans seem to indicate a threshold dose of asbestos in relation to the development of asbestosis.

Pathogenesis of Asbestosis

In Vitro Cellular Responses. In vitro effects of asbestos dusts are clearly dependent on the type of asbestos fiber; this is discussed in the section dealing with the degree of pathogenicity of different fibers. When using sublethal doses of asbestos dusts in vitro, it is possible to investigate the molecular mediators involved in the inflammatory reaction in cell and tissue injury and in the subsequent fibrogenesis of lung tissue. The alveolar macrophage is the key actor in these events (Fig. 3-4). Indeed, for many years asbestos fibers have been known to trigger the alveolar macrophage to release lysosomal enzymes[31,32] and to produce different mediators, which include chemotactic factors for polymorphonuclear neutrophils,[33] factors increasing fibroblast replication,[34] elastase,[35] plasminogen activator,[36] prostaglandins, and phospholipase.[37] The response of polymorphonuclear neutrophil leukocytes to asbestos fibers has been investigated less. However, Doll et al.[38] showed that polymorphonuclear neutrophils incubated with asbestos-released toxic oxygen metabolites and lysosomal enzymes. Finally, in culture, the response of fibroblasts to asbestos exposure was variable, showing either an increase or a decrease in collagen synthesis, depending on the state of the culture (growing or confluent cells).[39]

In Vivo Responses. The presence of polymorphonuclear neutrophils in bronchoalveolar lavage fluid from fibrotic patients with asbestosis and idio-

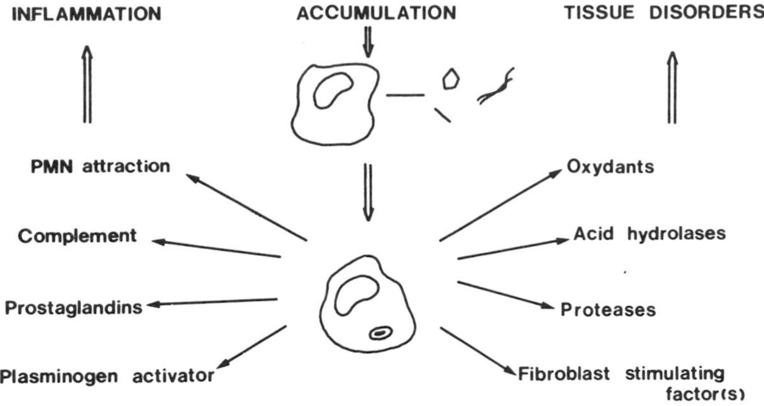

Fig. 3-4 Diagram showing how mineral dusts act on alveolar macrophages to contribute to lung inflammatory reaction, cell and tissue injury, and subsequently lung fibrosis.

pathic pulmonary fibrosis[15,16,40,41] suggests identical pathogenetic mechanisms for both diseases.[42] Asbestos fibers deposited at the surface of the airways are phagocytized by alveolar macrophages, which could be stimulated in vivo in the same manner as in in vitro. In fact, alveolar macrophages from asbestos-dusted rats have an increased number of complement and immunoglobulin receptors on their surface, suggesting a state of activation.[43] As shown in animals after intratracheal injection of asbestos dusts, these activated alveolar macrophages secrete a chemotactic factor for polymorphonuclear neutrophils.[44,45] The macrophage-derived chemotactic factor for polymorphonuclear neutrophils is extractable in ethyl acetate[33] and probably lipidic.[46] Subsequently, oxygen metabolites and proteases derived from polymorphonuclear neutrophils could damage the alveolar epithelium and the underlying connective tissue. The proteases involved are not yet well identified. Collagenase has been reported to be present in bronchoalveolar lavage fluid from patients with asbestosis.[47] The release of a fibroblastic growth factor by the activated alveolar macrophages could stimulate the collagen synthesis leading to lung fibrosis.[48,49] Modifications of cell-mediated and humoral immunity also have to be taken into account as discussed above and summarized by De Shazo.[50] Immunologic events are not, however, totally understood in asbestos-related diseases.

Nonmalignant Pleural Disease

Nonmalignant pleural diseases caused by asbestos, reviewed by Hillerdal,[51] can be divided into exudative pleurisy and pleural fibrosis types.

Asbestos-Related Pleurisy. Asbestos-related pleurisy has been recognized only recently. The exudative inflammatory reaction related to asbestos rarely gives a symptomatic disease. In that case, pleural effusion is usually bilateral.[52]

Pleural Fibrosis. Pleural fibrosis is a very common stigma of asbestos exposure.[4,5,51,53] As already emphasized,[54] pleural fibrosis takes two main forms: diffuse thickening of the parietal and visceral pleural and localized parietal and diaphragmatic pleural plaques. Both lesions can be identified by chest roentgenograms. An oblique roentgenogram (45°), computerized axial tomography, and more recently thoracoscopy are helpful adjuncts to diagnosis.

Gross examination of the pleura during surgery or at autopsy confirms these two pathologic entities. Diffuse pleural thickening is sometimes associated with a symphysis of the pleural cavity, which may represent the scar of a latent bilateral exudative pleurisy. By contrast, pleural plaques appear as irregular fibrohyaline areas, more or less necrotic and calcified, and are scattered at the bases of the thorax and on the diaphragm.

Dose–Response Relationship. In humans, no clear-cut relationship between the intensity and/or the duration of asbestos exposure and the extent of fibrogenic response of the pleura has been shown. However, pleural plaques seem to be time-related, increasing in number, size, and radiographic density with years.[55] Pleural fibrogenesis is possibly related to fiber types, but so far there is no definite proof for this view.

Measurements of asbestos dusts in human tissue samples does confirm the presence of asbestos fibers in pleural tissues. Some evidence in human and animal studies shows that asbestos fibers accumulate in the peripheral areas of the lung that are in close contact with visceral pleura.[56,57] This finding could explain why we were able to find a significant number of asbestos fibers in pleural fluids (Bignon, unpublished data). Coated and uncoated asbestos fibers, mostly short chrysotile microfibrils, have been found in samples taken from parietal pleura or pleural plaques, but no correlation between the pleural and the parenchymal fiber concentrations was found.[58] This lack of correlation could be explained by an irregular distribution of asbestos dusts with high concentrations of short and thin chrysotile fibers in some focal areas. The significance of these "hot spots" in relation to the pathogenesis of mesothelioma is still unknown.[54]

Pathogenesis of Nonmalignant Pleural Disease

Without doubt, asbestos fibers can be transported specifically from subcutaneous tissues to submesothelial regions and induce secondary histologic changes and mesothelioma.[59] Such migration must follow inhalation of asbestos fibers.

Fiber Migration. The mechanisms for migration of asbestos fibers to the pleura are still hypothetical. Three routes[60] are possible: (1) across the visceral pleura; (2) following the lymph flow; (3) through the systemic bloodstream. Pleural plaque formation could be related either to an inflammatory reaction induced by asbestos fibers at the level of the lymphatic pores of the pleura[54] or to the embolization of circulating fibers into the capillaries of the intercostal

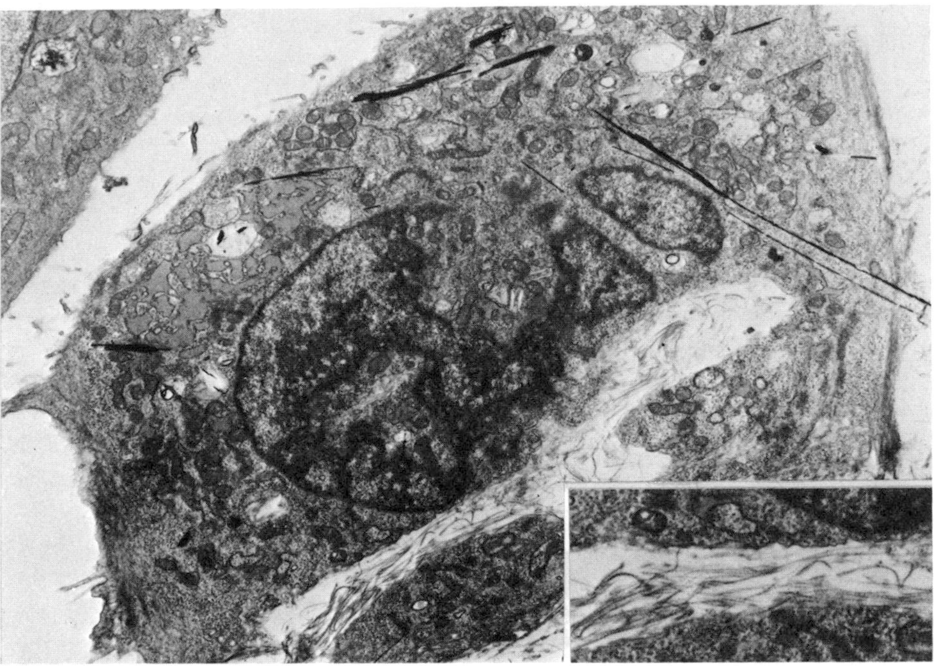

Fig. 3-5 Pleural mesothelial cells in culture treated with chrysotile fibers: numerous fibers are seen inside the cell and collagen fibrils are produced and released outside the cells (inset: high magnification of the collagen fibrils produced by mesothelial cells).

arteries. Subsequently, focal necrosis and fibrosis develops in contact with trapped foreign bodies. This migration has been confirmed by subcutaneous and intravenous injection of asbestos into mice.[61] By contrast, diffuse pleural thickening could be due to a pleural effusion and related to high concentration of fibers in neighboring parenchyma.[60]

Fibrogenicity. Experimentally, asbestos is known to be fibrogenic to the pleura in several species, even after inhalation.[24,25] Davis[62] injected various dusts into the pleural cavities of mice and found that all of the injected materials stimulated the production of collagen. Specimens rich in long fibers quickly produced cellular granulomas, while those rich in short fibers elicited a much weaker reaction. It is our opinion that the amount of fibrous tissue produced is not only related to asbestos fiber size but also to fiber type. In one study using a rat model, we injected intrapleurally 20 mg of different fibers and found the magnitude of the pleural inflammation and fibrogenic reaction was the greatest in the group injected with chrysotile. In contrast, the same chrysotile sample treated with 0.1 N oxalic acid produced a minor inflammatory reaction, with no pleural adhesions and no subsequent mesothelioma.[63] This in vivo response correlated well with the in vitro responses in red blood cells and alveolar macrophages incubated with chrysotile samples.[32] (Cf. the section on fiber gradient in pathogenic potential.)

The fibrogenic response to asbestos fibers could occur indirectly as a result of the action of different mediators released by stimulated macrophages[33] or after a direct stimulation of fibroblasts[39] or mesothelial cells.

Response of Mesothelial Cells to Fibers. Rat mesothelial cells in culture are able to synthesize different connective tissue components, such as Type I, Type III, and Type IV collagen, laminin, elastin, and fibronectin.[64] During the phagocytosis of asbestos fibers, these cells, as well as submesothelial fibroblasts, are possibly stimulated to synthesize collagen components (Fig. 3-5) and cooperate to induce fibrosis of the pleura.[65] Aalto et al.[66] have shown that mesothelial cells responded to silica in a manner similar to macrophages and produce a factor that promoted collagen synthesis not only by fibroblasts but also by mesothelial cells. In this regard, the mesothelium appears to possess the properties of both macrophages and fibroblasts. However, the early biologic events taking place in the pleura under the stimulation of asbestos dusts retained in lung parenchyma have not been so far investigated.

MALIGNANT ASBESTOS-RELATED RESPIRATORY DISEASES

Past occupational exposure to asbestos is associated with an increased risk of cancer in several organs.[4,5] The carcinogenic potential of all commercial varieties of asbestos has been irrefutably established in animals either by inhalation or by intrapleural or intraperitoneal inoculation.[24,25,63,67–69] Asbestos-related bronchogenic carcinoma and pleural mesothelioma are presently of particular concern from a public health standpoint because we still do not know if low-dose exposure to asbestos is hazardous to the general population. This is why intensive research is being carried out in order to advance our understanding of the mechanisms of fiber carcinogenesis. After a review of relevant epidemiologic and animal data, we will discuss the possible biologic events related to the pathogenesis of lung and pleural cancers induced by mineral fibers.

Epidemiologic Data

Although the mortality by lung cancer and mesothelioma is universally increased in different cohorts of workers exposed to asbestos dusts, several different epidemiologic features have been identified in mesothelioma by comparison to lung cancer.

The Latency Period. The time from first exposure to the development of disease is longer for mesothelioma (mean 40 years) than for lung cancer (mean 20 years).[4,5,70]

Dose–Response Relationship. Data obtained from heavily exposed asbestos workers[71–76] showed a linear dose–response relationship for lung cancer. A linear trend has also been found between exposure and the response for the incidence of pleural mesothelioma in a cohort of Australian crocidolite miners and millers. The occurrence of mesothelioma has been noted even in workers briefly exposed (less than 3 months).[77] This finding is consistent with a linear nonthreshold dose–response relationship. In other cohorts of workers heavily exposed to mixed types of asbestos (chrysotile, crocidolite, amosite),[71,75] death due to mesothelioma approached 7–10% and related clearly to the degree and length of exposure. By contrast, in other industries, such as chrysotile mining and milling, mesothelioma was found to be a rather rare disease.[76] These differences could be related to factors other than dose, such as size and type of fibers, and will be discussed later on. However, as scattered cases are reported in association with domestic and neighborhood exposure,[4] it is particularly important to better identify the level of past asbestos exposure. Again, we must stress the indispensable help provided by asbestos dust measurements in biologic samples.[17,56,58]

Cofactor. Regarding the role of a possible cofactor in respiratory carcinogenesis caused by asbestos, the combined effect of asbestos and cigarette smoking appears to multiply the chances for developing lung cancer.[71,72] By contrast, no cocarcinogenic agent has been identified in association with asbestos exposure in relation to mesothelioma. It does, however, appear that about 20–30% of mesothelioma occur in unexposed people, raising the question of whether other carcinogens are working alone or in association with an environmental exposure to fibrous dusts.[78,79]

Time Dependence. According to Peto et al.,[80] time dependence is different for asbestos-related lung cancer and mesothelioma. The lung cancer risk is not dependent on the age at first exposure to asbestos. This is in striking contrast to mesothelioma where the incidence increases by the third or fourth power of time since first asbestos exposure. One implication of this fact is that asbestos exposure during childhood, for instance in school buildings sprayed with asbestos, could increase the risk of mesothelioma much later in life. However, this model is derived from the mortality data of cohort studies of workers heavily exposed to crocidolite, amosite, or chrysotile, irrespective of duration of exposure. Thus, mesothelioma is the cancer most powerfully related to asbestos exposure. By contrast, lung cancer is mostly related to smoking and only slightly linked to asbestos exposure alone. These epidemiologic differences between lung cancer and mesothelioma could be due either to the lag-time necessary for fibers to reach the pleura or to some unknown specific response of mesothelial cells to carcinogens.

Animal Data

Experiments in animals also have shown discrepancies in the carcinogenic response of the lung and the pleura to asbestos. Wagner et al.,[24] in inhalation studies in the rat, found a dose–response relationship for lung cancer. By contrast, mesothelioma was observed even after as brief an exposure as one day. Intrapleural or intraperitoneal inoculation of dusts, although not a realistic model, allows the study of the influence of different fiber variables such as type, size, and physiochemical states in relation to the induction of pleural sarcoma or mesothelioma. From such studies, Stanton et al.[68] and Pott et al.[69] have suggested that the most carcinogenic fibers were the longest (length >8 μm) and the thinnest ones (diameter <0.25 μm). However, as discussed later, this statement is now controversial because it has not been confirmed by several recent animal experiments comparing chrysotile, acid-leached chrysotile,[63,81] fibrous and amorphous crocidolite,[82] and other fibrous dusts (such as erionite, attapulgite) and man-made mineral fibers.[83]

In Vitro Cell Responses

During the last past years, there has been an effort to develop in vitro assays for the evaluation of the carcinogenic potential of mineral dusts.[7,8] Asbestos fibers have been used in different systems in order to discover whether their mode of action is genetic or epigenetic. The absence of mutation when treating prokaryotic cells (Ames test) with asbestos fibers[84] does not necessarily indicate the lack of mutagenic potency because asbestos fibers are probably not ingested by bacteria. In eukaryotes the presence of asbestos fibers inside the nucleus of intermitotic cells has not been reported in spite of the presence of fibers sandwiched between membranes at the nuclear level (Fig. 3-6). An interaction between the genetic material and the asbestos fibers can occur inside dividing cells, as asbestos fibers are easily observed in mitotic cells.[85] Using Chinese hamster lung cells and the HGPRT system, Huang et al[86,87] found only a slight increase in the number of mutants when the cells were treated with asbestos dusts. Asbestos fibers were generally found to have clastogenic effects, documented either by the induction of chromosome abnormalities[86,88–90] or by a slight increase in the number of sister chromatid exchanges.[91,92] However, these exchanges were not always increased,[93,94] and these results indicate that asbestos is not a strong mutagen. In fact, its action could be more epigenetic than genetic.

Because of the enhancing effect of cigarette smoke on the incidence of lung cancer among asbestos workers,[71,72] investigators have suggested that asbestos fibers could potentiate the in vitro mutation and transformation of various cell lines treated with chemical carcinogens. Several investigators have reported the morphologic transformation of cell lines under the synergistic effect of polycyclic aromatic hydrocarbons and asbestos. An increased transformation of fibroblastic cell lines has been observed when cell cultures are treated with both benzo-a-pyrene and crocidolite fibers, as compared with benzo-a-pyrene alone.[95] Mutagenic studies performed on liver-derived epithelial cell lines showed an increase in the number of mutant colonies in the HGPRT system following treatment with chrysotile and benzo-a-pyrene.[96] These studies seem to indicate that asbestos may act as a promoter and allow the expression of cell changes initiated by chemical carcinogens. However, promoters have various in vitro effects and different sites of action within the cell,[97–100] and so far the site(s) of action of asbestos remains unknown.

Some other data do not support a tumor-promoting action of asbestos. For instance, amosite fibers did not inhibit the metabolic cooperation between hamster lung cells,[101] and plasminogen activator was not secreted by chick embryo cells when incubated with asbestos.[102] However, there is no absolute in vitro

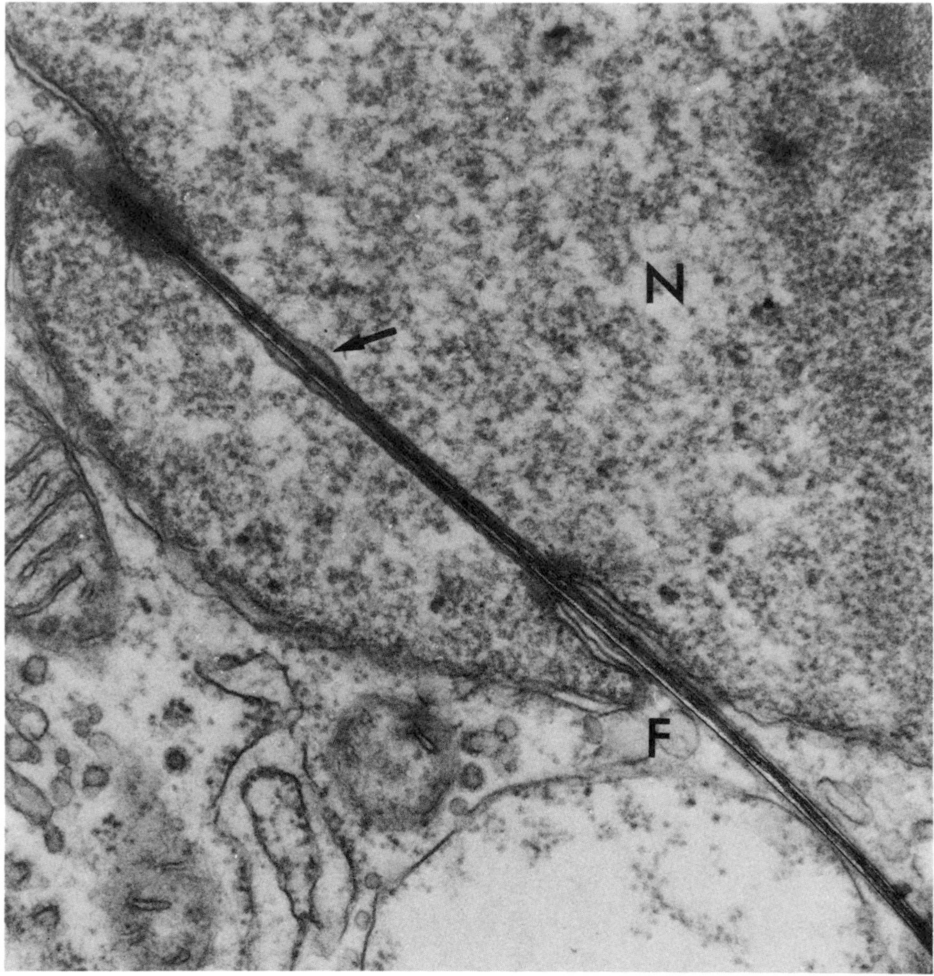

Fig. 3-6 Location of a fiber inside a mesothelial cell, in contact to the nuclear membrane (↓), after in vitro exposure to 5 μg/ml of chrysotile (F, fiber; N, nucleus).

test to demonstrate a promoter effect, so published data are sometimes conflicting as discussed recently by Trosko et al.[103] We must also point out the in vivo experiment of Topping and Nettesheim,[104] which suggests that asbestos could work more as a promoter than as an initiator.

Asbestos fibers exert a cytotoxic effect on fibroblastic cells,[105,106] as well as on epithelial cell lines.[85,107–109] The effect is characterized by a decrease in the plating efficiency, a cell death, and a decrease in the growth rate. At low concentrations, chrysotile fibers induce intense morphologic changes (binucleation, vacuolation), indicating a potent effect at the physiologic level. It would be interesting to study the cell pathology in order to know more about the mechanisms of action of asbestos fibers which could have some influence on the metabolic rate of polycyclic aromatic hydrocarbons. In this area, different results have been reported. Some have reported an enhancement of the cellular uptake of polycyclic aromatic hydrocarbons by asbestos fibers[110] and, instead of an increase of polycyclic aromatic hydrocarbon metabolism, an increase of DNA binding to metabolic products.[111] Others report a decrease in the conjugated metabolites.[112]

In opposition to the nonspecific carcinogenic effect of asbestos fibers on the lung, it seems that asbestos dusts act specifically at the pleural site. The absence of synergy between smoking and mesothelioma indicates that the effect of asbestos fibers may be direct and related to their own properties and their ability to reach the pleural tissue. Investigators have cultured rat mesothelial cells[113–115] and provided a useful tool for studying how asbestos fibers work in vitro on target cells. The metabolism of benzo-a-pyrene by rat pleural mesothelial cells has been studied with and without a concomitant treatment by chrysotile fibers.[116] The metabolites and the conjugates were not qualitatively or quantitatively different when compounds were added to confluent cells; however, a decrease in the percentage of conjugated metabolites was observed when the cells were treated during the exponential growth phase. Other studies, using isolated hepatic microsomal membranes showed an inhibition of the monooxidase detoxication system,[117] which could correlate with such an effect and might be related to the absence of synergy between smoking and asbestos in producing mesothelioma.

These different results suggest that asbestos fibers act at least as a cocarcinogen, increasing the effect of carcinogens,[118] and possible as a complete carcinogen. Then the question arises whether this phenomenon is specific to asbestos fibers or whether it is due to solid particulates inducing a foreign body reaction and secondarily promoting an effect on tumorigenesis.[119] Moreover, some host characteristics may influence the carcinogenic response to fibers.

PATHOGENIC POTENTIAL GRADIENT OF DIFFERENT FIBERS

Controversy still exists concerning the differential carcinogenic potential of different types of fibers. In a recent review[120] we tried to correlate the experimental data (in vitro and in vivo responses) with epidemiologic results. A relatively fair correlation between in vitro cell responses and the incidence of tumors and survival times in rats exposed by inhalation to different types of fibers has been found by comparing doses weight to weight. The most reactive fibers in vitro were also the most fibrogenic and the most carcinogenic in vivo. The pathogenic potential of the fibers was, in decreasing order, chrysotile, crocidolite, amosite, leached chrysotile, and glass fibers. Results could be different when adjusting for the number of fibers, since the number of fibers was not identical in the different types of asbestos studied. Chamberlain et al.[121] showed a relationship between the number of fibers and the biologic in vitro responses. However, other naturally occurring fibers, such as erionite-zeolite, have been found to be more carcinogenic than all forms of asbestos. Erionite gave a very high percentage of mesothelioma, even after inhalation.[83,122]

In humans the interpretation of epidemiologic data is not definitive and remains controversial. From mortality studies of cohorts of asbestos workers exposed to only one type of fiber, several authors believe that the carcinogenic potential for the mesothelium was the strongest with crocidolite, followed by amosite and chrysotile.[123] Two case-control studies of mesothelioma in the United Kingdom and North America have shown that an excess of amphiboles was found in the lungs of subjects with mesothelioma, whereas the chrysotile contents were similar in mesothelioma and in control cases.[124,125] As mentioned by Becklake,[123] there are scientists who think that this difference is also observed for lung carcinoma and lung fibrosis. Others are not convinced that the evidence for this difference is strong enough, even for mesothelioma.

The difference in pleural carcinogenicity between chrysotile and amphiboles, if it does exist, could be due to the fibers' difference in durability. Chrysotile is known to be largely eliminated from the lung, as documented by animal experiments[24] and by human measurements.[126] Moreover, there is evidence that magnesium and trace metals are leached from chrysotile asbestos in vivo, as well as in vitro.[127,128] This leaching within the lungs may reduce the hazardous effect of the remaining material, particularly if the duration of exposure is brief. By contrast, crocidolite and amosite persist in the lung. Thus a brief exposure to chrysotile might not be associated with an increased risk of mesothelioma, whereas a brief exposure to amphibole could produce a substantial risk for mesothelioma many years later.[78]

The high incidence of peritoneal tumors relative to pleural tumors found in several cohorts exposed mainly to amosite or crocidolite indicates that amphiboles are more responsible for asbestos-related peritoneal mesothelioma than chrysotile.[78] So far, no peritoneal mesothelioma has been found among Australian crocidolite miners.[77]

The difference in the incidence of mesothelioma in relation to fiber types has been recently validated by the discovery that fibrous erionite-zeolite from Turkey gave the highest incidence of pleural tumors ever seen in humans.[12] This discovery demonstrates the importance of knowing the nature, mechanisms, and pathogenic differences of different fibers, particularly new ones, if we are to avoid future health hazards associated with asbestos.

CONCLUSION

Although a lot of work has been done, the mechanisms of asbestos fibrogenesis and carcinogenesis remain poorly understood. Among the several outstanding questions, one is particularly intriguing: Why is the mesothelium a specific target for inhaled fibrous dusts? There also are no firm conclusions from the present evidence concerning the relative carcinogenic activities of short and long fibers and of the different types of asbestos. Moreover, recent studies have revealed that other fibrous or even nonfibrous materials are responsible for fibrosis and cancer, particularly of the mesothelium. The surface properties and the durability of mineral dusts seem at present to be important variables in the pathogenicity of fibers.

Our experience with asbestos implicates that we must allow new substitutes for asbestos to be commercially used only after extensive long-term inhalation studies in rodents and after short-term in vitro tests of cytotoxicity, genotoxicity, and carcinogenicity. In this area there is a need for improved in vitro methods, using specific target cells, such as pulmonary, mesothelial, and fibroblastic cells and developing different systems of cell cooperation adapted to the study of the inflammatory, fibrogenic, and carcinogenic potential of mineral dusts.

REFERENCES

1. Michaels L, Chissick SS: Asbestos: Properties, Applications and Hazards, vol 1. Chichester, Wiley, 1979.
2. Zoltai T: Asbestiform and acicular mineral fragments. Ann NY Acad Sci 330:621, 1979.
3. Zielhuis RL: Public health risks of exposure to asbestos. In: Report of Working Group of Experts Prepared for the Commission of the European Communities, Directorate-General for Social Affairs, Health and Safety Directorate. Oxford, Pergamon Press, 1977.
4. Selikoff IJ, Lee PHK: Asbestos and Disease. New York, Academic Press, 1978.
5. Becklake MR: Asbestos-related diseases of the lung and other organs: Their epidemiology and implication for clinical practice. Am Rev Respir Dis 114:187, 1976.
6. Wagner JC: Biological effects of mineral fibers, 2 vol. IARC Sci Publ 30, 1980.
7. Brown RC, Gormley IP, Chamberlain M, Davies R: The in Vitro Effects of Mineral Dusts, vol 1. New York, Academic Press, 1980.
8. Second International Workshop on the in Vitro Effects of Mineral Dusts. Environ. Health Perspect. vol 51 1983.
9. Sebastien P, Bignon J, Martin M: Indoor airborne asbestos pollution: From the ceiling and the floor. Science 216:1410, 1982.
10. Gillam JD, Dement JM, Lemen RA, et al: Mortality patterns among hard rock gold miners exposed to an asbestiform mineral. Ann NY Acad Sci 271:336, 1976.
11. Yazicioglu S, Ilcayto R, Balci K, et al: Pleural calcification, pleural mesotheliomas and bronchial cancers caused by tremolite dust. Thorax 35:564, 1980.
12. Artvinli M, Baris YI: Malignant mesothelioma in a small village in the Anatolian region of Turkey: An epidemiological study. J Natl Cancer Inst 63:17, 1979.
13. Becklake MR: Asbestos related diseases of the lungs and pleura. Am Rev Respir Dis 126:187, 1982.
14. Bignon J, Brochard P, Sebastien P: Pathologie de l'amiante aspects cliniques, données épidémiologiques et prévention. Schweiz Med Wochenschr 112:177, 1982.
15. Crystal RG, Fulmer JD, Roberts WC, et al: Idiopathic pulmonary fibrosis: Clinical histologic, radiographic, physiologic, scintigraphic, cytologic and biochemical aspects. Ann Intern Med 85:769, 1976.

16. Bignon J, Atassi K, Jaurand MC, et al: Etude cytologique et biochimique du liquide de lavage broncho-alvéolaire (LBA) dans la fibrose pulmonaire idiopathique et l'asbestose. Rev Fr Mal Respir 6:353, 1978.
17. Sebastien P: Possibilités actuelles de la biométrologie des poussières sur échantillons de liquide de lavage broncho-alvéolaire. Ann Biol Clin 40:279, 1982.
18. Lange A: An epidemiological survey of immunological abnormalities in asbestos workers. II. Serum immunoglobulin levels. Environ Res 22:176, 1980.
19. Turner-Warwick M, Parkes WR: Circulating rheumatoid and antinuclear factors in asbestos workers. Br Med J 3:492, 1970.
20. Wagner MMF, Campbell M, Edwards RE: Sequential immunological studies on an asbestos-exposed population. Factor affecting peripheral blood leukocytes and T-lymphocytes. Clin Exp Immunol 38:323, 1979.
21. Kagan E, Solomon H, Cochrane JC, et al: Immunological studies of patients with asbestosis. II. Studies of circulating lymphoid cell numbers and humoral immunity. Clin Exp Immunol 28:268, 1977.
22. Rola-Pleszczynski M, Lemaire I, Sirois P, et al: Asbestos related changes in pulmonary and systemic immune responses—Early enhancement followed by inhibition. Clin Exp Immunol 49:426, 1982.
23. Barbers RG, Wendy WHS, Saxon A: In vitro depression of human lymphocyte mitogen response (phytohaemagglutinin) by asbestos fibers. Clin Exp Immunol 48:602, 1982.
24. Wagner JC, Berry G, Skidmore JW, Timbrell V: The effects of the inhalation of asbestos in rats. Br J Cancer 29:252, 1974.
25. David JMG, Beckett ST, Bolton RE, et al: Mass and number of fibers in the pathogenesis of asbestos-related lung disease in rats. Br J Cancer 37:673, 1978.
26. McDonald JC, Becklake MR, Gibbs GW, et al: The health of chrysotile asbestos mine and mill workers in Quebec. Arch Environ Health 28:61:1974.
27. Weill H, Zikind MN, Waggensperck C, Rossiter CE: Lung formation corresponding to dust exposure in an asbestos cement manufacturing plant. Arch Environ Health 30:88, 1975.
28. Berry G, Gilson JC, Holmes S, et al: Asbestosis: A study of dose-response relationship in an asbestos textile factory. Br J Ind Med 36:98, 1979.
29. Begin R, Rola-Pleszczynski M, Masse S, et al: Asbestos-induced lung injury in the sheep model: The initial alveolitis. In: Occupational Lung Disease, eds. Gee JBL, Morgan WKC, Brooks SE. New York, Raven Press, 1983.
30. Lemaire F, Sirois P, Rola-Pleszczynski M, Masse S: Early biochemical reactions in the lung of sheep exposed to asbestos: Evidence of cyclic AMP accumulation in bronchoalveolar lavage fluids. Lung 159:323, 1981.
31. Davies P, Allison AC, Ackerman J, et al: Asbestos induces selective release of lysosomal enzymes from mononuclear phagocytes. Nature 251:423, 1974.
32. Jaurand MC, Magne L, Boulmier JL, Bignon J: In vitro activity of alveolar macrophages and red blood cells with asbestos fibers treated with oxalic acid, sulfur dioxide and benzo-3,4-pyrene. Toxicology 21:323, 1981.
33. Schoenberger C, Hunninghake GW, Gadek JE, Crystal RG: Inflammation and asbestos; characterization and maintenance of alveolitis following acute asbestos exposure. Chest 80(Suppl):705, 1981.
34. Bitterman P, Rennard S, Schoenberger C, Crystal RG: Asbestos stimulates alveolar macrophages to release a factor causing human lung fibroblasts to replicate. Chest 80(Suppl):38, 1981.
35. White R, Kuhn CH: Effects of phagocytosis of mineral dusts on elastase secretion

by alveolar and peritoneal exudative macrophages. Arch Environ Health 35:106, 1980.

36. Hamilton J, Vassalli JD, Reich E: Macrophage plasminogen activator: Induction by asbestos is blocked by anti-inflammatory steroids. J Exp Med 144:1689, 1976.
37. Sirois P, Rola-Pleszczynski M, Begin R: Phospholipase A activity and prostaglandin release from alveolar macrophages exposed to asbestos. Prostagl Med 5:31, 1980.
38. Doll JN, Stankus RP, Goldbach S, Salvaggio JE: The in vitro effects of asbestos fibers on polymorpho-nuclear leukocyte function. Int Arch Allergy Appl Immunol 68:17, 1982.
39. Hext PM, Richards RJ: Biochemical effects of asbestiform minerals on lung fibroblast cultures. Br J Exp Pathol 57:281, 1976.
40. Jaurand MC, Gaudichet A, Atassi K, et al: Relationship between the number of asbestos fibres and the cellular and enzymatic content of bronchoalveolar fluid in asbestos exposed patients. Bull Eur Physiopathol Respir 16:595, 1980.
41. Haslam PL, Turton CWG, Lukoszek A, et al: Broncho-alveolar lavage fluid cell counts in cryptogenic fibrosing alveolitis and their relation to therapy. Thorax 35:328, 1980.
42. Keogh BA, Crystal RG: Alveolitis: The key to the interstitial lung disorders. Thorax 37:1, 1982.
43. Miller K, Kagan E: The in vivo effects of asbestos on macrophage membrane and population characteristics of macrophages: A scanning electron study. J Retic End Soc 20:159, 1976.
44. Gadek JE, Hunninghake GW, Zimmerman RL, Crystal RG: Regulation of the release of alveolar-derived neutrophil chemotactic factors. Am Rev Respir Dis 121:723, 1980.
45. Bignon J, Le Maho S, Lambre C, et al: Cellular and biochemical acute alveolar responses to asbestos and quartz dusts in rats. In: Occupational Lung Disease, eds. Gee JBL, Morgan WKC, Brooks SE. New York, Raven Press, 1983.
46. Schoenberger CI, Hunninghake GW, Kawanami O, et al: Role of alveolar macrophages in asbestosis: Modulation of neutrophil migration to the lung following acute asbestos exposure. Thorax, 37:803, 1982.
47. Gadek J, Hunninghake GW, Schoenberger CI, et al: Pulmonary asbestosis and idiopathic pulmonary fibrosis: Pathogenetic parallels. Chest 80(Suppl):635, 1981.
48. Heppleston AG, Styles JA: Activity of a macrophage factor in collagen formation by silica. Nature 214:521, 1967.
49. Kulonen E, Aalto M, Aho S, et al: The SiO_2-liberated fibrogenic macrophage factors with reference to RNA. In: The in Vitro Effects of Mineral Dusts, eds. Brown RC, Gormley IP, Chamberlain M, Davies R. New York, Academic Press, 1980, pp 218.
50. De Shazo RD: Current concepts about the pathogenesis of silicosis and asbestosis. J Allergy Clin Immunol 70:41, 1982.
51. Hillerdal G: Nonmalignant asbestos pleural disease. Thorax 36:669, 1981.
52. Chahinian PH, Hirsch A, Bignon J, et al: Les pleurésies asbestosiques non tumorales (à-propos de 6 observations). Rev Fr Mal Respir 1:5, 1973.
53. Kiviluoto K: Pleural calcification as a roentgenologic sign of nonoccupational endemic anthophyllite asbestosis. Acta Radiol 194(Suppl):5, 1960.
54. Bignon J, Bernaudin JF, Jaurand MC, Pinchon MC: The pleura: Mesothelial cells and mesothelioma. In: Cellular Biology of the Lung, eds. Cumming G, Bonsignore G. New York, Plenum Press, 1981, pp 149.

55. Hillerdal G, Lindgren A: Pleural plaques: Correlation of occurrence at autopsy to radiographic findings and occupational history. Eur J Respir Dis 61:395, 1980.
56. Sebastien P, Fondimare A, Bignon J, et al: Topographic distribution of asbestos fibers in human lung in relation to occupational and nonoccupational exposure. In: Inhaled Particles IV, ed. Walton WA. Oxford, New York, Pergamon Press, 1977, pp 435.
57. Evans JC, Evans RJ, Holmes A, et al: Studies on the deposition of inhaled fibrous material in the respiratory tract of the rat and its subsequent clearance using radioactive tracer technique. I. UICC crocidolite asbestos. Environ Res 6:180, 1973.
58. Sebastien P, Janson X, Bonnaud G, et al: Translocation of asbestos fibers through respiratory tract and gastrointestinal tract according to fiber type and size. In: Dusts and Disease, eds. Lemen R, Dement JM. Park Forest South, IL, Pathotox Publishers, 1979, pp 65.
59. Roe FJC, Carter RL, Walters MA, Harington JS: The pathological effects of subcutaneous injections of asbestos fibers in mice: Migration of fibers to submesothelial tissues and induction of mesotheliomata. Int J Cancer 2:628, 1967.
60. Bignon J, Jaurand MC, Sebastien P, Dufour G: Interaction of pleural tissue and cells with mineral fibers. In: Diseases of the Pleura, eds. Chrétien J, Hirsch A. Masson, New York, in press.
61. Kanazawa K, Birbeck MSC, Carter RL, Roe FJC: Migration of asbestos fibers from subcutaneous injection sites in mice. Br J Cancer 24:96, 1970.
62. Davis TMG: The fibrogenic effects of mineral dusts injected into the pleural cavity of mice. Br J Exp Pathol 53:190, 1972.
63. Monchaux G, Bignon J, Jaurand MC, et al: Mesotheliomas in rats following inoculation with acid-leached chrysotile asbestos and other mineral fibers. Carcinogenesis 2:229, 1981.
64. Rennard S, Jaurand MC, Bignon J, et al: Connective tissue production by pleural mesothelial cells. Am Rev Respir Dis 123:24a, 1981.
65. Jaurand MC, Kaplan H, Thiollet J, et al: Phagocytosis of chrysotile fibers by pleural mesothelial cells in culture. Am J Pathol 94:529, 1979.
66. Aalto M, Kulonen E, Pentinnen R, Renvall S: Collagen synthesis in cultured mesothelial cells in response to silica. Acta Chim Scand 147:1, 1981.
67. Wagner JC, Berry G, Timbrell V: Mesotheliomata in rats after inoculation with asbestos and other materials. Br J Cancer 28:173, 1973.
68. Stanton MF, Layard M, Tegeris A, et al: Relation of particle dimension to carcinogenicity in amphibole asbestos and other fibrous minerals. J Natl Cancer Inst 67:965, 1981.
69. Pott F, Friedrichs KH, Huth F: Results of animal experiments concerning the carcinogenic effect of fibrous dusts and their interpretation with regard to the carcinogenesis in humans. Zentralbl Bakteriol [Orig A] 162:467, 1976.
70. Selikoff IJ, Hammond EC, Seidman H: Latency of asbestos disease among insulation workers in the United States and Canada. Cancer 46:2736, 1980.
71. Hammond EC, Selikoff IJ, Seidman H: Asbestos exposure, cigarette smoking and death rates. Ann NY Acad Sci 330:473, 1979.
72. McDonald JC: Asbestos and lung cancer: Has the case been proven? Chest 78(Suppl):374, 1980.
73. Peto J: Dose-response relationships for asbestos-related disease. Implications for hygiene standards; Part II: Mortality. Ann NY Acad Sci 330:195, 1979.

74. Enterline PE: Attributability in the face of uncertainty. Chest 78(Suppl):377, 1980.
75. Newhouse ML, Berry G: Reductions of mortality from mesothelial tumors in asbestos factory workers. Br J Ind Med 33:147, 1976.
76. McDonald JC, Lidell FDK, Gibbes GW, et al: Dust exposure and mortality in chrysotile mining 1910–1975. Br J Ind Med 37:11, 1980.
77. Hobbs MST, Woodward SD, Murphy B, et al: The incidence of pneumoconiosis, mesothelioma and other respiratory cancer in men engaged in mining and milling crocidolite in western Australia. IARC Sci Publ 30(1):615, 1980.
78. Peto J, Henderson BE, Pike MC: Trends in mesothelioma incidence in the United States and the forecast epidemic due to asbestos exposure during World War II. In: Banbury Report 9: Quantification of Occupational Cancer, eds. Peto R, Schneiderman MS. Cold Spring Harbor Laboratory, 1981, pp 51.
79. Hirsch A, Brochard P, De Cremoux H, et al: Features of asbestos exposed and unexposed mesothelioma. Am J Ind Med, 3:413, 1982.
80. Peto J, Seidman H, Selikoff IJ: Mesothelioma mortality in asbestos workers: Implications for models of carcinogenesis and risk assessment. Br J Cancer 45:124, 1982.
81. Morgan A, Davies P, Wagner JC, et al: The biological effects of magnesium-leached chrysotile asbestos. Br J Exp Pathol 58:465, 1977.
82. Kolev K: Experimentally induced mesothelioma in white rats in response to intraperitoneal administration of amorphous crocidolite asbestos: Preliminary report. Environ Res 29:123, 1982.
83. Wagner JC: Health hazards of substitutes. Proc of the World Symposium on Asbestos Canadian Asbestos Information Centre 1982, p 266.
84. Chamberlain M, Tarmy EM: Asbestos and glass fibers in bacterial mutation tests. Mutat Res 43:159, 1977.
85. Jaurand MC, Bastie-Sigcac I, Bignon J, Stoebner P: Effect of chrysotile and crocidolite on the morphology and growth of net pleural mesothelial cells. Environ Res 30:255, 1983.
86. Huang SL, Saggioro D, Michelmann H, Malling HV: Genetic effects of crocidolite asbestos in Chinese hamster lung cells. Mutat Res 57:225, 1978.
87. Huang SL: Amosite, chrysotile and crocidolite asbestos are mutagenic in Chinese hamster lung cells. Mutat Res 58:265, 1979.
88. Lavappa KS, Fu MM, Epstein SS: Cytogenetic studies on chrysotile asbestos. Environ Res 10:165, 1975.
89. Sincock A, Seabright M: Induction of chromosome changes in Chinese hamster cells by exposure to asbestos fibres. Nature 257:56, 1975.
90. Babu KA, Lakkad BC, Nigam SK, et al: In vitro cytological and cytogenetic effects of an Indian variety of chrysotile asbestos. Environ Res 21:416, 1980.
91. Livingston GK, Rom WN, Morris MV: Asbestos-induced sister chromatid exchanges in cultured Chinese hamster ovarian fibroblast cells. J Environ Pathol Toxicol 3:373, 1980.
92. Jaurand MC, Bastie-Sigeac MJ, Renier A, Bignon J: Possibility of using rat mesothelial cells in culture to test cytotoxicity, clastogenicity and cancerogenicity of asbestos fibers. Ann NY Acad Sci, 407:409, 1983.
93. Price-Jones MJ, Gubbings G, Chamberlain M: The genetic effects of crocidolite asbestos; comparison of chromosome abnormalities and sister chromatid exchanges. Mutat Res 79:331, 1980.
94. Kaplan H, Renier A, Jaurand MC, Bignon J: Sister chromatid exchanges in me-

sothelial cells cultured with chrysotile fibers. In: The in Vitro Effects of Mineral Dusts, eds. Gormley IP, Chamberlain M, Davies R. New York, Academic Press, 1980, pp 251.

95. Poole A, Brown RC, Fleming GTA: A study of the cell transforming ability of mineral dusts and the ability to induce changes in the metabolism on macromolecular binding of benzo(a)pyrene in C3H 10T 1/2 cells. Environ Health Perspect 51:319 1983.
96. Reiss B, Tong C, Telang S, Williams GM: Enhancement of benzo(a)pyrene mutagenicity by chrysotile asbestos in rat liver epithelial cells. Enivorn Res, 31:100, 1983.
97. Blumberg PM: In vitro studies on the mode of action of the phorbol ester, potent tumor promoters. Crit Rev Toxicol (Part 1) 8:153, 1980.
98. Blumberg PM: In vitro studies on the mode of action of the phorbol ester, potent tumor promotors. Crit Rev Toxicol (Part 2) 8:199, 1981.
99. Berenblum I, Armuth Y: Two independent aspects of tumor promotion. Biochim Biophys Acta 651:51, 1981.
100. Yotti LP, Chang CC, Troko JE: Elimination of metabolic cooperation in Chinese hamster cells by tumor promoter. Science 206:1089, 1979.
101. Chamberlain M: The influence of mineral dusts on metabolic cooperation between mammalian cells in tissue culture. Carcinogenesis 3:337, 1982.
102. Wigler M, De Feo D, Weinstein IB: Induction of plasminogen activator in cultured cells by macrocyclic plant diterpene esters and other agents related to tumor promotion. Cancer Res 38:1434, 1978.
103. Trosko JE, Jone C, Aylsworth C, Tsuchimoto G: Elimination of metabolic cooperation associated with the tumor promoters, oleic acid and anthralin. Carcinogenesis 9:1101, 1982.
104. Topping DC, Nettesheim P: Two-stage carcinogenesis studies with asbestos in Fischer 344 rats. J Natl Cancer Inst 65:627, 1980.
105. Richards RJ, Jacoby F: Light microscope studies on the effects of chrysotile asbestos and fiber glass on the morphology and reticulin formation of cultured lung fibroblast. Environ Res 11:112, 1976.
106. Chamberlain M, Brown RC: The cytotoxic effects of asbestos and other mineral dust in tissue culture cell lines. Br J Exp Pathol 59:183, 1978.
107. Neugut AI, Eisenberg D, Silverstein M, et al: Effects of asbestos on epithelial cell lines. Environ Res 17:256, 1978.
108. Reiss B, Solomon S, Weisburger JH, William GM: Comparative toxicities of different forms of asbestos in a cell culture assay. Environ Res 22:109, 1980.
109. Mossman BT, Kessler JB, Ley BW, Craighead JE: Interaction of crocidolite asbestos with hamster respiratory mucosa in organ culture. Lab Invest 36:131, 1977.
110. Mossman BT, Eastman A, Landesman JM, and Bresnick E: Effects of crocidolite and chrysotile asbestos on cellular uptake and metabolism of benzo(a)pyrene in hamster tracheal epithelial cells. Environ Health Perspect 51:331, 1983.
111. Daniel FB, Beach CA, Hart RW: Asbestos induced changes in the metabolism of polycyclic aromatic hydrocarbons in human fibroblastic cell cultures. In: The in Vitro Effects of Mineral Dusts, eds. Brown RC, Gormley IP, Chamberlain M, Davies R. New York, Academic Press, 1980, pp 255.
112. Brown RC, Fleming GTA, Knight AI: Asbestos affects the in vitro uptake and detoxification of aromatic compounds. Environ Health Perspect 51:315, 1983.
113. Thiollet J, Jaurand MC, Kaplan H, et al: Culture procedure of mesothelial cells from the rat parietal pleura. Biomed Express 29:69, 1978.

114. Jaurand MC, Bernaudin JF, Renier A, et al: Rat pleural mesothelial cells in culture. In Vitro 17:98, 1981.
115. Aronson JF, Cristofalo WJ: Culture of epithelial cells from the rat pleura. In Vitro 17:61, 1981.
116. Bastie-Sigeac I, Hubert-Habart M, Jaurand MC, Bignon J: Interaction des fibres d'amiante sur le metabolisme du benzo(a)pyrene dans les cellules pleurales en culture. VDI-Berichte vol 475 pp 283 VDI-Verlag GmbH-Dusseldörf 1983.
117. Kandaswami C, O'Brien PJ: Effects of asbestos on membrane transport and metabolism of benzo(a)pyrene. Biochem Biophys Res Commun 97:794, 1980.
118. Craighead JE, Mossman BT: The pathogenesis of asbestos-associated diseases. N Engl J Med 306:1446, 1982.
119. Brand KG, Buoen LC, Johnson KH, Brand I: Etiological factors, stages and the role of the foreign body in foreign body tumorigenesis: A review. Cancer Res 35:279, 1975.
120. Bignon J, Jaurand MC: Biological in vitro and in vivo responses of chrysotile versus amphiboles. Environ Health Perspect 51:73, 1983.
121. Chamberlain M, Brown RC, Davies R, Griffiths DM: In vitro prediction of the pathogenicity of mineral dusts. Br J Exp Pathol 60:320, 1979.
122. Suzuki Y: Carcinogenic and fibrogenic effects of zeolites: preliminary observations. Environ Res 27:433, 1982.
123. Becklake MR: Exposure to asbestos and human disease. N Engl J Med 306:1480, 1982.
124. McDonald AD, McDonald JC, Pooley FD: Mineral fiber content of the lung in mesothelial tumors in North America. Ann Occup Hyg, in press.
125. McDonald JC: Asbestos related disease: An epidemiological review. IARC Sci Publ 30(2):587, 1980.
126. Bignon J, Sebastien P, Gaudichet A, Bonnaud G: Measurement of asbestos retention in humans related to health effects. In: Definitions and Measurement Methods, eds., Gravatt CC, Lafleur PD, Heinrich KFJ. National Bureau of Standards Special Publication, 506:95, 1978.
127. Jaurand MC, Bignon J, Sebastien P, Goni J: Leaching of chrysotile asbestos in human lungs. Environ Res 14:245, 1977.
128. Jaurand MC, Gaudichet A, Halpern S, Bignon J: In vitro biodegradation of chrysotile fibres by alveolar macrophages and mesothelial cells in culture. Br J Indust Med, in press.

4 Health Implications of Nonasbestos Fibers

James E. Lockey
Farhad Moatamed

The medical implications of asbestos exposure are well documented in animal experiments and human epidemiologic studies. There is a significant financial impact on people with asbestos-related disabilities and on asbestos manufacturing companies being named as defendents in litigation involving exposure to asbestos. Manville Corporation, a diversified mining and manufacturing concern involved with the production and manufacturing of asbestos-related products, recently filed for reorganization under the protection of the Federal bankruptcy laws. The reason cited by Manville for this action was the pending and potential asbestos-related liability suits, which in the company's estimation could number 52,000 and cost more than 2 billion dollars. While the courts and Congress try to untangle this legal quagmire the majority of asbestos victims remain uncompensated.

This experience makes it imperative to establish whether the biologically active properties of asbestos that cause pulmonary disease in humans are shared with the more prevalent man-made vitreous fibers, synthetic crystalline fibers, and other naturally occurring fibrous minerals. This chapter is a review of mineralogical terminology, factors associated with fiber toxicity, and those nonasbestos fibrous minerals that have been studied in relation to human exposure.

MINERALOGICAL TERMINOLOGY

The terms fiber, fibrous, asbestos, and asbestiform have been used inconsistently by medical and industrial hygiene professionals and mineralogists. This inconsistency has caused difficulties in evaluating and comparing studies on the health effects of inorganic fibers. Mineralogists have been concerned that the improper use of mineralogical nonmenclature may adversely affect the nonasbestos mining and mineral processing industries. The current regulatory criteria used to identify asbestos within the environment is nonspecific enough to include particles derived from nonasbestos minerals.[1,2]

Mineralogists regard a particle as a fiber when the aspect ratio (length : diameter ratio) is ≥10 : 1. In general an acicular (needlelike) or prismatic cleavage fragment would fail to meet the mineralogic criteria for a fiber but would still be considered as subject to regulation by the asbestos criteria. The Occupational Safety and Health Administration has defined an asbestos fiber to mean a fiber >5 μm in length with an aspect ratio of ≥3 : 1. For the purpose of regulation, asbestos includes chrysotile, amosite, crocidolite, tremolite, anthophyllite, and actinolite. These criteria were established for air sampling in an occupational setting where commercial asbestos was being mined, milled, fabricated, or installed. Therefore, all chrysotile, amosite, crocidolite, tremolite, anthophyllite, and actinolite silicate particles with aspect ratio ≥3 : 1, whether a true fiber by the mineralogic definition or a prismatic or acicular cleavage fragment, are classified as fibers. This implies that these silicate fibers are asbestos under the OSHA asbestos standard. In actuality, the amphiboles, anthophyllite, tremolite, and actinolite occur in prismatic crystalline form far more commonly than in the fibrous form.[1,2] The Mine and Safety Health Administration has listed over 150 minerals that may occur in fibrous form or be generally expected to contain fibrous minerals. Proper morphologic identification of these fibers and determination of their biologic activity is a primary concern of professional in the occupational and environmental health field.[3]

A mineral *fiber* is an elongated crystalline or polycrystalline unit that resembles in shape organic fibers such as cotton or animal hair. Morphologically a fiber has a circular cross section and a high aspect ratio. The term *fibrous* refers to the occurrence of minerals in bundles of parallel, radiating, or interlaced fibers from which individual fibers can usually be separated. *Asbestos* is a collective term for the commercial fibrous, silicate minerals of the serpentine and amphibole groups. The asbestos variety of the mineral silicates have high tensile strength and extreme aspect ratios, are flexible and heat resistant, and have parallel or radiating bundles that can be aggregated into easily separated filamentous strands. A silicate mineral can be called asbestos when it meets these properties as measured on a megascopic level or if the silicate mineral being examined microscopically is derived from a known source of asbestos. The term *asbestiform* denotes a commercial variety of silicate fiber that meets the above criteria. Asbestiform is sometimes used as a synonym for asbestos and should not be used for *asbestoslike* fibers.[4–7]

The amphibole minerals range in form from the commercial asbestos variety to the more common nonasbestos variety. The size and shape of a silicate mineral is strongly dependent on the mineral's original crystallization. The mining and milling of a mineral containing a nonasbestos variety of amphibole such as tremolite can produce various types of short cleavage fragments that

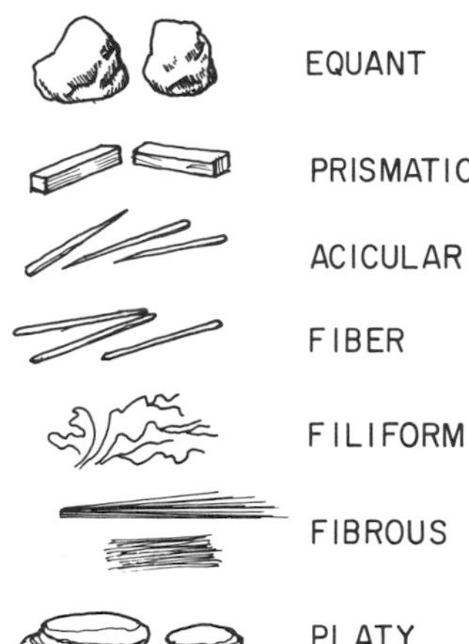

Fig. 4-1 Mineralogical terminology. (From: United States Dept. of the Interior, Bureau of Mines, Report No. 8751, 1977.)

fall within the current regulatory criteria for asbestos. The term *cleavage fragment* is defined as a fragment produced by the breaking of crystals in directions that are related to the crystal structure and are always parallel to possible crystal faces. The majority of cleavage fragments in the mineralogic view should not be called fibers. However, a cleavage fragment can take various configurations ranging from equant to a fiber shape. At times it is impossible to determine the difference between a cleavage fragment and a true fiber. The final particulate configuration is dependent on the primary crystalline structure of the mineral and locally controlled secondary factors. *Equant* is the shape of a single crystal with three approximately equal space dimensions. A *prismatic* crystal has one elongated dimension and two shorter, approximately equal dimensions. An *acicular* crystal resembles a short fiber with a small cross-sectional diameter. They can be pointed (needlelike) or have blunt ends. The various types of mineralogical configurations are shown in Fig. 4-1. It is important to note that silicate minerals occur in many forms. For example, tremolite can occur as true asbestos, as a fibrous form (Fig. 4-2), or as prismatic and acicular cleavage fragments (Fig. 4-3). The health impact of these different morphologic forms of tremolite may be substantially different.[4–7]

FIBER TOXICOLOGY

Current knowledge of the biologic activity of fibers is derived from human epidemiologic studies on asbestos exposure and from animal and in vitro cellular studies with asbestos and nonasbestos fibers. These studies indicate that the important determinants of the disease-producing potential of fibers are the dose delivered to the target organ, the dimensions of the fiber, and the biologic durability of the fiber. The degree of importance of each of these parameters, however, may not be equal for all fibers or for all disease entities.[5,8–10]

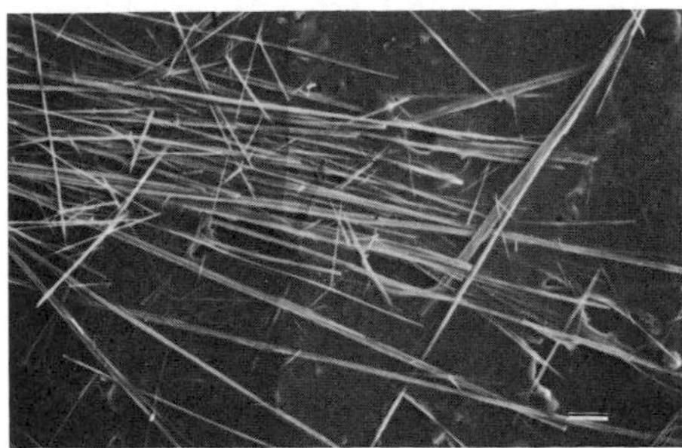

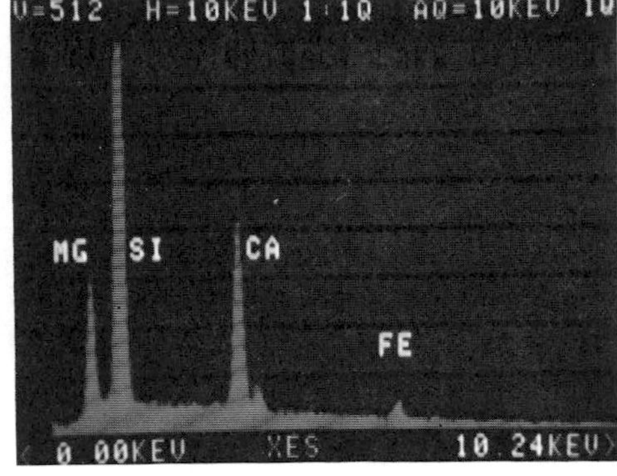

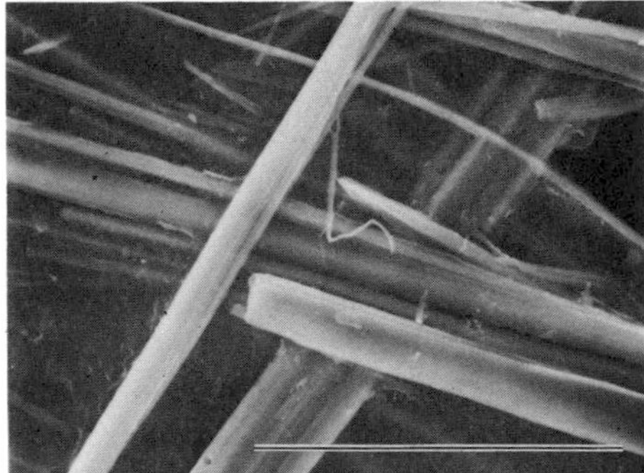

Fig. 4-2 Scanning electron micrograph of fibrous tremolite with Energy dispersive x-ray (EDX) analysis of the ore showing 25% magnesium, 56% silicon, 16% calcium, and 3% iron. The bars indicate 50 μm.

The dose delivered to the respiratory system is dependent on the number of fibers of respirable size, and the fiber's ability to penetrate and remain within the respiratory system. The aerodynamic behavior of fibers helps determine whether they are respirable. Experimental studies have demonstrated that fibers with the diameter of ≤ 3 μm and lengths up to 200 μm can penetrate the respiratory system.[11] Clearance of fibers is dependent on the mucociliary system and the alveolar macrophages. The mucociliary clearance mechanism effectively removes most particulate matter regardless of the size and shape of the particle. Once the particle reaches the alveoli, it is cleared mainly by alveolar macrophages. Short fibers (<5 μm) can be completely engulfed by alveolar macrophages. Longer fibers are either incompletely phagocytosed or not phagocytosed at all. The incomplete or "frustrated phagocytosis" may cause the release of cellular lysozomal enzymes and reactive oxidants that, in turn, may cause an inflammatory reaction, and possibly parenchymal scarring.[12] The biologic activity of the completely engulfed short fiber needs intensive investigation. Short fibers are the predominant fiber found within lung parenchyma. Crocidolite, which is found with the greatest number of short fibers per unit mass of material, is capable of producing marked fibrosis, as well as mesotheliomas and lung cancer.[5]

The biologic activity of fibers in animal studies has been demonstrated to be related to diameter and length. Fibers ≤ 1.5 μm in diameter and >8 μm in

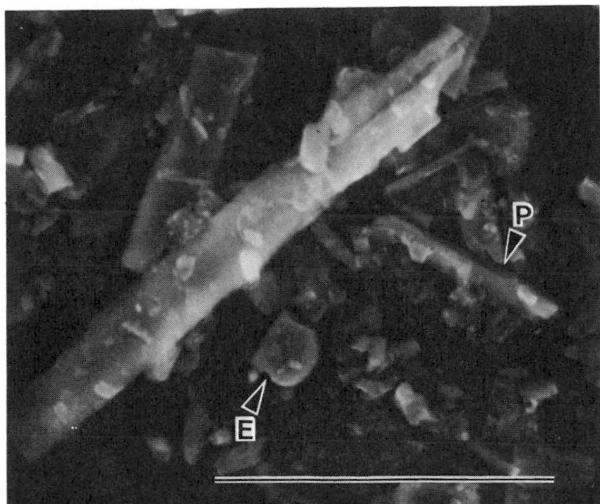

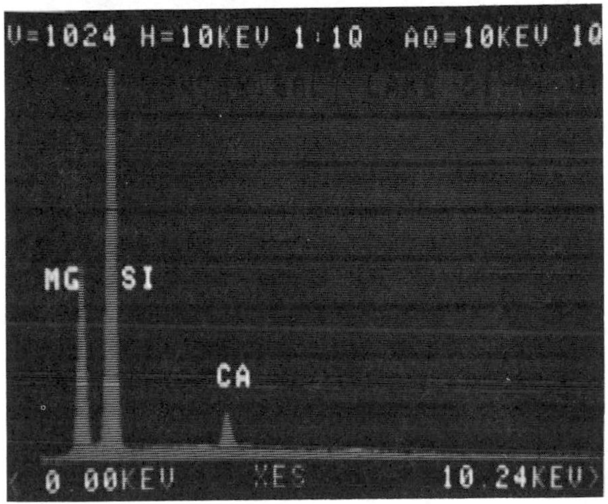

Fig. 4-3 Scanning electron micrograph of nonfibrous tremolite containing prismatic (P) and equant (E) cleavage fragments. EDX analysis of the ore shows 32% magnesium, 64% silicon, and 4% calcium. The bar represents 50 μm.

length have high probability of producing pleural sarcomas in rats.[13] The fibrogenic potential of glass fibers in animals exposed by intratracheal instillation appears also to be related to fiber diameter and length.[14] Fibers that have produced tumors in animals by pleural or peritoneal injections include amosite, anthophyllite, chrysotile, crocidolite, tremolite, borosilicate glass, aluminum silicate glass, mineral wool, aluminum oxide, potassium titanite, silicon carbide, sodium aluminum carbonate, wollastonite, attapulgite, and the zeolite erionite.[9,10,15]

Biologic durability is the third major component of fiber toxicity. In theory, the longer a biologically active fiber is retained unaltered within a target organ, the more likely a disease state will result. Fibers that go into solution or fracture perpendicular to their longitudinal plane most likely are not as toxic as more durable fibers. Little scientific information, however, is available that adequately addresses this theory.[9,10]

TALC

Talc is a soft, flexible, platelike crystalline magnesium-silicate with the chemical formula $3MgO \cdot 4SiO_2 \cdot H_2O$. Talc frequently exists in mineralogically complex deposits with varying amounts of other minerals of which quartz (SiO_2), the amphiboles, tremolite and anthophyllite, and the serpentines, antigorite, lizardite, and possibly chrysotile, are the most significant. Talc can roll into a scroll configuration and appear as a fiber. The complexity and variability of talc deposits is important when considering the potential health effect of the mineral.[2,16,17]

Within the United States, Vermont, Montana, New York, Texas, and California accounted for more than 75% of the talc production in 1979.[18] The talc from some areas are associated with a wide variety of minerals. The talc in New York State from the Gouverneur Talc District may contain in excess of 50% impurities, including significant amounts of tremolite (37–59%), anthophyllite (4.5–15%), and quartz (0.25–2.6%). The tremolite and anthophyllite appear as prismatic and acicular cleavage fragments and as true fibers. Environmental exposure studies have revealed mean airborne concentration of fibers of 4.5 to 5.0 fibers/cm^3 by phase contrast microscopy. Electron microscopy showed that 7% of the >5-μm fibers were tremolite and 65% were anthophyllite.[19] Talc from Ontario is very similar in composition to the talc from New York State. Talc from Death Valley, California is associated with nonfibrous tremolite and quartz. Montana and Vermont talc is free of any significant mineral contamination.[2,20] Figures 4-4 and 4-5 show pure platy talc and talc contaminated with tremolite.

Talc is a very versatile mineral with multiple commercial and industrial applications. Important properties include softness, smoothness, color, lubricating power, chemical inertness, heat and electrical conductivity, and absorption capacity. The largest use is in the ceramic industry, and as fillers in the paint and plastics industries. Talc is also used in paper, as a carrier for insecticides, in roofing material, and as a dusting agent for numerous products. The majority of the talc used in these processes is of an industrial grade containing mixtures of talc, tremolite, anthophyllite, and minor amounts of quartz. The cosmetic grade talc is more of a pure form of the mineral, free of most of the contamination found in the industrial grades. In consumer products it is found in pottery, chalk, crayons, cosmetic talcum powder, deodorants, condoms, coating for polished rice, food processing, and as fillers in pills and tablets.[18,21] There has been some evidence that cosmetic talcum powder marketed prior to 1973 contained varying amounts of quartz (2–5% with one sample containing 35%) and tremolite and anthophyllite (0.1–14% by weight).[22] The Cosmetic Toiletry and Fragrance Association of the United States has set higher specifi-

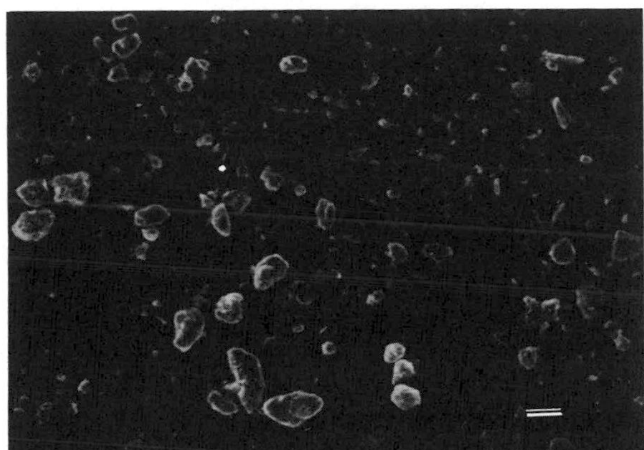

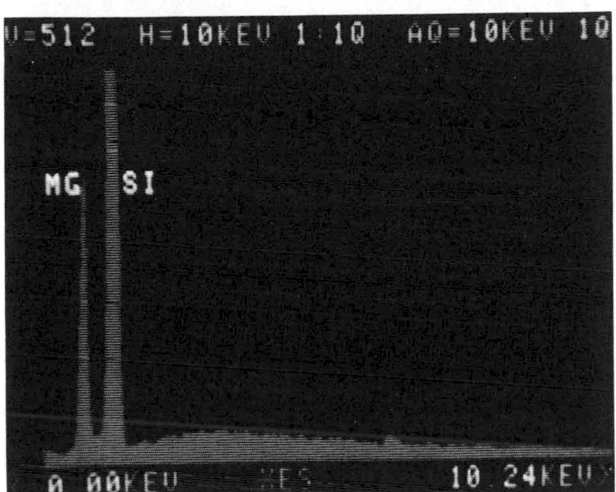

Fig. 4-4 Pure platy talc by scanning electron microscopy. EDX analysis of the ore shows 27% magnesium and 73% silicon. The bar represents 50 μm.

cations to ensure the purity of cosmetic talc.[23] Consumer grade talc now comes from sources of uncontaminated raw material. Subsequent analyses of cosmetic talcum powder manufactured between 1975 and 1978 have demonstrated lower fiber content.[16]

The pulmonary abnormalities seen with talc exposure are closely related to the amount of silica and/or tremolite and anthophyllite fibers within the mineral. Three forms of talc pneumoconiosis have been described: talcoasbestosis, talcosilicosis, and pure talcosis.[24] The term talcoasbestosis refers to pulmonary abnormalities commonly associated with asbestos exposure. In this case, however, the abnormalities are from exposure to talc contaminated with fibrous tremolite and anthophyllite. The use of these terms reflects the type of minerological exposure.

Morbidity studies on miners and millers from the talc district in New York State have generally revealed an increased prevalence of pulmonary abnormalities. Among 35 workers exposed to talc contaminated with tremolite and antho-

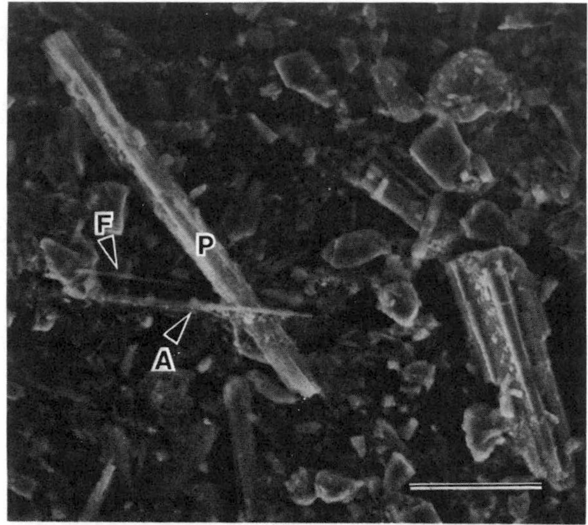

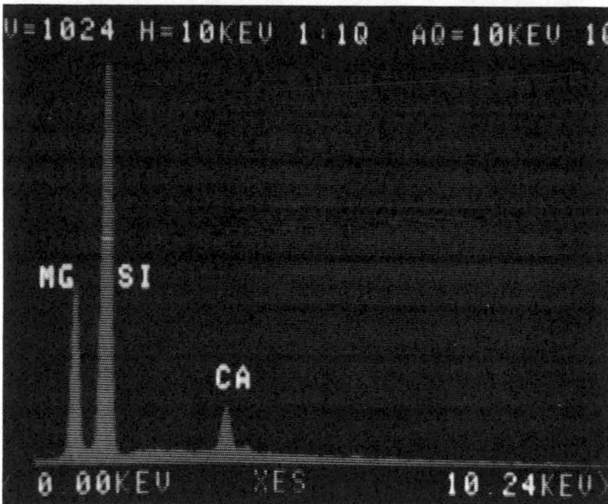

Fig. 4-5 Talc with acicular (A) and prismatic (P) cleavage fragments of tremolite. Occasional amphibole fibers (F) are also seen. EDX of tremolite fragments show 31% magnesium, 64% silicon, and 5% calcium. Compare the analytical results with Fig. 4-3. The bar indicates 50 μm.

phyllite for a mean duration of 17 years, 12 (34%) had radiographic findings consistent with pneumoconiosis, 63 percent had dyspnea and 22% had lung crepitations. The average dust count was 23 mppcf and 159 fibers/cm^3, >5 μm in length. A similar group of workers with the same mean duration of exposure, but at a lower dust and fiber exposure level (18 mppcf and 43 fibers/cm^3), had one case of pneumoconiosis and a significant increase in the prevalence of dyspnea (23%).[25,26] More recent studies revealed increased prevalence of pleural thickening (31%) and significantly lower spirometric values in talc-exposed workers when compared to potash miners. The mean total particulate and fiber exposure level, which most likely underestimates past exposure, was 10.62 mg/m^3 and 1.28 fibers/cm^3, >5 μm in length.[27,28]

Mortality studies from the talc district of New York State have demonstrated a fourfold increase in proportional mortality from pulmonary and pleural malignancies in the 60 to 79 age group with 15 years or longer exposure to talc. The mortality from pneumoconiosis or its complications, cor pulmonale, tuberculosis, and bronchopneumonia, were also inceased. The mean duration of exposure was 24.7 years (range 15 to 47 years) with the total dust exposure averaging 340 mppcf before 1945 and 27.6 mppcf between 1946 and 1965.[29] A follow-up study of the same group extended to 1969 revealed a significant decrease in death due both to pneumoconiosis and pulmonary and pleural cancers. Improved environmental controls resulting in decreased respirable dust levels is probably responsible for the decreased mortality.[30] A similar study of miners and millers in the same talc district looking at a cohort employed between 1947 to 1959 found a significant increase in malignant and nonmalignant respiratory disease.[31] Another study demonstrated increased mortality due to respiratory cancer and nonmalignant respiratory disease which was significantly increased when correlated with the presence of a previous occupational history.[32] It is apparent that past occupational exposure to talc contaminated with tremolite and anthophyllite can cause significant respiratory disorders. Recent control of exposures, however, appears to have reduced the risk.

Talcosilicosis is pneumoconiosis caused by exposure to talc containing significant amounts of silica. Studies of miners and millers of Italian talc revealed a threefold excess of mortality due to silicosis and silicotuberculosis. The free silica content in the air of the mine was measured as high as 18% during mine-drilling operations. The mortality was related to cumulative dust exposure. No increase in respiratory malignancy was noted in either miners or millers.[33,34]

The prevalence of pure talcosis in workers occupationally exposed to talc free of tremolite and anthophyllite or significant amounts of silica is not well defined. Increased symptoms of bronchitis and significantly decreased FEV_1 values were found in rubber workers using "pure" talc as a dusting agent.[35] A French study of 176 talc millers found 46 (26.6%) with pneumoconiosis of which 10 (5.6%) had "heavy radiological symptoms."[36] Bilateral pleural thickening has been found to be significantly related to exposure estimates in Montana, South Carolina, Texas, and New York talc miners and millers.[20] A mortality study of Vermont talc millers demonstrated a significantly increased rate of nonmalignant respiratory deaths.[37] A recent review of the pathology on seven men employed in the mining and milling of talc from Vermont demonstrated extensive focal and diffuse fibrosis. The three workers with the longest duration of exposures (26 to 27 years) had radiographic changes consistent with pneumoconiosis and had the heaviest dust loads within the lungs. There were no radiographic changes for workers with shorter duration of exposure (4 to 19 years) even though the lungs exhibited focal and diffuse fibrosis.[38] It appears that talcosis may be a complication of occupational exposure to pure talc exposure and may be associated with an increase in nonmalignant respiratory mortality.

Talc has been associated with other health abnormalities not associated with occupational exposure. Habitual use of excessive amounts of cosmetic talc in adults and accidental aspiration of talc in infants can cause significant pulmonary disease. When suspended in water and injected intravenously by drug addicts, a foreign body pulmonary granulomatous reaction can occur.[21]

An interesting relationship between talc and ovarian cancer has been postulated for a number of years. Talc particles have been found in the ovaries of patients with ovarian cancer.[39–42] A recent case-control study found a significant correlation between genital exposure to talc and epithelial ovarian cancer.[43] Ovarian cancer has been induced in guinea pigs with asbestos and it has been suggested there is a similarity between mesotheliomas and ovarian cancer.[44] If there is a relationship between talc and ovarian cancer, it is probably due to the uniqueness of the ovarian tissue and the durability of pure talc and/or associated mineral contaminants. After ovulation the surface epithelium along with any foreign particulate become incorporated in the ovarian stroma. An important observation is the lack of pleural or parenchymal lung tumors in patients who have undergone talc pleurodesis.[45]

The health implications of talc exposure can be summarized as follows:

1. The talc from New York State has significant amounts of tremolite and anthophyllite. The majority of these amphiboles exist as particles ≤ 5 μm in length. Fibrous forms of these amphiboles, however, have been identified in airborne dust samples from these mines.
2. Occupational exposure to talc from New York State in the past has been associated with an increased respiratory morbidity and mortality, including malignancies of the lung and possible the pleura. The increased rates are most likely related to previous cummulative exposures and do not reflect current exposure levels.
3. Exposure to talc with significant amounts of free silica has been associated with increased nonmalignant respiratory mortality.
4. Exposure to pure talc in an occupational setting may be associated with an incease in nonmalignant respiratory mortality. Pathologic studies have demonstrated significant focal and diffuse fibrosis in Vermont talc workers.
5. The possible association between talc and ovarian cancer is an important observation that needs further study. If an association exists, it is probably secondary to the uniqueness of the ovarian tissues and the persistence of a foreign substance within the ovarian stroma.

VERMICULITE

Vermiculite is the name given to a family of hydrated magnesium-aluminum-iron silicates in sheet form derived from hydrothermally altered biotite. So far, 19 varieties of this mineral have been identified. Vermiculite has the unique property of expanding up to 12 times its original size with the application of heat at 800–2000°F. This expanding property depends on the conversion of the intrinsic water content to steam. The steam forces apart the laminal plates at right angles of the cleavage planes to form an accordianlike or "wormlike" structure. Hence the name vermiculite from *vermicular* meaning "to produce worms."[46,47]

The main domestic deposits of vermiculite are located in Montana, Virginia, and South Carolina. One of the world's largest reserves is located in South Africa. The unexpanded ore is shipped to approximately 47 regional expander plants located in 30 states. Accessory minerals in vermiculite deposits include quartz, feldspar, apatite, corundum, chlorite, talc, and clay. Recent analysis of the Montana ore has found it to be contaminated with a fibrous form of the amphibole, tremolite (Fig. 4-6). The ore from Virginia and

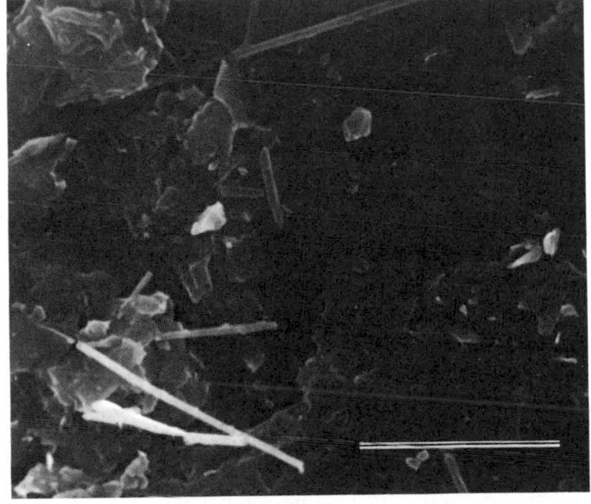

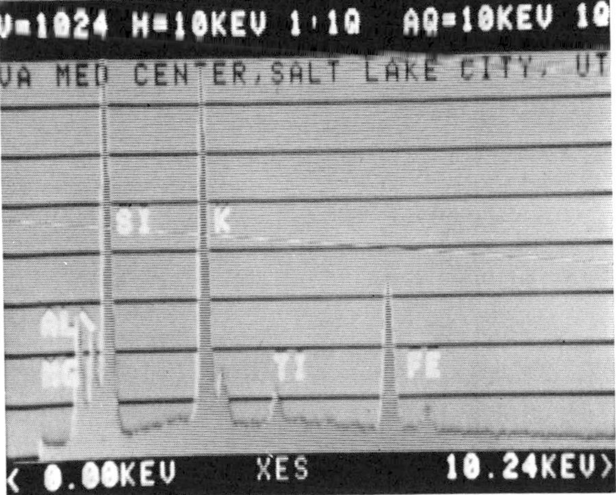

Fig. 4-6 Montana unexpanded vermiculite ore with fibrous amphibole by scanning electron microscopy. EDX analysis of the ore shows 19% magnesium, 10% aluminum, 30% silicon, 19% potassium, 3% titanium, and 19% iron, basically magnesium-aluminum-silicate. The bar indicates 10 μm.

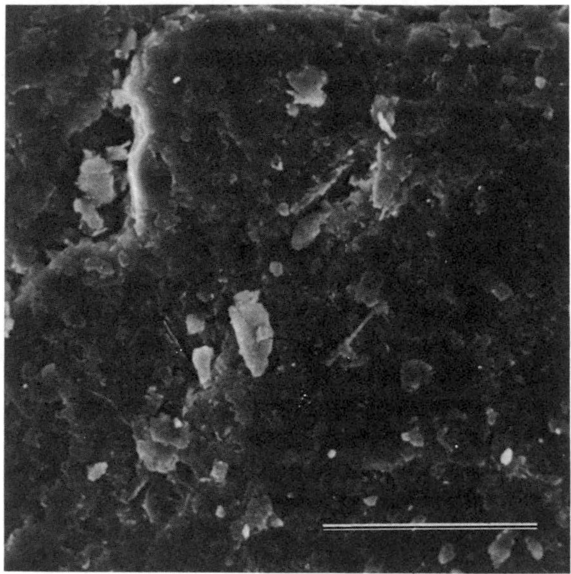

Fig. 4-7 South African unexpanded vermiculite ore. (Note almost complete lack of fibrous structure.) EDX analysis of ore showed a similar composition to that in Fig. 4-6. The bar indicates 22 μm.

South Carolina appears to contain a variety of tremolite that, when milled, tends to form cleavage fragments. The South African ore is currently felt to be free of amphibole or serpentine contamination (Fig. 4-7).[3,47–49]

The main domestic uses of vermiculite are related to its fire resistance, insulation, and ion exchange properties. Other uses include aggregates in cement and hard boards, fillers for paint, plasters, and rubber, loosefill insulation for attics and hollow masonry walls, ion-exchange agents for various applications in chemistry, including water purification, soil additives, an animal feed bulking agent, and a carrier for herbicides, insecticides, fungicides, fertilizers, and seeds.[47]

Recently a company processing mainly Montana ore to its expanded form reported an apparently unusual number of benign bloody pleural effusions of unknown etiology among their employees. Environmental sampling of the work area revealed airborne fibers resembling tremolite. A subsequent epidemiologic study revealed a significant association between cumulative tremolite fiber exposure and pleural abnormalities noted on chest radiography. The mean cumulative fiber exposure for employees with abnormal chest radiographs was approximately threefold greater than for age-matched controls with normal chest radiographs. There were no associations between cumulative fiber exposure and spirometry or single-breath diffusion capacity results. This finding was probably due to the relatively low cumulative fiber exposure of these employees compared to the relatively high fiber exposure levels associated with the parenchymal fibrotic manifestations of asbestos. Bloody pleural effusions, however, have been documented to be early manifestations of asbestos exposure.[49]

Vermiculite is an example of a mineral that can be contaminated with fibrous particles depending on the source of the ore. The health implications of vermiculite exposure are probably related to the degree of contamination with fibrous tremolite. Significant exposure to fibrous tremolite could occur in vermiculite mining, milling, and expanding operations. The National Institute for Occupational Safety and Health is currently reviewing the available health data from the vermiculite mine in Montana. The animal studies on vermiculite are limited and need to be expanded to include studies on vermiculite contaminated with the various forms of tremolite.[50,51]

ZEOLITES

Zeolites are a group of crystalline, hydrated aluminum silicate minerals with worldwide distribution. The name is derived from the ancient Greek word meaning "boiling stone." Zeolites "boil" at 200°C, giving off water that is reabsorbed at room temperature without disrupting the basic mineral structure. The commercial uses of zeolite are related to the hydrophilic nature and selective absorption and ion exchange capabilities of the mineral. The mineral is used in petrochemical, water-waste treatment, and water filtration industries. Domestic production of nonfibrous synthetic zeolites currently meets the majority of the commercial needs.[52]

Approximately 40 distinct fibrous and nonfibrous zeolite species have been identified. Two fibrous zeolites, mordenite and erionite, resemble commercial asbestos fibers. Mordenite fibers are thin, curved, and delicate with aspect ratios of 100 or greater. Erionite fibers average 10 to 20 μm in length and less than 1–3 μm in diameter (Fig. 4-8). The main deposits of natural zeolites in the United States are along the margins of the great basins in the West. There is currently little commercial mining of the mineral. The construction of the MX missile system within these western basins might expose workers to these naturally occurring fibrous zeolites.[52,53]

Erionite, has recently been identified as a naturally occurring fibrous mineral that may induce pulmonary disease in humans. A high incidence of malignant pleural mesotheliomas and nonmalignant pleural and parenchymal pulmonary disease has been identified in the villages of Karain and Tuzköy, located in an area of central Anatolia known as Cappadocia. Karain is known for picturesque rock dwellings called "fairy chimneys" carved from volcanic tuffs locally composed largely of erionite. The significance of the mesothelioma problem is reflected by the local saying, "the peasant of Karain falls ill with pain in the chest and belly, the shoulder drops, and he dies."[54–57]

Since the initial reports describing these clusters of malignant pleural mesotheliomas, two distinct mesothelioma groups in Turkey have been identified. Group 1 consists of cases from the villages of Karain (51), Tuzköy (10), and Ürgüp (2). The occurrence of the tumors at an early age (mean age 50 with a range of 27–71) and the large number of females (41%) are different from previous experience with occupational exposure to asbestos. The earlier occur-

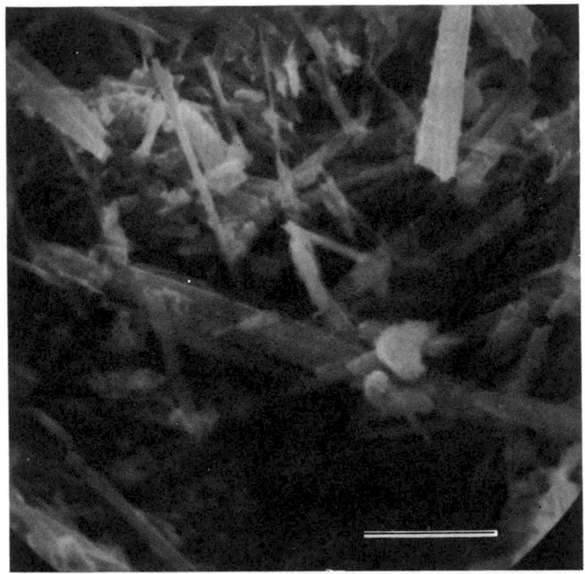

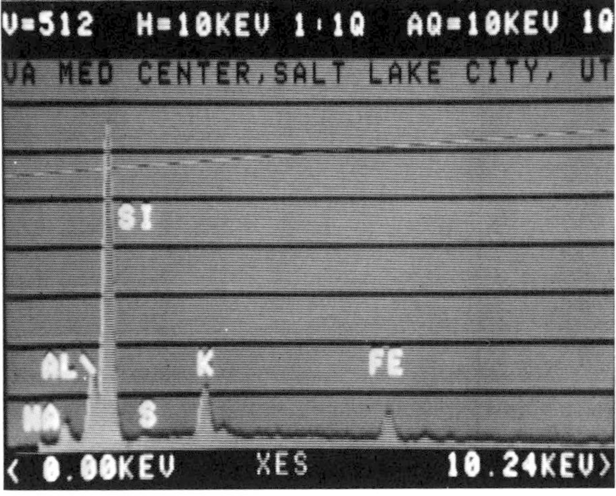

Fig. 4-8 Scanning electron micrograph of zeolite fibers (erionite), a sample obtained from near Elko, Nevada. EDX analysis of the ore shows 22% sodium, 13% aluminum, 52% silicon, 6% potassium, and 7% iron, an aluminum-silicate. The bar represents 10 μm.

rence of mesothelioma is probably related to exposure since birth.[58] A chest radiographic survey of Karain revealed 7.9% of the population had pleural calcifications and 5.3% had diffuse fibrosis.[55] In Tuzköy the prevalence of calcified pleural plaques (17%), pleural thickening (10.5%), pulmonary fibrosis (12.5%), and obliteration of the costophrenic angle (15%) was increased in comparison to a control population.[56] Mineralogical surveys of these villages have revealed respirable-size erionite fibers within the volcanic tuffs, street dust, and in their homes. Until recently no other mineral fibers have been identified in the environment, although chrysotile fibers were found in the pleural tissue of two of the five cases initially investigated.[54,59] Tremolite and chrysotile fibers have recently been identified in small amounts in the environment and in additional pleural and lung parenchymal tissue samples. It appears that the epidemic of mesotheliomas within Group 1 probably represents the result of a mixed environmental fiber exposure.[60]

Group 2 consists of mesothelioma cases from other rural parts of Central Anatolia. There were 122 cases of mesothelioma of which 5 could have been of an occupational origin; 33% of the population were females. The mean age for males was 42.8 (range 15–71) and for females 48.5 (range 12–69). The most plausible etiologic agent within this group is the fibrous tremolite and possible chrysotile found in the whitewash stucco for local homes and in local soil and air samples.[58] A study around the town of Cermik in southeast Turkey revealed a cluster of 22 mesotheliomas. Of a population of 7000, 6.5% had pleural thickening and calcification and 1.47% had interstitial pulmonary fibrosis. The whitewash and stucco contain fibrous tremolite. Tremolite fibers, asbestos bodies, and a few chrysotile fibers were found in the lung of a patient with bronchogenic adenocarcinoma.[61]

The Turkish experience with pleural and parenchymal disease and malignant mesothelioma in relation to fibrous erionite and tremolite exposure is significant for the following reasons:

1. There is a strong indicator that the natural zeolite fiber, erionite, causes disease in humans previously recognized only with asbestos exposure. Animal experiments have demonstrated that erionite is capable of producing tumors.[15]
2. The available airborne fiber counts for fibers at Karain indicates an average fiber contamination at or below 0.01 fiber/cm^3. The peak level obtained during cleaning of a family cave was 1.38 fiber/cm^3. These levels are significantly lower than the current standard for asbestos fibers (2 fibers/cm^3) and, if substantiated, indicate a previously unrecognized hazard for low-level airborne fiber exposure.[62]
3. It is apparent that environmental exposure to fibrous tremolite can cause pulmonary abnormalities currently associated with commercial asbestos.

WOLLASTONITE

Wollastonite is a naturally occurring monocalcium silicate. The natural cleavage of the mineral causes it to form acicular, prismatic, and fiber cleavage fragments (Fig. 4-9). It has been mined in upper New York State since 1952. Other deposits are found in Finland, Mexico, and Australia. Its largest use is as a filler and flux in the ceramic industry. High resistance to heat and insulating properties make it useful as an asbestos substitute in wallboard, insulation, and brake linings.[2,63]

Health and environmental studies in the mine of northern New York have not revealed any significant correlation between wollastonite exposure and the

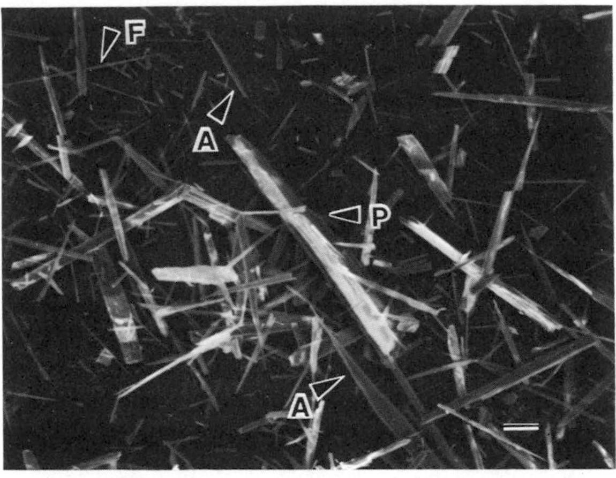

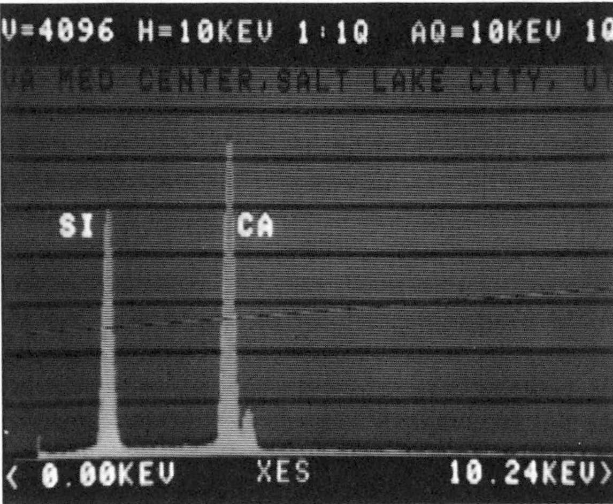

Fig. 4-9 Scanning electron micrograph of wollastonite with acicular (A), prismatic (P), and fiber (F) cleavage fragment. EDX analysis of ore shows 43% silicon, 56% calcium, and 1% or less iron. The bar represents 50 μm.

prevalence of bronchitis, abnormal spirometry, abnormal diffusion, or radiographic abnormalities. The average airborne concentration at the mine was 1 fiber/cm^3 and 20 fibers/cm^3 at the mill. The median fiber diameter was 0.22 μm (range 0.1–5.2 μm) and the median length was 2.5 μm (range 0.3–41.0 μm). As the New York mine has only been in production since 1952, only 43% of the workers had more than 10 years of exposure.[64,65]

The preliminary results of a Finnish study looking at workers with exposure of 10 years or more in a limestone-wollastonite quarry found 30% with "slight fibrosis" and 28% with "slight pleural thickening." Dust and fiber concentrations were said to be high.[66]

Additional animal and human data are needed before assessing the biologic activity of wollastonite in humans. The demonstration of a tumorigenic potential in animals, and the preliminary results of the Finnish study warrants more intensive study with this naturally occurring silicate fiber.

MAN-MADE MINERAL FIBERS

Man-made mineral fibers or vitreous fibers are amorphous silicates made from glass, natural rock, and fusible slag. They include rock and slag wool as mineral wool, fibrous glass wool, and refractory or ceramic fibers. They are produced in large quantities throughout the world by spinning, pulling, or blowing molten raw material. Glass fibers are commonly combined with a phenolic resin as a binder, which is normally fully polymerized and chemically inert in the final product. The multiple uses of these fibers are related to their high tensile strength, resistance to chemicals, and insulating properties. They have been effective in many uses previously reserved for asbestos and now have over 35,000 applications.[67,68]

The type of production process for man-made mineral fibers determines the degree of variability in the fiber diameter. Mineral wool and fibrous glass wool used as insulation are mainly produced by a blowing or spinning process. The nominal (specific) fiber diameter is usually 4.0–6.0 μm. The production process results in a wide fiber diameter distribution around the nominal diameter (Fig. 4-10).[68,69] Man-made mineral fibers produced by a continuous filament process and used in textile fabrics and as plastic reinforcement usually range from 2.5 to 15 μm in diameter. The continuous filament production process narrowly limits any variation in size from a predetermined nominal diameter.[70] Continuous filament fiber can range from 0.05 to 25.40 μm in diameter depending on production specifications.[71] Microfiber production has occurred in the United States since the 1940s and makes up a very small percentage of total continuous filament production (Fig. 4-11). The high aspect ratios and small diameters of these microfibers (<1 μm diameter) have generated a significant amount of scientific interest concerning the possible adverse long-term health implications.[68]

Ceramic fibers are made from alumina (Al_2O_3) and silica (SiO_2). These fibers are used in industrial processes requiring high-temperature thermal insu-

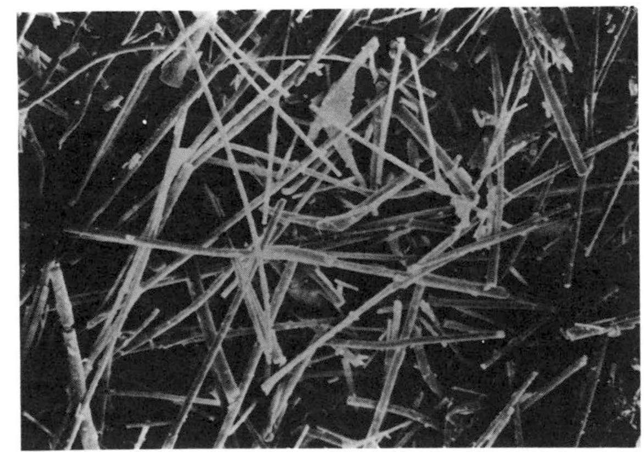

Fig. 4-10 Scanning electron micrograph of mineral wool fibers. Notice the variability in fiber diameter. (Courtesy of Manville Corporation.) Original magnification 250 X.

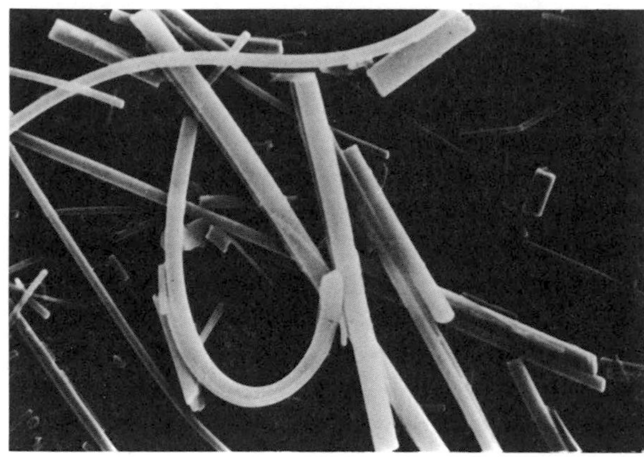

Fig. 4-11 Scanning electron micrograph of glass microfibers. (Courtesy of Manville Corporation.) Original magnification 5000 X.

lation beyond the capacity of glass fibers. The production process for ceramic fibers usually involves blowing or spinning molten material.[71]

Other types of synthetic crystalline fibers have been manufactured for certain specialty applications. This includes alumina, silicon carbide, sodium aluminum carbonate, potassium titanate, and graphite. The graphite fibers have been especially important to the aerospace industry. As mentioned previously, some of these fibers have shown biologic activity in animals.[9]

Occupational exposure to man-made mineral fibers during the production process has been under intensive study. Depending on the production process and the type and nominal diameter of the fiber being manufactured, a significant portion of the resultant airborne fibers are of respirable size (<3 μm diameter). A review of 16 man-made mineral fiber production facilities within the United States (slag and rock wool, and fiberglass wool) demonstrated an average total suspended particulate matter concentration of 1.0 mg/m³ with a range of 0.1–8 mg/m³. Average fiber concentrations <1 μm in diameter ranged from 0.003 to >6 fibers/cm³ with a median of 0.013 fiber/cm³. Fibers <1 μm in diameter represent about 25% of the total fiber count. As the nominal fiber diameter decreased the percentage of fibers <1 μm in diameter increased.[72] It has also been demonstrated that, as the nominal fiber diameter decreases, the total number of airborne fibers increase.[73] Another survey of United States plants demonstrated that mean fiber counts, in facilities producing fibers <1 μm in diameter, ranged from 1.0 to 21.9 fibers/cm³ with 40–80% ≤0.5 μm in diameter. Mean fiber counts in facilities producing large diameter fibers ranged from 0.06 to 0.13 fibers/cm³ and over 50% of the fibers were <3.5 μm in diameter.[69] At five production plants in Europe (glass and rock wool) the highest concentration of respirable fibers (defined as aspect ratio of 3 : 1 with length >5 μm and diameter <3 μm) was 1.9 fibers/cm³ and was found in the secondary processes of the production plants (molding, cutting, sawing, etc.).[74] In facilities manufacturing man-made mineral fibers, average exposure concentrations expressed in fibers/cm³ can be summarized as follows: continuous filament 0.00X–0.0X, insulation fibrous glass wool 0.0X–0.X, fine specialty fiber 0.X–X, mineral wool 0.0X–0.X, and ceramic fiber 0.X–X.[71] The National Institute for Occupational Safety and Health has recommended that exposure to fibrous glass be limited to 3 fibers/cm^3, $\leq$3.5 μm in diameter, and $\geq$10 μm in length. The recommended time weighted average for total fibrous glass is 5 mg/m^3.[73]

Commonly recognized health problems caused by man-made mineral fibers are secondary to mechanical irritation. Fibers generally larger than 5 μm in diameter can cause a chronic dermatitis. Newly exposed workers can develop transient burning and itching of the skin, which usually resolves spontaneously. Individuals with dermographism, however, may be unable to tolerate continued exposure because of lower itch thresholds. Eye, nasal, and throat irritation are uncommon manifestations of man-made mineral fiber exposure and usually occur only after exposure to unusually dusty situations.[21]

Morbidity studies on man-made mineral fibers have generally not demonstrated any significant increase in pulmonary abnormalities as measured by chest radiographs or pulmonary function tests.[75–78] Preliminary results of a recently completed study of seven fibrous glass and mineral wool facilities demonstrated a 10% prevalence of small radiographic opacities with profusion $\geq$0/1–1/1. The radiographic changes were related to exposures to fibers <1 μm in diameter. The relationship becomes weaker if only profusion 1/0 and 1/1 are counted as evidence of pneumoconiosis.[79] Mortality studies on workers exposed to rock and slag wool fibers have been limited. A study of a manufacturing facility in production for over 70 years showed increases in the standardized mortality ratio for digestive tract and respiratory cancer and nonmalignant respiratory disease. None of the results, however, were at a statistically significant level. The mean airborne fiber size was 2.1 μm in diameter and 15.1–17 μm in length, with 75% considered respirable.[80] Studies sponsored by the Thermal Insulation Manufacturers' Association (TIMA) with the University of Pittsburgh demonstrated a significant increase in respiratory cancer and possibly digestive tract cancer in a group of workers whose first exposure was 20 or more years earlier. The standardized mortality ratio for respiratory cancer was also increased in mineral wool workers with 20 years of exposure 30 years or more after onset of exposure, but not at a statistically significant level. There was no clear correlation between cumulative exposure to respirable fibers and respiratory cancer deaths.[81] It was subsequently noted that many of the mineral wool plants previously used asbestos, and the increased standardized mortality ratios may have been a reflection of that previous exposure.[82] The disclosure of the possible previous use of asbestos and the lack of worker smoking information makes this aspect of the Thermal Insulation Manufacturers' Association's epidemiologic data difficult to interpret.

Three mortality studies on fibrous glass wool workers have demonstrated no significant increases in mortality from malignant or nonmalignant respiratory disease.[83–85] One study did demonstrate a significant increase in nonmalignant respiratory mortality (19 observed cases versus 10 expected). However, subsequent review of the individual cases revealed other plausible causes of nonmalignant respiratory deaths in five (bronchiectasis and silicosis).[86–88]

Studies sponsored by the Thermal Insulation Manufacturers' Association have revealed a significant increase in nonmalignant respiratory deaths (excluding influenza and pneumonia) in fibrous glass workers and in a total cohort of fibrous glass and mineral wool workers. There was no clear correlation, however, between nonmalignant respiratory deaths and cumulative fiber exposure. Fibrous glass workers exposed to fine fiber (<1.5 μm diameter) had a significant increase in nonmalignant respiratory deaths, but not in respiratory cancer.[81]

The results of the 17-plant study sponsored by the Thermal Insulation Manufacturers' Association and the 72-plant study sponsored by the European Insulation Manufacturers' Association will add significant information concerning the health effects of man-made mineral fiber exposure. These cohorts should continue to be followed before definitive conclusions can be reached.

The majority of the currently available information on the human health effects of man-made mineral fibers demonstrates no (or minimal) fibrogenic and tumorigenic effect in humans. Additional scientific studies are needed, however, before reaching any definitive conclusions. This is particularly important with exposure to fibers <1.0 μm in diameter. The production of microfibers is a relatively recent event in view of the long latency for the development of respiratory cancer and mesothelioma. Epidemiologic studies following these populations over the next 20 years will help determine the safety of these fibers. The cytotoxic, fibrogenic, and tumorigenic potential of these thin fibers, as demonstrated in animal studies, makes it a necessity to monitor these populations very carefully. In the interim exposure to microfibers should be maintained at a minimal level.

ACKNOWLEDGMENT

This work in part has been supported by Veteran's Administration.

REFERENCES

1. Campbell WJ, Steel ER, Virta RL, Eisner MH: Relationship of Mineral Habit to Size Characteristics for Tremolite Cleavage Fragments and Fibers. Washington, DC, US Department of the Interior, Bureau of Mines, 1979 (Report of Investigations 8367).
2. Parkes WR: Occupational Lung Disorders, 2nd ed. London, Butterworth, 1982, p 31, 233.
3. Bank W: Asbestiform and/or Fibrous Minerals in Mines, Mills, and Quarries. Washington, DC, US Department of Labor, Safety and Health Administration, 1980 (Publication 1980-603-102/34).
4. Campbell WJ, Blake RL, Brown LL, et al: Selected Silicate Minerals and Their Asbestiform Varieties. Mineralogical Definition and Identification-characterization. Washington, DC, US Department of the Interior, Bureau of Mines, 1977 (Information Circular 8751).
5. Langer AM, Rohl AN, Wolff MS, Selikoff IJ: Asbestos, fibrous minerals and acicular cleavage fragments: Nomenclature and biological properties. In: Dusts and Disease, eds. Lemen RA, Dement JM. Park Forest South, IL, Pathotox Publishers, 1979, p 1.

6. Zoltai T: History of asbestos-related mineralogical terminology. In: Proceedings of Workshop on Asbestos: Definitions and Measurement Methods, eds. Gravatt CC, et al. Washington, DC, 1967 (NBS-SP-506).
7. Zoltai T: Asbestiform and acicular mineral fragments. Ann NY Acad Sci 330:621, 1979.
8. Harington JS: Fiber carcinogenesis: Epidemiological observations and the Stanton hypothesis. J Natl Cancer Inst 67(5):977, 1981.
9. Leineweber JP: Dust and chemistry and physics: Mineral and vitreous fibres. IARC Sci Publ 30:881, 1980.
10. Leineweber JP: Fiber toxicology. J Occup Med 23(6):431, 1981.
11. Timbrell V, Skidmore JW: The effect of shape on particle penetration and retention in animal lungs. In: Inhaled Particles III, ed. Walton WH. Surrey, England, Unwin, 1971, p 49.
12. Bitterman PB, Rennard SI, Crystal RG: Environmental lung disease and the interstitium. Clin Chest Med 2(3):393, 1981.
13. Stanton MF, Layard M, Tegeris A, et al: Carcinogenicity of fibrous glass: Pleural response in the rat in relation to fiber dimension. J Natl Cancer Inst 58:587, 1977.
14. Wright G, Kuschner M: The influence of varying lengths of glass and asbestos fibers on tissue response on guinea pigs. In: Inhaled Particles IV, ed. Walton WH. Oxford, New York, Pergamon, 1977, p 455.
15. Suzuki Y, Rohl AM, Langer AM, Selikoff IJ: (Abstract). Fed Proc 39:3, 1980.
16. Rohl AN, Langer AM: Fibrous mineral content of consumer talc-containing products. In: Dusts and Disease, eds. Lemen RA, Dement JM. Park Forest South, IL, Pathotox Publishers, 1979, p 393.
17. Rohl AN, Langer AM: Identification and quantitation of asbestos in talc. Environ Health Perspect 9:95, 1974.
18. Clifton RA: Talc and pyrophyllite. In: Mineral Facts and Problems. Washington, DC, United States Department of the Interior, Bureau of Mines, 1980 (Bulletin 671).
19. Dement JM, Zumwalde RD: Occupational exposures to talc containing asbestiform minerals. In: Dusts and Disease, eds. Lemen RA, Dement JM. Park Forest South, IL, Pathotox Publishers, 1979, p 287.
20. Gamble JF, Greife A: Health studies of miners and millers exposed to talc. In: Health Issues Related to Metal and Nonmetallic Mining, eds. Wagner W, Rom WN, Merchant J. Ann Arbor, MI, Ann Arbor Science, 1983, p 277.
21. Lockey, JL: Nonasbestos fibrous minerals. Clin Chest Med, 2:203, 1981.
22. Rohl AN, Langer AM, Selikoff IJ, et al: Consumer talcums and powders. Mineral and chemical characterizations. J Toxicol Environ Health, 2:255, 1976.
23. CTFA Specification. Talc, cosmetic: Cosmetic, Toiletry, and Fragrance Association, Inc. Issue 10–17, 1976.
24. Leophonte P, Fabre J, Pous J, et al: Les effets nocifs du talc: Plaidoyer pour un verdict nuance. Nouv Presse Med 4(30):2201, 1975.
25. Hildick-Smith GY: The biology of talc. Br J Ind Med 33:217, 1976.
26. Kleinfeld M, Messite J, Langer AM: A study of workers exposed to asbestiform minerals in commercial talc manufacture. Environ Res 6:132, 1973.
27. Gamble F, Fellner W, Dimeo MJ: An epidemiological study of a group of talc workers. Am Rev Respir Dis 119:741, 1979.
28. Gamble JF, Fellner W, Dimeo MJ: Respiratory morbidity among workers and millers of asbestiform talc. In: Dusts and Disease, eds. Lemen RA, Dement JM. Park Forest South, IL, Pathotox Publisher, 1979, p 307.
29. Kleinfeld M, Messite J, Kooyman O: Mortality among talc miners and millers in New York State. Arch Environ Health 14:663, 1967.

30. Kleinfeld M, Messite J, Zaki H: Mortality experience among talc workers: A follow-up study. J Occup Med 16:345, 1974.
31. Brown DP, Dement JM, Wagoner JK: Mortality patterns among miners and millers occupationally exposed to asbestiform talc. In: Dusts and Disease, eds. Lemen RA, Dement JM. Park Forest South, IL, Pathotox Publishers, 1979, p 317.
32. Stille WT, Tabershaw IR: The mortality experience of upstate New York talc workers. J Occup Med 24(6):480, 1982.
33. Rubino GF, Scansetti G, Piloatto G, et al: Mortality study of talc miners and millers. J Occup Med 18:186, 1976.
34. Rubino GF, Scansetti G, Piolatto G, et al: Mortality and morbidity among talc miners and millers in Italy. In: Dusts and Disease, eds. Lemen RA, Dement JM. Park Forest South, IL, Pathotox Publishers, 1979, p 357.
35. Fine LT, Peters JM, Burgess WA, et al: Studies of respiratory morbidity in rubber workers. IV. Respiratory morbidity in talc workers. Arch Environ Health 4:195, 1976.
36. Leophonte P, Fernet P, Pincemin J, et al: Epidemiological study on chronic respiratory disease among talc millers. Rev Fr Mal Respir August 1:43, 1980.
37. Selevan SG, Dement JM, Wagoner JK, et al: Mortality patterns among miners and millers of non-asbestiform talc: Preliminary report. In: Dusts and Disease, eds. Lemen RA, Dement JM. Park Forest South, IL, Pathotox Publishers, 1979, p 379.
38. Vallyathan NV, Craighead JE: Pulmonary pathology in workers exposed to nonasbestiform talc. Human Pathol 12(1):28, 1981.
39. Henderson WJ, Hamilton TC, Griffiths K: Talc in normal and malignant ovarian tissue. Lancet 1:499, 1979.
40. Henderson WJ, Joslin CAF, Turnbull AS, et al: Talc and carcinoma of the ovary and cervix. Br J Obstet Gynecol 78:266, 1971.
41. Longo DL, Young RC: Cosmetic talc and ovarian cancer. Lancet 2:349, 1979.
42. Lord GH: The biological effects of talc in the experimental animal: A literature review. Food Cosmet Toxicol 16:51, 1978.
43. Cramer DW, Welch WR, Scully RE, Wojciechowski CA: Ovarian cancer and talc. Cancer 50:372, 1982.
44. Graham J, Graham R: Ovarian cancer and asbestos. Environ Res 1:115, 1967.
45. Research Committee of the British Thoracic Association and the Medical Research Council Pneumoconiosis Unit: A survey of the long-term effects of talc and kaolin pleurodesis. Br J Dis Chest 73:285, 1979.
46. Otis LM: Vermiculite. In: Mineral Facts and Problems. Washington, DC, U. S. Department of the Interior, Bureau of Mines, 1960 (Bulletin 585).
47. Meisinger AC: Vermiculite. In: Mineral Facts and Problems. Washington, DC, U. S. Department of the Interior, Bureau of Mines, 1980 (Bulletin 671).
48. Chatfield EJ, Lewis GM: Examination of Vermiculite for the Presence of Asbestos Fibers. Mississauga, Ontario, Canada, Ontario Research Foundation, 1979 (Report No. 22056-2).
49. Lockey JL, Jarabek A, Carson A, et al: Pulmonary hazards from vermiculite exposure. In: Health Issues Related to Metal and Nonmetallic Mining, eds. Wagner W, Rom WN, Merchant J. Ann Arbor, Michigan, Ann Arbor Science, 1983, p 303.
50. Goldstein B, Rendall REG: The relative toxicities of the main classes of minerals. In: Pneumoconiosis, ed. Shapiro HA. Proceedings of the International Conference, Johannesburg, Cape Town, South Africa. London, Oxford University Press, 1969, p. 429.
51. Hunter B, Thompson C: Evaluation of the tumorigenic potential of vermiculite by intrapleural injection in rats. Br J Ind Med 30:167, 1973.

52. Sand LB, Mumpton, FA, eds: Natural Zeolites, Occurrence, Properties, Use. Oxford, Pergamon Press, 1978.
53. HDR Sciences: Draft of Environmental Impact Statement on the M-X Deployment Area Section and Land Withdrawl/Acquisition. Environmental Characteristics of Alternative Designated Deployment Areas: Mining and Geology. Santa Barbara, California, HDR Science, 1980 (M-X ETR-11 Prepared for U. S. Air Force, Ballistic Missile Office, Norton Air Force Base, California).
54. Baris YI, Sahin AA, Ozesmi M, et al: An outbreak of pleural mesothelioma and chronic fibrosing pleurisy in the village of Karain/Urgüp in Anatolia. Thorax 33:181, 1978.
55. Baris YI, Artvinli M, Sahin AA: Environmental mesothelioma in Turkey. Ann NY Acad Sci 330:423, 1979.
56. Artvinli M, Baris YI: Malignant mesotheliomas in a small village in the Anatolian region of Turkey: An epidemiologic study. J Natl Cancer Inst 63:17, 1979.
57. Lilis R: Fibrous zeolites and endemic mesothelioma in Cappadocia, Turkey. J Occup Med 23(8):548, 1981.
58. Baris Y: The clinical and radiological aspects of 185 cases of malignant pleural mesothelioma. IARC Sci Publ 30:937, 1980.
59. Sebastian P, Gaudichet A, Bignon J, Baris YI: Zeolite bodies in human lungs from Turkey. Lab Invest 44(5):420, 1981.
60. Rohl AN, Langer AM, Moncure G, et al: Endemic pleural disease associated with exposure to mixed fibrous dust in Turkey. Science 216:518, 1982.
61. Yazicioglu S, Ilcayto R, Balci K, et al: Pleural calcification, pleural mesotheliomas, and bronchial cancers caused by tremolite dust. Thorax 35:564, 1980.
62. Baris YI, Saracci R, Simonato L, et al: Malignant mesothelioma and radiological chest abnormalities in two village in central Turkey. Lancet 1:984, 1981.
63. Shasby DM: Medical survey of workers at the Interspace Corporation, Willsboro, New York. Morgantown, West Virginia, National Institute for Occupational Safety and Health, 1977.
64. Shasby DM: Respiratory morbidity of workers exposed to wollastonite through mining and milling. In: Dusts and Disease, eds. Lemen RA, Dement JM. Park Forest South, IL, Pathotox Publishers, 1979, p 251.
65. Boechlecke B: Cross-sectional medical study of wollastonite workers. In: Proceedings of the National Workshop on Substitutes for Asbestos. Washington, DC, U. S. Environmental Protection Agency, Consumer Product Safety Commission, and the Interagency Regulatory Liaison Group, 1980 (Publication EPA-560/3-80-001).
66. Huuskonen MS, Tossavainen A, Koskinen H, et al: Respiratory morbidity of quarry workers exposed to wollastonite. International Conference on Occupational Lung Disease, March 24–27, 1982, Chicago, IL.
67. Pundsack FL: Fibrous glass manufacture, use, and physical properties. In: Occupational Exposure to Fibrous Glass: Proceedings of a Symposium. Washington, DC, National Institute for Occupational Safety and Health, 1976, P. 11 (DHEW/PHS/CDC Publication (NIOSH) 76-151).
68. Hill JW: Health aspects of man-made mineral fibers: A review. Ann Occup Hyg 20:161, 1977.
69. Dement JM: Environmental aspects of fibrous glass production and utilization. In: Occupational Exposure to Fibrous Glass: Proceedings of a Symposium. Washington, DC, National Institute for Occupational Safety and Health, 1976, P. 97 (DHEW/PHS/CDC Publication No. (NIOSH) 76-151).
70. Smith HV: History, processes, and operations in the manufacturing and uses of fibrous glass: one company's experience. In: Occupational Exposure to Fibrous

Glass: Proceedings of a Symposium. Washington, DC, National Institute for Occupational Safety and Health, 1976, p 19 (DHEW/PHS/CDC Publication (NIOSH) 76-151).

71. Corn M: An overview of inorganic man-made fibers in man's environment. In: Dusts and Disease, eds. Lemen RA, Dement JM. Park Forest South, IL, Pathotox Publishers, 1979, p 23.
72. Esmen N, Corn M, Hammad Y, et al: Summary of measurements of employee exposure to airborne dust and fiber in sixteen facilities producing man-made mineral fibers. Am Ind Hyg Assoc J 40:108, 1979.
73. National Institute for Occupational Safety and Health: Occupational Exposure to Fibrous Glass: Criteria for a Recommended Standard. Washington, DC, US Department of HEW, 1977.
74. Dodgson J, Ottery J, Cherrie JW, Harrison GE: Fibre concentrations and size distributions of airborne fibres in several European man-made mineral fibre plants. IARC Sci Publ 30:913, 1980.
75. Hill JW, Whitehead WS, Cameron JD, et al: Glass fibers: Absence of pulmonary hazard in production workers. Br J Ind Med 30:174, 1973.
76. Nasr AN, Ditchek T, Schottens PA: The prevalence of radiographic abnormalities in the chest of fiber glass workers. In: Occupational Exposures to Fibrous Glass: Proceedings of a Symposium. Washington, DC, National Institute for Occupational Safety and Health, 1976, p 225 (DHEW/PHS/CDC Publication (NIOSH) 76-151).
77. Utidjian M, Cooper WC: Human epidemiologic studies with emphasis on chronic pulmonary effects. In: Occupational Exposure to Fibrous Glass: Proceedings of a Symposium. Washington, DC, National Institute for Occupational Safety and Health, 1976, p 223 (DHEW/PHS/CSC Publication (NIOSH) 76-151).
78. Wright GW: Airborne fibrous glass particles: Chest roentgenograms of persons with prolonged exposure. Arch Environ Health 16:175, 1968.
79. Hughes J, Hammad Y, Glindmeyer H, et al: Respiratory health in man-made vitreous fiber industry. Am Rev Respir Dis, Pt 2 127(4): 158, 1983.
80. Ness GO, Dement JM, Waxweiler RJ: A preliminary report of the mortality patterns and occupational exposures of a cohort of mineral wool production workers. In: Dusts and Disease, eds. Lemen RA, Dement JM. Park Forest South, IL, Pathotox Publishers, 1979, p 233.
81. Enterline P, Marsh G, Esmen N: Respiratory disease among workers exposed to man-made mineral fibers. Am Rev Respir Dis 128:1, 1983.
82. Enterline PE, March GM: Mortality of workers in the man-made mineral fibre industry. IARC Sci Publ 30:965, 1980.
83. Enterline PE, Henderson V: The health of retired fibrous glass workers. Arch Environ Health 30:113, 1979.
84. Enterline PE, March GM: Environment and mortality of workers from a fibrous glass plant. In: Dusts and Disease, eds. Lemen RA, Dement JM. Park Forest South, Ill., Pathotox Publishers, 1979. p 221.
85. Morgan RW, Kaplan SD, Bratsberg JA: Mortality study of fibrous glass production workers. Arch Environ Health 36(4):179, 1980.
86. Bayliss D, Dement JM, Wagoner JK, et al: Mortality patterns among fibrous glass production workers. Ann NY Acad Sci 271:324, 1976.
87. Saracci R: Introduction: Epidemiology of groups exposed to other mineral fibres. IARC Sci Publ 30:951, 1980.
88. Hill JW: Review of the epidemiology of man-made mineral fibres. IARC Sci Publ 30:979, 1980.

5 Airborne Free Silica: How Much?

W. K. C. Morgan

Silicosis has been recognized since antiquity as a disabling and sometimes fatal lung disease. It is customarily divided into the classical, acute, and subacute forms.[1] Descriptions of the clinical features, physiologic abnormalities, and radiographic characteristics of each of these forms of silicosis can be found in standard texts.[2,3] Classical silicosis usually occurs after ten or more years of exposure to dust containing free silica and presents as an abnormal chest radiograph. It is further subdivided into simple and complicated silicosis. The former is recognized by the presence of small rounded opacities and may be classified into categories 1, 2, and 3 according to profusion of such opacities. Generally, the more free silica in the lung, the higher the radiographic category. Simple silicosis is not associated with any significant decrement in lung function other than an occasional slight increase in lung stiffness.[2–4] The excellent preservation of lung function that is seen in this condition is best explained by the fact that the silicotic nodules are not located in the alveoli but around the pulmonary arterioles, with the result that the intervening gas exchanging surface is normal. Occasionally when there are numerous nodules present in simple silicosis, such as is seen in categories 2 and 3, the nodules aggregate and form a conglomerate mass. By definition this is the complicated form of the disease and is associated with both morbidity and premature death.

The above facts have been known for many years and are generally accepted. By the same token the scientific and medical communities are well aware of how to prevent silicosis, namely, by limiting exposure as far as possible to dust containing free silica. The only matters of dispute that remain to be decided are (1) on what data should a silica dust standard be based, and (2) what should the standard be.

PROPOSED STANDARD

In 1975 the National Institute of Occupational Safety and Health (NIOSH) published a recommended standard for occupational exposure to crystalline silica.[5] The document recommended that no worker be exposed to a time weighted average concentration of free silica greater than 50 $\mu g/m^3$ as determined for up to a 10-hour working day. The recommended level for free silica in the NIOSH Criteria Document is half what is permitted in United States coal mines. This anomalous recommendation receives no scientific justification, and appears to be a consequence of either lack of thought or sheer perversity. Aside from the proposed dust standard, certain medical examinations were to be made available to each employee who is exposed to free silica. These include a medical and occupational history, a standard posteroanterior chest radiograph, and measurement of the forced expiratory volume in one second (FEV_1) and the forced vital capacity (FVC). It was recommended that any employee with or without radiographic changes of silicosis who had respiratory distress or functional impairment should be evaluated by a physician qualified to advise the employee whether he or she should continue working in a dusty trade. Just what criteria were to be used by the so-called qualified physician in deciding who should continue working were not stated.

VERMONT GRANITE SHED STUDIES

The NIOSH Criteria Document for silica and the recommendations and opinions contained therein have to be judged in relation to what is known in regard to silicosis. The recommendations for pulmonary function testing were based on a series of studies from the Harvard School of Public Health.[6–8] These were carried out in the Vermont granite shed workers. Dust sampling has been carried out in the industry for limited periods in 1924 and 1937 to 1938, 1964, 1965 to 1966, and 1972. Different sampling techniques were used but all the early measurements depended on particle counts. From the dust data available, certain assumptions were made by Theriault and colleagues[6] in regard to the dust levels that prevailed between surveys. By manipulating these data with considerable panache and even greater ingenuity, the authors managed to concoct a lifetime dust exposure for each man employed in the Vermont granite sheds. This estimate came about by summing time spent in each job and multiplying by the current estimates of dustiness observed in each job. As such Theriault et al.[6] assumed no change in the dustiness of each job over a period of 37 years. There are compelling reasons for rejecting this assumption. Moreover, in their calculations, the authors arbitrarily rejected all values outside two standard deviations from the mean. The missing values were then replaced by a formula, the derivation of which was and continues to remain obscure. The reason for the authors rejecting certain of the data in question is unclear, but the substitution of artificially derived values reduced the variance of the measurements. There are other theoretical objections to the stepwise regression model used by the authors, but these are of a technical nature and will not be discussed here.

The ventilatory capacity of the various groups of granite shed workers exposed to silica was then related to the derived lifetime dust exposure data. Dust exposure was stated to cause a significant decrease in ventilatory capacity, and, in this context, the calculated excess decrement in FVC was stated to be 2 ml/dust year.[7] The authors state that the 2-ml decrement is statistically significant; moreover, they go on to state that pulmonary function is a more sensitive method of detecting silicosis and the effects of exposure to silica. The effect of the 2-ml annual decrement in FVC is best put into perspective by considering a man who is 20 years old and whose height is 68 inches. At the age of 20, his predicted FVC should be 5 liters. By the time he is 65 his FVC will have fallen to 4.0 liters from the effects of aging alone. Assuming that the Theriault predictions of a 2-ml decrement per year are correct, had this man been exposed and suffered the consequences of exposure to silica dust in the granite sheds, then at the age of 65, his FVC would be 3.91 rather than 4.0 liters. What sort of significance does a decrement in the FVC of this size have? Providing that he did not age any further after the age of 65, an unlikely possibility, he would still have to work for 300 years before he would collect Social Security benefits for ''premature'' disability.

In a follow-up study of the Vermont granite shed workers, again conducted by the Harvard School of Public Health, an excess decrement of 35 ml/year in the FEV_1 was found.[9] In contrast to the earlier cross-sectional studies, the later study was longitudinal. The disparity between decrement derived in the early cross-sectional studies and that obtained from the longitudinal study was pointed out by the author to the leading investigator, who responded by saying that his statisticians informed him that such differences were fairly frequent when comparing the results of cross-sectional and longitudinal studies.[10] Whatever the statistical justification for the disparity, it is clear that either the cross-sectional or the longitudinal study is grossly incorrect, or more probably both were in error.

The results obtained from the Vermont granite shed workers are completely out of line with all the previously published evidence concerning the effects of silicosis and lung function. Over the past 20 years my colleagues and I have seen and examined a fair number of nonsmokers with categories 2 and 3 simple silicosis. Although some of these subjects complained of cough and sputum, virtually all had normal or near-normal pulmonary function. The subjects had worked in a variety of industries ranging from metal mining and tunneling to the manufacture of silica flour. Some were referred by Workmen's Compensation Boards, others by local physicians. The most striking feature in this group of nonsmoking men with simple silicosis was their lack of impairment of lung function. The ventilatory capacity, blood gases, and diffusing capacity were all within the normal range. The data are shown in Table 5-1. The fact that subjects with established disease and, it can be assumed, a significantly elevated free silica content in the lungs, can have normal function, should cast some doubt on the validity of the Theriault studies.

Table 5-1. Silica Exposed Subjects, Nonsmokers[a]

	Category 0	Categories 2 and 3
No.	10	15
Mean age	48	54
Mean years exposed	17	30
Mean FVC (% predicted)	98.5	94
Mean FEV_1 (% predicted)	99	87
Mean TLC (% predicted)	101	92
Mean FEV_1/FVC%	73	69
Mean C stat (L.cm/H_2O)	0.210 (2.1 kPa^{-1})	0.182 (1.8 kPa^{-1})
Pel (cm H_2O)	33	40
Mean $DLco_{SB}$ (% predicted)	97	98
Mean Pao_2 mm (rest)	84 (11.1 kPa)	86 (11.47 kPa)
Mean $Paco_2$ mm (rest)	34 (4.53 kPa)	36 (4.8 kPa)
Mean (A-a)O_2 mm (rest)	14 (1.87 kPa)	22 (2.05 kPa)
Mean (A-a)O_2 mm (exercise)	13 (1.73 kPa)	18 (1.65 kPa)

[a] SI units in parentheses.

At the time of publication of the silica criteria document there were those who questioned the findings and conclusions contained in it, and these critics suggested that endorsement of pulmonary function tests as part of medical surveillance was unwise.[11,12] Even if the validity of the Theriault studies is granted, the conclusion that the 2-ml decrement was due to the deposition in the alveoli of dust containing silica was entirely unwarranted. Neither Theriault nor NIOSH in their document considered the possibility that industrial bronchitis could be responsible for the small decrement in ventilatory capacity. Industrial bronchitis is a nonspecific condition found in many dusty trades.[13] It is a consequence of the deposition of particles in the deadspace. Prolonged deposition of inert dust in the tracheobronchial tree will lead to mucous gland enlargement and to an increase in the number of goblet cells. It must be remembered that many dusts which, were they deposited in the alveoli, would be harmful and fibrogenic, are relatively inert when deposited in the tracheobronchial tree. Since those particles deposited in the deadspace are removed by the mucociliary escalator, industrial bronchitis is unassociated with radiographic abnormalities. It has also been noted that there is a poor correlation between the presence of silicosis as detected from the chest radiograph and industrial bronchitis, although both conditions may be present in the same subject. Industrial bronchitis does not lead to emphysema, but may be associated with a minor degree of large airways obstruction.[13,14] The lack of association between silicosis and industrial bronchitis is explained by the fact that the former is a consequence of the deposition of respirable particles in the gas-exchanging portion of the lungs with the most dangerous particles being those between 0.5 and 3 μm. In contrast, industrial bronchitis is due for the most part to the deposition in the tracheobronchial tree of particles between 4 and 10 μm, most of which are too large to enter the alveoli.

Aside from the conclusions reached by Theriault et al.[6–8] in regard to the effect of the inhalation of silica on ventilatory capacity, the Harvard School of

Public Health studies contain numerous other blemishes that should have been a warning signal to those in NIOSH who prepared the Criteria Document. On page 36 of the Criteria Document the following statement is to be found: "No cases of silicosis among workers in the granite industry whose span of employment began after 1937 were observed." By the time the Theriault studies were completed, many of the employers who started working in 1937 or shortly thereafter, had been working for 20 years or more. But on page 39 of the Criteria Document the statement occurs that no less than 233 of the 784 examined had some evidence of pneumoconiosis. The prevalence rate must have changed dramatically between 1965 and 1971, since it seems improbable that all the 233 men with silicosis started working before 1937. Such contradictory statements cannot be reconciled and must be considered in conjunction with Figure 1 of the study by Theriault et al.,[8] which shows no less than 30% of workers with no exposure having radiographic evidence of silicosis. Clearly the one interpreter who read the films was so deafened by noise that he could not hear the signal. The reported high frequency of category 1 with small rounded opacities likewise can be regarded as invalid.

The NIOSH Criteria Document based its recommendations on the Harvard School of Public Health Studies, and inherent in their thesis is the assumption that exposure to silica had a demonstrable effect on lung function before the onset of conglomerate silicosis. Besides the numerous anomalies alluded to in these studies, subsequent studies have completely refuted those from Theriault et al.[6–8]

FURTHER STUDIES

Since the publication of the Criteria Document a number of important studies have been published. These include an extensive well-controlled study of South African gold miners.[15] This study showed that when allowance was made for dust exposure, men with silicosis have the same degree of airways obstruction as those without. The FVC did not differ between the two groups, suggesting that any changes in lung stiffness must be minimal. This study emphasizes that the main problem in South African gold miners who do not have radiographic evidence of conglomerate silicosis is industrial bronchitis, and it is the latter which is responsible for their symptoms of cough and sputum.

A further study by Graham et al.[16] repeated the pulmonary function tests in the Vermont granite shed workers and showed an improvement in ventilatory capacity in many of them. This was particularly true for the FVC. Such an increment occurring over a span of years is out of the question were the original studies valid. It is now all too apparent that they were not, and the spirometer used was noted to have a leak. In addition, the average duration of many of the spirograms was only 2 to 3 seconds, an unduly short time that is completely unacceptable as far as quality control is concerned.

SECOND THOUGHTS FROM NIOSH

In October 1981 NIOSH brought forth "An Update of the Literature: Crystalline Silica".[15] The authors of this review, a review that, one might add, is more exhausting than exhaustive, referred to several papers from Europe, and apparently failed to recognize that many European authors use the term silicosis as synonymous with coal workers' pneumoconiosis. Of more concern was the suggestion by the authors of the review that silica is a cofactor in the development of lung cancer.

In reviewing recent studies of the effects of silica exposure in humans, the authors of "The Update in the Literature" chose to place significant emphasis on a paper of Navratil et al.[17] As mentioned above, Navratil and associates use the term "silicosis" as synonymous with coal workers' pneumoconiosis. The group of subjects selected for this study consisted almost entirely of smokers who happened to have what he terms silicosis, but which in reality was almost certainly coal workers' pneumoconiosis. The description of the study suggests that he was following the natural history of chronic airflow obstruction due to bronchitis and emphysema, rather than the course of silicosis. The NIOSH reviewers also quote a study of Teculescu et al.[18] relating to abnormal mixing as found in silica-exposed workers. This paper makes it clear that abnormal mixing was related to chronic bronchitis rather than silicosis, and indeed provides additional circumstantial evidence that it is not silicosis per se that is responsible for the symptoms of bronchitis. Moreover, the abnormal mixing time noted by Teculescu et al.[18] in those exposed to silica suggest an abnormal distribution of inspired gas due to small airways dysfunction, and cannot be equated with significant or disabling impairment of lung function. Later on in the "Update," based on the Graham et al.[16] study, the statement is made by the reviewers that current Vermont granite shed workers showed an annual decrement for the FEV_1 of 10 ml between 1970 and 1979, and for the workers with 20 or more years of experience there was a decrement of 7 ml. These figures are less than the expected annual decrement for the FEV_1, a fact on which the authors do not comment. By the same token, retired workers, many of whom probably retired because of illness unrelated to their job, showed an annual rate of decline of ventilatory capacity that is usual for elderly subjects.[19]

Later the NIOSH reviewers turn to the studies of Ohman[20] and endorse them with much enthusiasm. Unfortunately, Ohman's data came from Sweden, a country that does not use the International Labour Organization Radiographic Classification for pneumoconiosis, and instead relies on its own classification, for which there is little scientific justification and which lacks validation that the radiologic abnormalities bear any relationship to dust retention. Moreover, Ohman's conclusions are based on a series of assumptions made in regard to cumulative silica exposure, which in the main appear to be based on average readings of particle counts in Swedish industry between 1950 and 1970. Conversion of particle counts into gravimetric values has been shown to be notoriously unreliable, and to endorse a gravimetric standard that is based on data derived from particle counts to which a conversion factor has been applied should under few circumstances be accepted as wise. The review also endorses the study by Nelson et al.[21] conducted in Ontario in which the population consisted of workers exposed to silica flour. The NIOSH reviewers apparently failed to realize that the silica particles to which Nelson's population was exposed were much smaller than usually encountered in the workplace. Such smaller particles are appreciably more dangerous. It is well accepted that a few larger particles have a greater effect on the gravimetric estimation of dust levels than they do when the dust levels are measured by particle counting. Thus one particle of 3 μm weighs as much as 200 particles of 0.5 μm, and yet the latter are infinitely more hazardous.

SILICA EXPOSURE AND LUNG CANCER

The NIOSH reviewers also implied that silica is a cofactor in the etiology of lung cancer. Their conclusions appear to be based on one or two studies of which the methodology and conclusions are suspect. Retrospective studies in which mortality statistics are compiled from death certificates fail to take into account the effects of cigarette smoking unless a detailed cigarette smoking history is available. Differences in smoking habits between the reference population and the industrial group under study often exist. In this context it is not sufficient to know whether the subject was a smoker or not; it is essential to know the lifelong cigarette consumption and, if an ex-smoker, exactly when the habit was given up, and how many cigarettes were smoked prior to giving up the habit. The NIOSH reviewers quote a Russian study that claimed to show that underground gold miners had a higher relative risk of lung cancer than surface miners.[22] Such findings are more likely to be due to exposure of the underground miners to radon daughters rather than exposure to silica. In this study standardization was not carried out for social class; however, even allowing for the fact that equality reigns supreme in a Communist society, the investigator will probably perceive that some are more equal than others. The Decennial Supplement on Occupational Mortality[23] published by Her Majesty's Stationery Office makes one realize that, at least in Great Britain, standardization for social class will often eliminate excess death rates for lung, esophageal, and stomach cancers. Similarly, the increased lung cancer rate in Canadian Foundry workers described by Gibson et al.[24] may be explained partly by differences in social class, partly by different cigarette smoking habits, and mostly by the fact that foundry workers are exposed to polycyclic hydrocarbons. A study of Registrar General's Decennial Supplement makes it quite clear that quarrymen have no excess of lung cancer, and yet quarrymen are heavily exposed to silica. Additional well-controlled studies have been carried out looking at the risk of lung cancer in silica-exposed workers in Switzerland and South Africa.[25,26] Although the NIOSH reviewers mention the excellent study conducted by McDonald et al.[27] in a South Dakota gold mine, they tend to dismiss it with the pejorative description that it is retrospective. No such epithet describes the several other retrospective studies that they endorse in their review.

The recent publication of a report describing several foundry workers who developed a rare form of pneumonia due to *Acinetobacter calcoaceticus* is of interest.[28] The paper originated from NIOSH and somewhat facilely attributed the development of this rare type of pneumonia to the fact that the foundry air to which the affected subjects were exposed, to use their phrase, "exceeded the standard of the National Institute of Occupational Safety and Health for free silica of 0.05 mgm/M^3." This phraseology implies that the proposed standard has been accepted and is in effect; moreover, had the standard been adhered to, the subjects would not have developed pneumonia. The paper[28] also contains a series of disingenuous remarks concerning the "potential" toxic effects of chromium, nickel, and other airborne contaminants. The authors seem to fail to realize that the various air quality standards for agents such as silica and coal have as their purpose the prevention of pneumoconiosis and other dust-related respiratory diseases and not the prevention of pneumonia, least of all by such a rare organism. Such far-fetched justifications of the proposed silica standard have no scientific basis.

DERIVATION OF THE SILICA STANDARD

The quantification of the risk of a particular hazard requires deriving a dose–response relationship. In humans this can be effected by relating biologic measurements, for example, radiographic or pulmonary function changes, to environmental measurements of the hazardous agent, be the latter a particulate, gas, or vapor. In the case of silica, quantitation of the risk necessitates relating the development of radiographic abnormalities to the dust levels that have prevailed over the period of observation. Pulmonary function tests are of no value in this situation. The method whereby this can be effected is to calculate the radiographic attack rate of silicosis in previously unexposed workers.[29] When the term "attack rate" is used in this context, it refers to the percentage of previously unexposed workers who develop silicosis over a certain period, for example, ten years. The percentage will vary according to the dust levels that workers have been exposed to over the period of observation. If dust measurements are available it should be possible to calculate the attack rate for various levels of exposure. A second and complementary approach is to relate radiographic progression of silicosis to measured dust levels over a period of observation. Of necessity, in slowly developing diseases such as silicosis and coal workers' pneumoconiosis, the period of observation must be measured in years. It is most unlikely that any man would develop silicosis without at least five years of exposure, and were he to do so, this would imply that the dust levels to which he had been exposed were far above the present standard. Radiographic progression can be assessed by two methods, side by side and independent reading.[29,30] The former involves placing paired films side by side with the dates known, with the interpreter comparing the abnormalities present in each film. Side-by-side reading is influenced by chronological sequence of the films, since the reader knows, or assumes the silicosis and coal workers' pneumoconiosis do not regress.[31] It also permits compensation for varying films techniques. The independent method involves reading paired films in such a way that both films are read without any knowledge of the other. This method eliminates the bias introduced by a knowledge of the chronological sequence of the film, but makes it difficult for the reader to compensate for changes in film technique, that is, over- and underpenetrative films known to have a marked effect on interpretation. In general, the independent method yields a progression index about half of that obtained with the side-by-side method.[29,30] Nevertheless, it has been shown by the National Coal Board of Great Britain,[32] and by Reisner[33] in Germany, that it is possible with these methods to quantitate progression fairly accurately. Comparable studies have not been carried out for exposure to silica-containing dust, although the necessary dust measurements and also the necessary serial chest films are available in both Ontario metal miners and in the Vermont granite shed workers. With the availability of these data, it is incongruous, and indeed completely unjustified for NIOSH to publish a proposed standard for silica based on irrelevant and inaccurate pulmonary function data. Moreover, to persist with the proposed standard when the studies on which it is based have been shown to be invalid can only be regarded as folly. That the appropriate dust and radiologic data are available to derive a dose–response relationship has been known to NIOSH for some time, and one can only wonder the reasons why this agency has not encouraged and funded a study to settle this issue once and for all.

The pronouncements and criteria documents published by NIOSH relate to all sorts of hazards and are widely regarded as disinterested and scientifically valid documents. They are frequently quoted by the media and often influence legislation and regulations in other countries. That such pronouncements should be based on the best available scientific evidence stands to reason, but too frequently in this context "the emperor has no clothes." Nowhere has this been more evident than in the formulation of the proposed silica standard. NIOSH and OSHA have been dickering over the 50 $\mu g/m^3$ for about ten years. Despite all the contradictory hard evidence which has been generated in the past several years, both agencies apparently persist in proposing a standard for which there is no scientific justification. It seems that NIOSH shares with Lewis Carroll and Edward Lear that marvelous propensity to generate nonsense stories, lacking only these poets' ability to make their nonsense rhyme. Lewis Carroll preceded OSHA by many years in recognizing the hazard when he wrote:

> The Walrus and the carpenter
> Were walking close at hand,
> They wept like anything to see
> Such quantities of sand.
> If only this were cleared away,
> They said, it would be grand.

A further verse is likewise apropos, since it points out the need and the means to eliminate the hazard:

> If seven maids with seven mops
> Swept it for half a year,
> Do you suppose, the walrus said,
> That they could get it clear?
> I doubt it said the Carpenter,
> And shed a bitter tear.

One assumes that in the end good sense and science will prevail, but as far as the silica standard is concerned, only after everything else has been tried first.

In conclusion, data are available from which a satisfactory dose–response relationship for free silica can be derived; and the appropriate analysis of these data is long overdue. Lacking an analysis of such data, there is at present no scientific basis for changing the present standard for silica, an opinion that can be amply justified by the low attack rate noted in the Vermont granite shed workers who have been employed there for many years under the current standard,* and who in doing so have developed almost no silicosis.

REFERENCES

1. Guidelines for the Use of the ILO International Classification of Radiographs of Pneumoconioses, Rev. Ed. Occupational Safety and Health Series, No. 22, International Labour Office, Geneva, Switzerland, 1980.
2. Seaton A: In: Occupational Lung Diseases, ed. Morgan WKC, Seaton A. Philadelphia, Saunders, 1975, chap 7.
3. Morgan WKC, Sargent N. Silicosis. In: Induced Disease, ed. Preger L. New York, Grune & Stratton, 1979, chap 16.
4. Ziskind M, Jones RM, Weill H: Silicosis: State of the art. Am Rev Respir Dis 113:643, 1976.
5. Criteria for Recommended Standard Occupational Exposure to Crystalline Silica. National Institute of Occupational Safety and Health. U.S. Department of Health, Education and Welfare. Publication 75-120, Washington, DC, 1974.
6. Theriault GP, Burgess WA, DiBerardinis LJ, Peters JM: Dust exposure in Vermont granite sheds. Arch Environ Health 28:12, 1974.
7. Theriault GP, Peters JM, Fine LJ: Pulmonary function in granite shed workers of Vermont. Arch Environ Health 28:18, 1974.
8. Theriault GP, Peters JM, Johnson WM: Pulmonary function and roentgenographic changes in granite dust exposure. Arch Environ Health 28:23, 1974.
9. Musk AW, Peters, JM, Wegman DG, Fine LJ: Pulmonary function in granite dust exposure: A four year follow-up. Am Rev Respir Dis 115:769, 1977.
10. Peters JM: Personal communication. 1980.

---

* 0.1 mg/m^3.

11. Morgan WKC: The walrus and the carpenter, or the Silica Criteria Standard. J Occup Med 17:782, 1975.
12. Wright GW: A critique of the recommendations and supporting data contained in the NIOSH Criteria Document for a Recommended Standard for Occupational Exposure to Crystalline Silica. Submitted to NIOSH July 17, 1975.
13. Morgan WKC: Industrial bronchitis. Br J Ind Med 35:285, 1978.
14. Hankinson JH, Reger RB, Morgan WKC: Maximal expiratory flow rates in coal miners. Am Rev Respir Dis 116:175, 1977.
15. Irwig L, Rocks P: Lung function and respiratory symptoms in silicotic and nonsilicotic gold miners. Am Rev Respir Dis 117:429, 1978.
16. Graham WBG, O'Grady RV, Dubuc B: Pulmonary function loss in Vermont granite workers: A long term follow-up and critical reappraisal. Am Rev Respir Dis 123:25, 1981.
17. Navratil M, Koval Z, Spacilova M: Development of radiological and functional changes in silicosis during a long-term follow-up. Int Arch Arbeitsmed 34:301, 1975.
18. Teculescu D, Muica N, Prader N: Impairment of pulmonary mixing in simple and complicated silicosis. Bull Physiopathol Respir 11:447, 1975.
19. Milne JS: Longitudinal respiratory studies in older people. Thorax 33:547, 1978.
20. Ohman JKG: Prevention of silica exposure in elimination of silicosis. Am Ind Hyg Assoc J 39:847, 1978.
21. Nelson HM, Rajans GS, Morton S, Brown JR: Silica flour exposures in Ontario. Am Ind Hyg Assoc J 39:261, 1978.
22. Katsnelson BA, Mokronosova KA: Nonfibrous mineral dusts and malignant tumours. An epidemiological study of mortality. J Occup Med 21:15, 1979.
23. Occupation and Mortality, 1970–1972. Decennial Supplement. London, Her Majesty's Stationery Office, 1978.
24. Gibson FS, Martin RH, Lockington JN: Lung cancer mortality in a steel foundry. J Occup Med 19:807, 1977.
25. Ruttner JR: Proceedings International Conference on Pneumoconioses. Johannesburg, 1969. London, Oxford University Press, 1970, 512.
26. Chatgidakis CB: Silicosis in South African white gold miners. Med Proc 9:383, 1963.
27. McDonald JC, Gibbs GW, Liddell FDK, McDonald AD: Mortality after long exposure to cummingtonite grunerite. Am Rev Respir Dis 118:271, 1978.
28. Cordes LG, Brink EW, Checko PJ, et al: A cluster of *Acinetobacter* pneumonia in foundry workers. Ann Intern Med 95:688, 1981.
29. Liddell FDK, Morgan WKC: Methods of assessing serial films for the pneumoconioses. A Review. J Soc Occup Med 28:6, 1978.
30. Amandus HE, Reger RB, Pendergrass EP, et al: The pneumoconioses: Methods of measuring progression. Chest 63:736, 1973.
31. Reger RB, Butcher DF, Morgan WKC: Assessing change in the pneumoconioses using serial radiographs. Am J Epidemiol 98:243, 1973.
32. Jacobsen M: New data on the relationship between simple pneumoconiosis and exposure to coal mine dust. Chest 78(Suppl):408, 1980.
33. Reisner MTR: Results of epidemiologic studies in the progression of coal workers pneumoconiosis. Chest 78(Suppl):406, 1980.

6 Occupational Asthma: Identification of the Agent

Brian T. Butcher
Yehia Y. Hammad
David J. Hendrick

Occupational asthma can be defined as reversible airways obstruction induced by inhaled sensitizing agents encountered in the workplace. It should be distinguished from preexisting asthma, which is exacerbated by exposure to industrial irritants. Legislatively, this is an important distinction. In much of Europe occupational asthma is already accepted as a compensable disease. In the United States it is the basis of numerous individual legal actions and is of much legislative concern at state and federal levels. While exposure concentrations are rarely so high that they pose a significant threat to the consumer population, this potential exists and, occasionally, industrial agents do induce asthma in nonoccupational settings. Also, individuals living in the neighborhood of manufacturing processes have been shown to develop asthma following exposure to factory-emitted dusts or vapors.[1]

Most surveys suggest that 2–6% of the general adult population has asthma, and it is estimated that 2–15% of this may be of occupational origin.[2] Prevalence varies according to potency of the agent and its respirable concentration in the workplace. Similar prevalences may therefore be observed from agents of high potency at low concentration and agents of low or moderate potency at high concentration. While prevalences of greater than 50% have occasionally been observed, these are, fortunately, the exception. In general, prevalence of the disease in most occupational environments is no more than 5–10% of the exposed workforce.

In the majority of cases there is a latent or sensitizing exposure period of some months before symptoms arise, although this can vary from days to many years. Environmental factors, such as exposure to accidental heavy spills or coincidental viral infections of the upper respiratory tract, may be important etiologic factors, although their role in disease pathogenesis remains to be confirmed. In most industries, however, reduction in levels of exposure through improved industrial hygiene is effectively reducing incidence of occupational asthma.

The response of the worker following exposure to potential asthma-inducing agents also depends on a number of host factors. Individuals with personal or family history of hay fever, eczema, or asthma have an increased tendency to develop sensitivity to certain environmental agents. These atopic subjects give immediate wheal and flare responses when skin is tested with common inhalant allergens, and they usually have high serum IgE levels. This immunoglobulin is predominantly bound to mast cells in tissues and is frequently present in greater concentrations in atopic than in nonatopic individuals. In general, atopic subjects have been shown to be at greater risk of developing asthmatic hypersensitivity to occupational agents, although this has not been a uniform observation. In some cases IgE antibodies with specificity for certain asthma-inducing agents are demonstrable.

Other host factors of possible etiologic relevance are nonspecific bronchial hyperreactivity and altered adrenergic tone. The importance of these has been the subject of much discussion and controversy. It is tempting to believe that asthma, whether occupational or not, is a likely consequence if either preexists, but current evidence suggests that they are more commonly a result of occupational asthma rather than its cause.

When individuals with asthma are exposed to relevant provoking agents, two major response patterns are seen: an immediate type, which begins and reaches a peak within minutes, and is usually resolved in the first hour following exposure; and a late type, which does not begin for at least one hour after the provoking exposure, reaches a peak after a period of some hours, and often requires long periods to resolve. Both types are sometimes observed in the same individual, who then shows a dual type of response. Late responses can sometimes show a prominent circadian rhythm that may last for a number of days or even weeks, and may be manifested solely as recurrent nocturnal exacerbations. In most cases dose dependence of the response can be shown if exposure conditions are controlled.

A number of mechanisms have been shown to be of importance in occupational asthma. Many individuals, when exposed to sufficiently high levels of irritating substances such as isocyanates, develop reversible airways narrowing, suggesting that one possible mechanism of occupational asthma may involve irritant receptors and reflex vagal pathways.

Some types of occupational asthma are thought to be mediated by antibodies. Type I hypersensitivity, mediated by mast cell bound specific IgE antibodies and the subsequent release of pharmacologic mediators that cause bronchoconstriction, is more frequently seen in atopic subjects. It should, however, be emphasized that everyone is capable of mounting an IgE antibody response so that occasionally nonatopic individuals respond to sensitizing occupational agents with Type I hypersensitivity responses. Recent evidence that late skin test reactions can be mediated by IgE antibodies raises the possibility that this antibody class may play a role in late asthmatic responses also.

IgG- or IgM-mediated hypersensitivity responses have also been shown to mediate late asthmatic reactions. These responses usually involve complement, development of immune complexes, and subsequent release of a variety of mediators. Complement-triggered responses may also be activated via the antibody independent, alternative pathway. Although intuitively appealing, there is little evidence that Type IV cellular hypersensitivity is relevant in occupational asthma.

Pharmacologic mechanisms may also play a role in certain types of asthma. Some occupational agents are known to stimulate release of histamine, although the clinical importance of this reaction is unclear. Asthma provoked by idiosyncrasy to ingested aspirin suggests that interference with prostaglandin synthesis may be etiologically important. The demonstration that the asthma-inducing agent toluene diisocyanate can diminish the cyclic adenosine monophosphate (cAMP) response of blood mononuclear leukocytes to beta agonists and prostaglandin E_1 suggests that this chemical may act, at least partially, as a blocker of beta adrenergic and prostaglandin receptors.[3] It is also conceivable that reactive industrial agents could activate cholinergic receptors or produce acetylcholine esterase inhibition.

The variety of agents currently recognized to induce or provoke asthma in the workplace is already large (Table 6-1) and is increasing rapidly as more and more reactive chemicals are introduced by industry. The identification of the specific agent responsible in a particular workplace (or a particular worker) may involve complex interdisciplinary research. It begins with the identification of the individual workers who are affected.

CLINICAL EVALUATION OF THE PATIENT

Once it is established that affected workers truly exist, attention can be directed to the agent responsible. Suspicion of occupational asthma may arise for a variety of reasons. Most commonly, characteristic symptoms develop in a working environment known to be associated specifically with this risk, and the affected workers are quick to appreciate their significance. It is when there is no previously recognized risk that an occupational cause may not be considered, particularly if the hypersensitivity response is not of the immediate type. Asthma is, after all, a common disease in the population at large. Coincidence alone may therefore be responsible when it arises in an industrial setting.

Clues that an occupational agent may be responsible include onset (or recurrence) of symptoms within months of starting a new job or using a new

Table 6-1. Agents Causing Occupational Asthma

Natural Organic
Animal proteins
Bean dusts (castor, coffee beans)
Colophony
Enzymes (alkalase, papain)
Flour (grain, soybean)
Insect and arthropod dusts
Organic dyes
Plant dusts (cotton, devil's tongue, grain, psyllium)
Vegetable gums
Wood dusts
Pharmaceuticals
Cimetidine
Penicillins (natural, semisynthetic)
Phenylglycine acid chloride
Piperazine
Spiramycin
Sulfathiazine
Tetracycline
Organic Chemicals
Amines
Formaldehyde
Isocyanates
Phthalic anhydride
Plexiglas dust
Sulfone chloramides
Trimellitic anhydride
Inorganic Chemicals
Chromium salts
Nickel salts
Platinum salts

industrial process/agent; worsening of symptoms on Mondays (i.e., the first workday each week) with improvement during weekends and vacations; and relationship to a specific industrial process that generates dusts, gases, or vapors—particularly the relationship of accidental heavy exposures to isolated asthmatic attacks. While the presence of such clues strongly supports the possibility of occupational asthma, their absence does not always exclude it. Occupational asthma occasionally arises after a decade or two of unchanging exposure to the inducing agent. Also, occupationally provoked exacerbations may persist so that significant recovery is not evident after a weekend or even a vacation away from work. Often there are similar, even stronger, clues relating rhinitis to the working environment; and it may be known that fellow workers have become similarly affected. The latter is, of course, an important clue, but may be distorted by bias. In general, workers tend to change jobs (or are removed from them) when it becomes suspected that these are responsible for ill health. This leaves disproportionate numbers of unaffected subjects in the "survivor" population. By contrast, disproportionate emphasis may occasionally be placed on one or two former workers whose wheezing and undue breathlessness were neither asthmatic nor occupational in origin.

Once the history suggests asthma with occupational triggering factors, the clinician needs to consider whether these are specific (i.e., sensitizing agents primarily responsible for inducing the asthmatic state) or merely nonspecific irritants, inevitably triggering worsening airway obstruction in any subject with preexisting bronchial hyperreactivity. Smoke, oxides of nitrogen and sulfur, and inert dusts could all be considered in this category, as could occupational exertion, especially when the ambient air is cold and dry. If nonspecific irritants do not appear to be responsible, the search for a specific sensitizing agent begins. Most likely this will be a reactive chemical or an organic dust that is intimately related to the industrial processes of the plant concerned.

Occasionally, however, the source is more subtle, and may not be directly related to the particular industry involved. "Occupational" asthma has, for instance, been described in office workers with no obvious exposure to asthma-inducing agents.[4] Their building proved to be ventilated via a roof duct which ensnared isocyanate fumes from the exhaust vents of a neighboring factory. A situation such as this is not easily uncovered from the history alone, and at times a site visit may prove necessary—particularly when more than one worker appears to be affected. When only one worker complains of asthmatic attacks occurring predominantly in the workplace, the clinician must be careful to exclude the possibility that the inducing or triggering agent is actually nonoccupational in origin. For example, a worker may previously have developed asthmatic hypersensitivity to molds, house dust, mites, or animal danders, and then was exposed to these allergens at work at levels sufficient to provoke symptoms. This is asthma occurring at work, but it is not strictly "occupational" in origin. Similarly, a worker may show late hypersensitivity reactions in the workplace to allergens encountered on the way to work (microbial contaminants in a car air conditioner provide an interesting, recently reported example),[5] or this individual may be accustomed to use aspirin or tartrazine-containing beverages more commonly at work than at home. A careful history is consequently an essential starting point, and requires both experience and sound knowledge of the agents currently recognized to induce and trigger asthma.

By the time the affected worker consults a physician or is referred for a specialist's advice, he or she may have left the workplace, either temporarily or permanently. Evidence of active asthma may therefore have subsided. This is, of course, supportive historical evidence that the occupational environment was to blame, but in a litigious world a claimant's story alone is unlikely to satisfy all parties involved. Evidence of personal or family atopy might encourage the belief that the subject concerned was a likely candidate to develop occupational asthma, as may a previous personal or family history of asthma itself; but neither factor deserves undue emphasis. Although there is evidence in some industries that both atopy and previous asthma may be predisposing factors, occupational asthma usually arises among the great majority of the "at risk" workforce who are without personal (or family) history of either.

Irrespective of whether clinical evidence of airways obstruction persists, spirometric measurements may reveal significant abnormalities which reverse following the use of a bronchodilator. This provides adequate confirmatory evidence of asthma. When spirometry shows no abnormality, demonstration of nonspecific bronchial hyperreactivity may provide alternative supporting evidence of an asthmatic history. This may be done by a variety of recently developed techniques, including exercise, cold (dry) air hyperventilation, and inhalation challenge with nebulized distilled water. The most useful method, however, remains pharmacologic inhalation challenge with histamine or a cholinergic agent (methacholine or carbachol). It must be emphasized that such tests relate to a fundamental characteristic of asthma in general, bronchial lability, and do not address the question of whether specific occupational agents are responsible. The degree of hyperreactivity varies with the severity of asthma, and is influenced by a number of factors that are known to influence asthma. In particular, ''colds'' provoke a temporary increase in bronchial reactivity, while cessation of exposure to an inducing agent leads to lessening reactivity. In an occupational setting, bronchial hyperreactivity (and clinical asthma) has been noted to regress completely within as short a period as a few weeks without exposure, though more commonly, bronchial reactivity can be demonstrated for months or even years afterward. A negative methacholine test a year after symptoms (and occupational exposure) ceased would consequently be of limited significance. When a negative result is obtained within days or weeks of symptoms, however, the validity of the history could be questioned.

When worker and employer are prepared to cooperate and allow the effects of a return to work to be monitored, the need for measurement of bronchial reactivity diminishes. A safe, practical, and inexpensive procedure is the comparison of multiple readings of peak expiratory flow (PEF) between days spent in a normal work environment, and control days spent elsewhere. A number of cheap and portable devices are now available with which a worker can record PEF at frequent intervals. Ideally, measurements are made every 1 to 2 hours, throughout the waking hours of one or more work and control days, and graphs are drawn to illustrate the results. Appreciable changes in PEF indicate active asthma, and when these are convincingly related to the day or days spent at work, occupational asthma is strongly suggested. If the accuracy of the readings obtained is questioned, the whole procedure can be readily repeated under the investigating physician's intermittent supervision. It is particularly important in these circumstances that the worker be admitted to hospital for the evening and night of each 24-hour test period, because late asthmatic reactions may be manifested only after the worker has left the workplace. Once the extra expense of surveillance is accepted, lung function could be monitored more accurately by a skilled technician. If a spirometer is taken to the workplace and a technician is engaged to use it, the same spirometer then accompanies the worker to the hospital for continuing measurements during the ensuing evening and night. Ideally, environmental hygiene studies are carried out concurrently, allowing the challenge exposure itself to be quantified. Such sophisticated arrangements are time-consuming and substantially more costly, but they increase validity. Willful fraud is less readily countered, and there is little the physician can do to ensure that a worker with nonoccupational asthma does not use bronchodilators on his control day while omitting them from a workday(s):

or take a known provoker such as aspirin when work-related asthma is to be simulated.

Overall, the monitored workplace challenge is likely to produce convincing evidence that occupational asthma does or does not exist. This assumes that relevant exposure levels on the test day(s) closely resemble those which were responsible for earlier attacks. If previous occupationally related attacks occurred only with high exposures associated with accidents, or at times when bronchial reactivity had been increased by a recent viral infection, then a normal working day exposure may be insufficient to provoke a significant change in ventilatory function. Few workers present themselves for investigation when asthmatic symptoms occur rarely, so this is not a serious limitation to this investigative procedure.

A major limitation does, however, exist, and this is of particular importance to the theme of this chapter. A positive response to a return-to-work challenge confirms that occupational asthma exists, but it does little, if anything, to identify the specific agent responsible. If different processes or different industrial agents are used on different workdays, the choice of potentially responsible agents will be narrowed appreciably by showing differences in ventilatory function on different days. Ultimately, more sophisticated investigations will be required if a previously unrecognized cause of occupational asthma is to be identified; or when a number of possible (and recognized) causes are present in the workplace and it becomes important to identify the one of specific relevance to the worker concerned. The initial responsibility of the evaluating physician is completed when he or she has demonstrated beyond reasonable doubt that occupational asthma truly exists. If resources permit epidemiologic studies of the workplace concerned, further clinical evidence may be obtained that a particular process or a specific agent should be subjected to the industrial hygiene and immunologic investigations that are described below.

INDUSTRIAL HYGIENE

Industrial hygiene encompasses the recognition, evaluation, and control of potential occupational health hazards. For the purpose of this chapter only, the recognition and evaluation aspects of industrial hygiene will be discussed for their application in identification of the agent(s) of occupational asthma.

Recognition and evaluation of worker exposure is achieved by two types of surveys: preliminary and comprehensive. The preliminary survey, conducted to familiarize the hygienist with the industrial processes, raw materials, products, and by-products, is best accomplished by following the industrial process through the plant from raw materials to finished products. It identifies locations in the plant where workers' exposures are later to be evaluated, and the apparatus necessary for the comprehensive survey.

In the comprehensive survey, evaluation of all potential exposures is attained by measuring concentrations of airborne contaminants from the emission sources. Individual worker exposure is also determined by personal sampling equipment that, in many cases, provides a complete profile of the worker's exposure over the entire work shift. All shifts of the same process should be evaluated since exposure during night shifts may change due to different work practices. Where possible, representative samples should be obtained during normal and the most unfavorable conditions, especially in the petroleum and chemical industries where processing is carried out in closed systems and workers are usually stationed in "exposure-free" control rooms and booths. When the system is shut down for inspections and maintenance operations, gross exposures are frequently encountered that differ sharply from those encountered under continuous production schedules. Other important factors to be evaluated during the comprehensive survey are exposure control measures, including engineering control, ventilation exhaust systems, respiratory protective equipment, and work practices.

Recently, emission inventory, a well-established procedure in the field of air pollution control, has been incorporated into industrial hygiene practice. It is utilized for identification of agents and emission sites and provides a record of the variability of utilization of chemicals over time. Sources for emissions inventory estimates are found in the records of process and production, plant engineering, industrial engineering, accounting, and personnel.

Sampling of Airborne Contaminants

The procedures used for sampling airborne contaminants depend primarily on the physical state (i.e., particulates or gases and vapors) of the agent. There are several factors to be considered for sampling. Statistically, an adequate number of samples is required to estimate the mean (or other measures of central tendency) and standard deviation (or measures of dispersion) of the airborne concentration. Biologically, the sampling duration should be short enough to determine individual concentration peaks, determined on the basis of the biologic half-life of the contaminant. Equally, the sampling duration (and air sampling flow rate) should provide adequate amounts of the airborne contaminant for subsequent physical and chemical analysis and the collection media utilized for sampling should be compatible with analytical techniques. Analytical techniques must, where possible, be specific and not suffer from interferences of other chemicals that may be present in the working environment.

Gases and Vapors. Airborne contaminants in the gaseous phase are usually divided into gases and vapors; a vapor being defined as readily condensable at ambient temperature, whereas a gas has a boiling point far removed from normal room temperature.

There are several methods available for sampling gaseous phase pollutants. In direct reading methods, the sampling and analysis steps occur simultaneously and are usually indistinguishable. Samplers may be simple hand-operated pumps connected to detector tubes, or they may be completely automated, battery-operated, personal or area monitors capable of continuous measurements with digital readout. Since chemical and physical properties of gases are utilized for quantitation, most instruments are designed to measure specific gases and vapors, but few are capable of measuring more than one gas. Physical properties on which direct reading instruments are designed include electrochemical (electrical conductivity, potentiometry, and coulometry), thermal (flame ionization, thermal conductivity, and heat of combustion), and spectroscopic or spectrophotometric (infrared, ultraviolet, and visible light absorption).

In many cases, only indirect reading methods are available. In these a representative sample is collected in the field on some solid or liquid substrate and transported to the laboratory, where desired species are separated and concentrations determined by conventional qualitative and quantitative analytical techniques.

A variety of collection devices are available for gas sampling. They include (1) air displacement using glass evacuated flasks and sampling bags made of Teflon, Mylar, PVC, Saran, etc.; (2) condensation, where air is passed through a condenser cooled below the boiling or freezing point of the sampled gas or vapor; (3) absorption of the gas in a suitable solvent or reaction with a chemical dissolved in a solvent (usually contained in bubblers, scrubbers, and impingers); or (4) adsorption of gas molecules on surfaces of activated charcoal, silica gel, alumina, zeolite, or other suitable materials.

Particulate Matter. Airborne particulates, usually referred to as aerosols, can be in either solid or liquid form and may include gases and vapors absorbed on airborne particles. The most important properties of particles are shape, density, surface area, and size. No other category of toxic substances exhibits the degree of interdependence of physical characteristics and toxicity as do aerosols.

Aerosol deposition in the human respiratory tract depends primarily on particle aerodynamic properties. Because most particles involved in occupational exposure are irregular in shape and have variable densities, it is important to define particle size in relation to aerodynamic behavior. The parameter used, Stoke's diameter, is defined as the diameter of a sphere having the same settling velocity as the particle and a density equal to that of the bulk material from which the particle was formed. Estimation of Stoke's diameter requires preknowledge of the particle density, but this is not always known, and in some cases particles are formed from materials of many densities (grain dust, cotton dust). To overcome this problem, a new concept has been introduced, which describes particle size in terms of aerodynamic equivalent diameter, defined as the diameter of a sphere having the same settling velocity as the particle and a density of 1 g/cm^3.

Airborne particles are usually classified into two types—viable or nonviable. Viable particles include pollen and microorganisms including viruses, bacteria, spores, rusts, molds, yeasts, fungi, protozoa, and algae, some of which are associated with disease. While most viable particles are of natural origin, others result from man-made processes such as sewage treatment. Viable particles can be redisseminated from accumulations in the dusts of rooms, air conditioning ducts, streets, sidewalks, and even the respiratory tract following sneezing and coughing.

Nonviable particles include (1) dispersion aerosols that can be generated by suspension of powders, grinding of solids, or atomization of liquids (dispersion aerosol with solid particles are usually called dusts), (2) condensation aerosols such as fog and metal fumes formed when saturated vapors are condensed, (3) condensation and dispersion aerosols with liquid particles (mists), and those with solid and liquid particles (smokes).

The following is a classification of the methods available for sampling of aerosols[6]:

1. Collection without size separation (total dust). In this mode, suspended particulate matter is collected with filters, impactors, electrostatic precipitators, or thermal precipitators. The mass of the collected dust can be indirectly determined by gravimetric methods or quantitative chemical analysis. Instruments are also available that provide direct readout of the collected mass either by light extinction, attenuation of β-particles, or frequency shift of a vibrating crystal. Size distribution of collected particles can subsequently be determined by light and electron microscopy, sieving, or elutriation.
2. Collection with size separation. Since the site of deposition of aerosols in the human respiratory tract depends on particle size, several sampling instruments are designed to separate an airborne dust cloud into fractions representing particles likely to be deposited in the nasopharyngeal, tracheobronchial, or pulmonary compartments (the last is usually called the respirable fraction); or into other convenient size fractions that allow the determination of the size distribution of the dust cloud. These instruments utilize gravitational, centrifugal, or impaction forces for size separation.
3. Particle size determination without collection. Instruments in this category have direct readout and determine the size distribution of particles in their airborne state by utilizing electrostatic or light scattering properties of the particles.

IMMUNOLOGIC STUDIES

A number of immunologic tests may be of use in the diagnosis of occupational asthma and the identification of the etiologic agent. Some tests can be done at the job site and some in the laboratory on samples collected from the work site. Others are only possible when the worker visits the physician's office or laboratory.

Determination of atopy by skin prick testing with common inhalant allergens, which can easily be performed at the work site, is important for identifying individuals who may be more prone to develop asthma. Skin testing using specific occupational materials is sometimes of use in identifying the causative sensitizing agent. The suspected agent is usually prepared for testing as an aqueous extract. In the case of small molecular weight chemicals, it is frequently necessary to attach these haptenic materials to a carrier protein, such as human serum albumin, to permit skin testing.

A typical preparation procedure for manufacture of extracts for skin testing entails extraction into pyrogen-free water, filtration and centrifugation to remove particulates, and lyophilization. Prior to testing, samples are reconstituted in physiologic buffered saline, sterilized with a bacterial filter, cultured to confirm sterility, and tested in animals for pyrogenicity or toxicity and mutagenicity (Ames test). In the case of human serum albumin-conjugated haptens, testing for hepatitis antigen is also performed. A series of dilutions are prepared and tested in normal volunteers to determine a nonirritative dose before use in test individuals.

Skin prick testing is usually a relatively harmless procedure, though uncomfortable late or even delayed responses may occur, and anaphylaxis has been described with agents of extreme potency such as penicillin derivatives. When in vitro testing is preferable, the radioallergosorbent test, although slightly less sensitive than the skin prick test, is the best available method for detecting specific IgE antibodies. The radioallergosorbent test is most suited to protein allergens and least suited to polysaccharides. In the case of small molecular weight chemicals, conjugation to protein carriers such as human serum albumin is usually necessary.

The radioallergosorbent test involves complexing the test antigen to a chemically activated solid carrier, such as Sepharose or a small filter paper disk. Specific antibodies react with the conjugated antigen when the disk is incubated with patient serum. Following washing to remove unreacted material, radiolabeled anti-IgE is added. This radiolabeled antiserum combines with specific IgE antibodies, which have reacted with the allergen conjugated to the disk, and can be measured semiquantitatively in a gamma counter.

The radioallergosorbent test is of use in epidemiologic surveys and can be invaluable for identification of specific agents that provoke IgE-mediated asthma. Using a modification of the radioallergosorbent test, inhibition studies can be performed. In such studies, serum is preincubated with specific or related antigen prior to use in the radioallergosorbent test to confirm specificity of the antibodies and to eliminate the possibility of cross-antigenicity. An example of this involved asthma occurring in workers roasting green coffee beans.[7] It was shown that they had skin reactivity to crude aqueous extracts of green coffee bean and coffee factory dust contaminated with small amounts of castor bean dust (some coffee bean sacks had been previously used to transport castor beans). Provocative inhalation challenge with the factory dust extract and with a purified green bean extract confirmed the etiologic relevance of the green coffee bean, but the possible relevance of castor bean could not be tested in this way because of the presence of the potent castor bean toxin, ricin. The radioallergosorbent test inhibition was used to demonstrate that in some cases immunologic specificity was also directed against castor bean antigen (Fig. 6-1).

In addition to performing skin prick tests, it can be important to measure total serum IgE levels. Frequently, a high total IgE level is associated with atopy, a finding of use in surveys where it is not practical to use skin testing. Also, serum from individuals with elevated total IgE levels show nonspecific

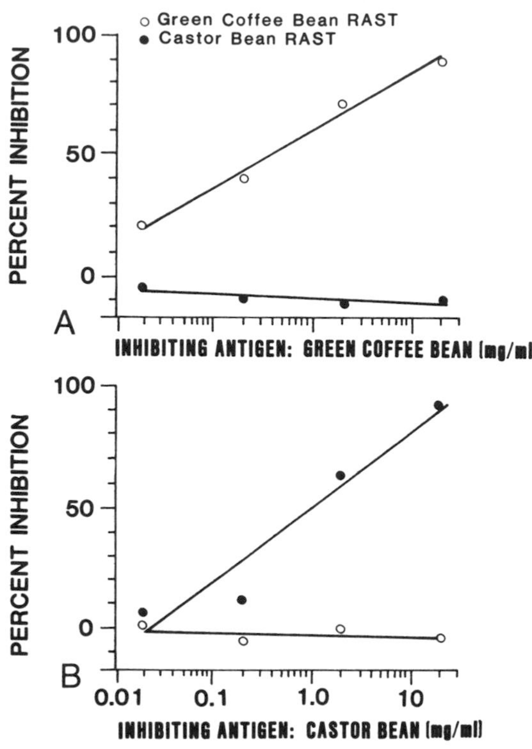

Fig. 6-1 Use of RAST inhibition to demonstrate bean specificity of coffee dust antibodies. (Karr RM, Lehrer SB, Butcher BT, et al:, Coffee workers' asthma: A clinical appraisal using the radioallergosorbent test. J Allergy Clin Immunol, 62:143, 1978).

binding to the allergen disk used in the radioallergosorbent test. Measurement of total IgE levels consequently allows correction factors to be applied which eliminate false positive results.

Quantitation of other immunoglobulins has proved of little value, although there are occasional reports of alterations in total immunoglobulin levels attributable to occupational exposure. Measurement of specific antibodies of the other immunoglobulin classes (IgG, IgM, IgA) on the other hand, is sometimes of use in identification of the etiologic agent(s) in occupational asthma. A variety of techniques are available for this.

One useful qualitative technique for detection of precipitating antibodies is the double diffusion gel technique for Ouchterlony. Other methods include counterimmunoelectrophoresis, where antigen and antiserum are driven together by an electric current, and crossed immunoelectrophoresis, where the antigen is first separated by electrophoresis, followed by electrophoresis at right angles into a gel containing specific antibodies. This latter technique may be of particular use where large numbers of antigenic materials are present in extracts. A modification of this method, crossed radioimmunoelectrophoresis, where patient serum is layered on the crossed immunoelectrophoresis plate and developed with radiolabeled anti-IgE antiserum, can be useful in identification of allergenic components in complex antigens such as vegetable dusts.

Radioimmunoassay methods have generally proved unsuitable for measurement of specific antibodies other than IgE. The polystyrene tube assay is a useful exception. In this test, antigen is conjugated directly to the polystyrene tube surface and use of radiolabeled immunoglobulins allows measurement of specific antibodies of other immunoglobulin classes, in addition to IgE. Using this assay, Patterson and colleagues[8] were able to demonstrate specific IgG and IgM antibodies to trimellitic anhydride and show that in some workers these may have been relevant in the pathogenesis of trimellitic anhydride asthma. The technique has also been used to demonstrate high levels of specific IgG antibodies against methylene bis(phenyl) isocyanate (MDI) in the serum of a worker with MDI asthma.

The enzyme-linked immunosorbent assay (ELISA) is a similar, but less sensitive test, used to quantitate specific antibodies of the different immunoglobulin classes. In this test, antiserum used to detect specific antibodies of the different classes is labeled with an enzyme such as horseradish peroxidase, which gives a color reaction when developed with specific substrate.

When specific IgG or IgM antibodies are present, there may be involvement of complement in the immune reaction. Complement can also be activated by the antibody independent alternative pathway. When the complement cascade is activated, a number of potent pharmacologic agents are formed, including anaphylatoxins, which can lead to bronchoconstriction. Studies of complement activity have rarely proved to be useful in the evaluation of occupational asthma, though there is evidence that complement may be involved in asthma induced by some vegetable dusts.

There are a number of immunologic tests available to demonstrate Type IV, cell-mediated hypersensitivity, but the relevance of this type of hypersensitivity has yet to be confirmed in asthma. In the lymphocyte transformation test, lymphocytes from the patient are incubated in the presence of the suspected etiologic agent, together with tritium-labeled thymidine. If there is specificity of the cell for the agent, blastogenesis occurs and there is increased uptake of the thymidine, which is easily measured in a beta radioactivity counter. There have been occasional reports that positive lymphocyte transformation tests may be useful in the diagnosis of occupational asthma, but most workers have failed to confirm this.

If it is established that pharmacologic mechanisms are responsible for some varieties of occupational asthma, a valuable role could emerge for pharmacologic tests in identifying the etiologic agent. The effect of isocyanates on mononuclear leukocyte cyclic AMP stimulation by isoproterenol and prostaglandin E_1 has already been discussed. Work with cotton dust and bract extracts indicates that some components in these extracts also act upon cyclic AMP production by lymphocytes. Since cotton dust and bract extracts are complex mixtures, measurement of cyclic AMP effects of purified extracts could help identify the active etiologic material in occupational asthma induced by cotton dust.

In addition to the methods described above, a number of immunologic and pharmacologic tests can be used in conjunction with provocative inhalation challenge studies. In general, their value is in the elucidation of underlying mechanisms, rather than in the recognition of positive asthmatic responses, although they can be of use when challenge produces equivocal results, especially upon repeated challenge.

Histamine is released into plasma during some types of response to provocative challenge, but, unless arterial samples are collected, measurement of plasma histamine levels is of little use since, in peripheral venous blood, catabolism occurs very rapidly. Release of 5-hydroxytryptamine and bradykinin into plasma does occur in some types of asthma, but these measurements have not been shown to be useful in study of the etiology of occupational asthma. The action of occupational agents on complement has already been discussed; measurement of complement consumption during challenge studies has not, however, proved to be of diagnostic value. Leukotrienes are potent mediators of bronchoconstriction but, at present, the techniques for measuring these compounds are difficult and await further refinement before they can be considered for use as tests for identifying agents of occupational asthma.

Eosinophil counts have been demonstrated to increase significantly in response to exposure to certain occupational agents which induce asthma. The diagnostic significance of eosinophilia is discussed below.

HUMAN INHALATION CHALLENGE SYSTEMS

The basic components of an inhalation challenge system are air purification and the generation and delivery of the challenge agent, whether aerosol or gas. The concentration of a gas or vapor in air is usually expressed in units percent (%) or parts per million parts of air by volume (ppm). The concentrations of aerosols and sometimes vapors are expressed in units of weight per unit of volume (usually milligrams/cubic meter, mg/m^3).

Air Purification

During inhalation challenge procedures, all air supplies utilized for generation or dilution (compressed air from cylinders, compressors, or air conditioning systems) must be purified to prevent contamination and possible chemical reactions. Common contaminants in usual sources of air are oil mist, carbon dioxide, carbon monoxide, and hydrocarbons. Particulates can also be present from rust and scale in the pipe system. Humidity in the air line may also be higher than ambient humidity because of condensation.

Excess water vapor is most conveniently removed using dry desiccants, such as Drierite (calcium sulfate), though a variety of methods are available, such as cooling coils immersed in Dry Ice/acetone mixture or liquid nitrogen. Removal of hydrocarbons and other organic vapors is usually accomplished by passing the airstream through activated charcoal filters. These have low efficiency for organic gases with low molecular weight, such as acetylene and methane, carbon monoxide, carbon dioxide, and other acid gases, which may require special absorption material. Particulate matter is usually removed by filtration through high efficiency glass fiber filters or membrane filters. Combinations of high efficiency filters and activated charcoal filters are available commercially.

Generation of Challenge Agent

Accuracy of the concentrations delivered during inhalation challenge procedures depends primarily on the accuracy of airflow measurement. Atmospheric pressure, airline pressure, and temperature should be continuously monitored to permit correction of measured volume. Air volume or flowrate metering devices are usually divided into primary standards and secondary standards. Primary standards, which include spirometers, aspirating bottles, and frictionless pistons such as soap bubble meters, are utilized for calibration of the secondary standards only. Secondary standards, which include wet and dry gas meters, rotameters, orifice meters, and critical orifices, are convenient to use, of relatively small size, and capable of operation over long periods of time without resetting, but are subject to corrosion of movable parts and need daily corrections for temperature and pressure changes.

Selection of an appropriate delivery system depends on the type of inhalation challenge system (static or dynamic) as well as the properties of the delivered agent.[9] In static systems, a known weight or volume of the contaminant is introduced into a chamber of fixed volume. If gaseous, it may be contained in a glass ampoule, which is either broken or fitted with a mechanism for displacing the gas with a liquid. If a volatile liquid, it may be placed in an evaporating vessel on a hot plate. After the test individual enters the chamber, a fan is operated briefly to ensure even distribution of the airborne agent.

Static exposure has a number of limitations. Since the test subject gradually consumes oxygen and excretes carbon dioxide and water vapor, concentration of oxygen and agent will decrease, while carbon dioxide and water vapor concentrations increase. Hence an unsatisfactory pattern of exposure, that is, concentration versus time, is obtained. This system is, however, of use when only a limited quantity of agents are available.

Because exposure to a uniform concentration is usually desirable, dynamic systems, which are capable of continuously producing and blending one or more agents (in a constant proportion) with a diluent, usually air, over the entire challenging period, are most frequently used. They can generate large volumes of reproducible and precise concentrations for extended time periods. This is especially important in the case of unstable gas mixtures, where undesirable products are continuously replaced by fresh unreacted mixtures. The disadvantages of the system are its complexity (and, consequently, high initial and operations costs) and the need for large quantities of the agent.

Gases and Vapors. Methods for generating gases and vapors include gas mixing, evaporation, permeation, diffusion, and injection. Gas mixing is utilized when the agent is available in bottled form (gas cylinders) at known concentration and the agent is diluted with air in predetermined and continuously measured proportions. The system consists of flowmeters, a mixing chamber, a source of the agent gas and a source of compressed air. When more than one step of dilution is utilized, some means for waste gas disposal is needed. All delivery lines should be constructed from inert materials such as Teflon, glass, or stainless steel to prevent chemical reactions.

In the evaporation method, diluent gas is passed through the liquid to be evaporated to produce a saturated gas mixture. The concentration of vapor in the gas mixture depends upon flowrate of diluent gas, the temperature, viscosity, and boiling point of the liquid, and properties of the bubbling bottle. To ensure a constant output concentration, the bubbler should be enclosed in a constant temperature bath and level of the liquid in the bubbler kept constant by connecting it to a large volume reservoir.

The permeation tube method uses liquefied gas sealed in a tube made from polymer resin. The gas dissolves in the polymer and permeates through the wall of the tube at a constant rate, which depends on properties of the gas, membrane area and thickness, and the pressures on both sides of the membrane. If the tube geometry is fixed, with all other variables constant, permeation will be governed by ambient temperature. Permeation tubes are used as primary standards for calibration of sampling instruments and provide stable concentrations during inhalation challenges, although their output is low.

The property of a gas or vapor at high concentration to diffuse into another at lower concentration is utilized to generate constant vapor concentrations of volatile liquids. The system is comprised of a constant temperature bath, a source of diluent gas, metering devices, and diffusion tubes consisting of a reservoir to contain the volatile liquid, connected to a long, narrow tube of known length and cross section.

In the injection system, volatile liquid or gas is injected into a moving stream of diluent by a mechanical device such as a syringe pump. This system generates precise concentrations over extended periods of time but some means of evaporation, such as atomization or the addition of heat at the point of injection, is required.

Aerosols. Aerosols can be divided into two categories: clouds of uniform size particles (monodispersed) and those associated with a wide size range (polydispersed). In practice, aerosol clouds with a geometric standard deviation ≤ 1.22 (or a coefficient of variation $\leq 20\%$) are considered to be monodispersed. Methods currently available for production of monodispersed aerosols[10] include condensation, vibrating orifice, and spinning disk.

Condensation aerosols can be generated in a narrow size range by controlled condensation of organic vapors on condensation nuclei in a system employing a nuclei source, a boiler, reheater, and cooling chimney. Particle size is controlled by the number of nuclei available for condensation and by the mass concentration of the vapor.

In the spinning disk and spinning top generators, uniform droplets are produced when a liquid that wets the disk surface is fed on the center of the disk at a constant rate. The liquid spreads over the disk in a uniform, thin film, which accumulates at the rim until the centrifugal force exceeds the capillary force holding the liquid together and a droplet is thrown off. Size of the droplet is controlled by the angular velocity and diameter of the disk, as well as density and surface tension of the liquid.

In the vibrating orifice generator, liquid is forced through a small orifice at a constant flowrate. Vibrating the orifice by a piezoelectric transducer breaks the stream into uniform droplets, with one droplet formed for each cycle. When flowrate and cycle frequently are kept constant, the generated droplets all have the same size with a very small geometric standard deviation.

Monodisperse aerosol generation procedures are tedious, difficult, and expensive. Great care must be paid to neutralization of electrostatic charge on the particle cloud, removal of satellite particles (in the spinning disk) and prevention of coagulation after dispersion.

Generation of polydisperse aerosols is somewhat easier than monodisperse aerosols and they can be generated from liquids or powders by one of the following methods.[10]

In the air nebulizer, air entering at a flowrate dependent on the diameter of the orifice and the pressure drop across it, expands when it passes across the mouth of the liquid inlet tube. The resulting drop in pressure brings about a flow of liquid into the airstream, which breaks up to form droplets of various sizes.

In ultrasonic nebulizers, the liquid is atomized by a vibrating piezoelectric crystal. The vibrations are transmitted through a coupling liquid to a nebulizer cup containing the solution to be aerosolized where a conical shaped fountain is formed, from the apex of which a jet of droplets is emitted.

Dry powder is most simply dispersed by blowing air through the loose mass of the powder, but neither concentration nor size distribution can be predicted and output of aerosol cannot be maintained at a constant level. To overcome this problem, a surface of a compact powder is abraded at a controlled rate, either by mechanical scrapers or air jets, as used in the Wright dust feed, the Timbrell generator, and National Bureau of Standards dust feed. Recently, the fluidized bed dust generator has been devised, consisting of an elutriation chamber in which large inert beads of stainless steel are fluidized by compressed air. Continuous movement of powder introduced to the fluidized bed at a constant rate causes dispersion of powder into single particles with very few agglomerates. The aerosol is removed from the elutriation chamber by compressed air at a flowrate that removes the fine powder but not the large beads of the bed.

Delivery Systems

For delivery, the challenge substance is introduced either via a mouthpiece or a face mask, or the test subject enters a chamber in which the challenge substance is introduced either previously (static system) or continuously (dynamic system).

In the face mask technique, a tightly fitting rubber mask is connected to the generation system with the mask inlet and outlet valved so that the respiratory movement of the subject acts as a demand system. This system is preferred when small amounts of challenge substance are required or when radioactive tracers are utilized for quantitation of dose. Disadvantages of the system are loss of the test substance by absorption or adsorption to, or chemical reaction with the tubing, valves, or mask, and inability of challenge subjects to tolerate the test conditions for extended time periods.

The advantage of the whole body chamber, which can be operated in the dynamic mode to attain a uniform concentration, is that the test subject is free to move and sit comfortably in the chamber. It allows prolonged testing procedures and more than one person can be challenged at the same time to the same concentration. There are disadvantages of the system. When operated dynamically, large quantities of agent are consumed during challenge. It cannot be used when radioisotopic labeling is necessary to quantitate exposure dose because the subject or his clothing would become contaminated. Contamination of the body or clothing may also be a problem with nonradioactive agents, but this can be overcome by showering or use of disposable gowns.

When dynamic generation of the agent commences, concentration increases exponentially from zero toward an equilibrium (C_{max}) (or theoretically, maximum) value which is the ratio of the agent flowrate (G) to total air flowrate in the chamber (Q). The concentration increases exponentially as shown in equation (i), Fig. 6-2, where C is the concentration of the agent at time T, and V is the volume of the chamber. This equation is followed if G and Q are kept constant and perfect mixing is achieved in the chamber. In reality, perfect mixing is not possible and a mixing factor (K) is added in the equation. Value of K ranges from 1 to 3 for well-designed chambers, and 3 to 10 for general room ventilation. When the agent generator is turned off, the concentration in the chamber decays exponentially. The concentration profile is exactly the same in shape as that for reaching equilibrium but inverted. The concentration decreases according to equation (ii) in Fig. 6-2.

Design and Safety Considerations—The Tulane Chamber

The Tulane University inhalation challenge chamber is shown in Fig. 6-3. It consists of a 4-foot wide, 6.2-foot high, and 7.2-foot long stainless steel chamber with an observation window through which the subject can be readily

$$C = \frac{G}{Q}\left[1 - e^{-\frac{QT}{KV}}\right] \rightarrow \text{i}$$

$$C = C_{MAX}\, e^{-\frac{QT}{KV}} \rightarrow \text{ii}$$

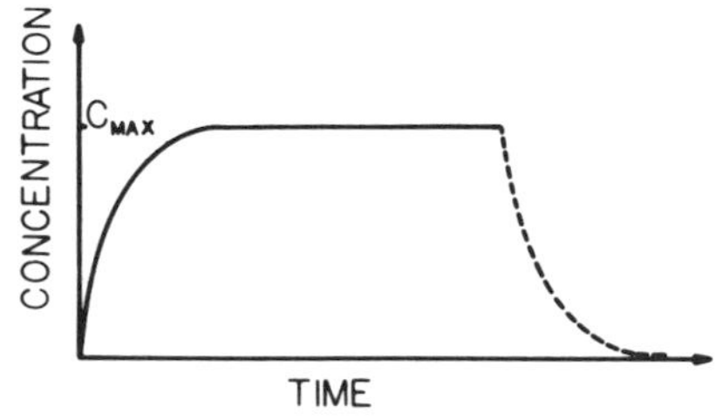

Fig. 6-2 Concentration–time relationships in a dynamic chamber.

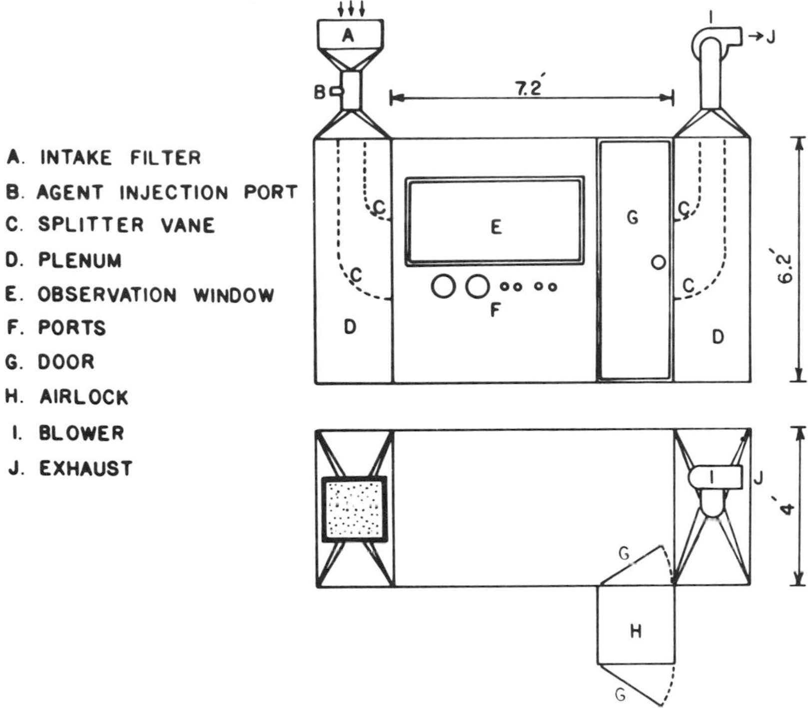

Fig. 6-3 Schematic drawing of the Tulane inhalation challenge chamber.

observed throughout exposure. Air entering the chamber through high efficiency particulate and charcoal filters is mixed with the test agent, enters the chamber through air splitter vanes to ensure even distribution, and sweeps the entire chamber. The air mixture is also exhausted through air splitter vanes by a blower capable of suction flowrates up to 250 cfm. The chamber is maintained at a slight negative pressure (1.5 inches of water) to prevent leakage of the agents from the chamber. Subjects enter the chamber through an air lock so that fluctuations in the concentration of agent in the chamber are reduced to a minimum. Access ports in the chamber allow monitoring of vital signs, measurement of pulmonary function, and blood sampling while the subject is in the chamber undergoing exposure. Some of the safety features include air sampling monitors with alarms that sound when the concentration reaches levels above predetermined settings and pressure sensitive switches capable of shutting off the agent delivery system and/or blower if pressure reaches a critical value.

For some challenge procedures, the agent is available in compressed cylinders. This carries the risk that a power failure could stop the exhaust blower while the agent, under pressure, continues to be introduced to the chamber. This would result in a sharp rise in concentration beyond acceptable limits. To prevent such circumstances, agent delivery is controlled by electric (solenoid) switches, which, in the case of a power failure, automatically shut off the agent delivery lines.

CHAMBER INHALATION TESTS

Once etiologic suspicion falls on a specific industrial agent (or mixture), the affected worker may elect to undergo formal inhalation provocation tests in the laboratory using an exposure chamber of the type described. Such tests serve two important functions. They may provide definitive evidence that the test subject does have occupational asthma, and they may establish that the test agent is indeed responsible. Their great advantage is that they test directly the question under consideration—does the test agent provoke asthma in the test subject? Both sensitivity and specificity should therefore approach 100%, providing appropriate exposure levels are used, and providing the subject's reactivity has not changed as the result of leaving the workplace. No other test (including local application of test agents to the nasal mucosa) can be expected to provide such definitive results, but other tests are correspondingly less time-consuming, less costly, and less hazardous.

Challenge Dose

Industrial hygiene measurements in the workplace will ideally provide a guide to the exposure levels necessary to provoke asthmatic reactions. The primary consideration is to avoid a challenge dose that could provoke an unduly severe response. Asthma can, albeit relatively rarely, be fatal, and tests designed to provoke attacks must be carried out with full awareness of the potential risks involved. These risks must also be appreciated by the subject and advisors, and written informed consent should be obtained. Knowledge that the subject concerned has previously been safely and repeatedly exposed for many hours to measured levels of the test agent in the workplace, makes laboratory challenge at a similar or lesser level of exposure acceptably safe, particularly as the laboratory exposure is likely to be of lesser duration. Convenient exposure times range from 5 to 60 minutes, though symptoms and lung function should be carefully monitored at 5- to 10-minute intervals during the first 30 to 60 minutes of any challenge, so that exposure may be discontinued as soon as a significant immediate asthmatic reaction is provoked.

If the initial challenge produces no response, the exposure dose may be increased on subsequent days by 2- to 5-fold increments until an unequivocally positive response is obtained, or a dose exceeding any likely to be experienced in the workplace is administered without response. When there is no historical suspicion of late asthmatic reactivity, it is reasonable to consider sequential tests with higher challenge doses on the same day; otherwise, the possibility of severe late responses precludes this, and in general it is better to regard each test as a 24-hour procedure with challenge increments being administered at the same time on different mornings. When an equivocal result is obtained, the choice of a 2-fold challenge increment is advisable for the next test. When no suspicion of reactivity is observed we recommend a 4- to 5-fold increment, though in many instances 10-fold increments have proved acceptably safe. Exposure dose is probably best expressed in cumulative terms, though it is by no means established that a 15-minute exposure at 4 ppm is, for example, clinically equivalent to a 60-minute exposure at 1 ppm. We find it convenient to use 15-minute exposures until test levels reach the current industrial standard or threshold limit value. We then increase the duration up to 4 hours, depending on the industrial exposure regulations pertaining to the agent involved.

There are occasions when the history suggests that asthmatic attacks occur only following exceptional (accidental) levels of exposure at work. In these circumstances, the above regimen is unlikely to be appropriate, and some consideration must be given to using exposure doses beyond those permitted legally in industry. These regulations do not apply outside the workplace, and there is no legal restriction preventing the physician from using higher exposure doses in tests he considers necessary for his patient's ultimate well-being. All parties should be aware of the special circumstances, however, and the physician should realize the potential litigious risks if any unduly severe reaction were to occur.

The foregoing assumes exposure levels have been measured in the test subject's workplace and regulatory standards are available for the test agent. When the former are not available, some guidance can be obtained from the latter and from published evidence of other investigators. If a 5-fold increment regimen is used, a dose range of 1–125× can be obtained from only 4 tests, while with 6 tests a range exceeding 3000× is obtained. With a 2-fold increment regimen these ranges would be reduced, respectively, to 8 and 32 only. Depending on the maximum dose chosen (the dose at which a negative result would be declared), the starting dose can be determined from the clinical history. If this suggests exquisite sensitivity, a regimen involving 4 to 6 incremental challenges should be considered; if not, 2 to 4 are likely to be acceptably safe. Knowledge of the level of nonspecific bronchial reactivity may be of additional value, high levels emphasizing the need for extra caution. Similarly, a skin test with worthwhile sensitivity and specificity might add further useful data regarding the degree of specific hypersensitivity.

Our own regimen regarding challenge tests with toluene diisocyanate, for example, involves a methacholine test and a starting challenge dose of 0.005 ppm for 15 minutes if moderate or high levels of bronchial reactivity are found. If the subject shows little or no reactivity to methacholine, and the history suggests reactions to heavy occupational exposures only, we begin with 0.01 ppm or the TLV of 0.02 ppm for 15 minutes. When no suspicion of an asthmatic response is noted, 4-fold dose increments are administered on subsequent days, the maximum challenge dose involving 0.02 ppm toluene diisocyanate for 4 hours.

When the agent concerned has not previously been recognized to induce asthma, regulatory exposure standards are likely to be lacking or inappropriate, and no guidance is available from past experience. In these circumstances, measurements or estimates of workplace exposure are particularly important before costly and potentially hazardous investigations of this type are embarked upon.

When tests are to be carried out with nebulized aerosols of antigenic solutions, challenge doses are less readily equated with occupational exposures. The principle is to create relatively high levels of exposure over short periods of time. It is assumed that the cumulative dose approximates that of an average day's work, but in practice the specificity of such tests depends more on showing that nonspecific responses do not follow similar challenges in clinically unaffected subjects. Soluble test extracts cannot be made in concentrations much above 10 mg/ml, and in general, exposure to this concentration for 10 to 30 minutes (tidal breathing through a mouthpiece or face mask) without response is taken to exclude hypersensitivity to the agent concerned. A convenient and safe protocol is to prepare serial 10-fold dilutions from 0.001 to 10 mg/ml. In ascending order of concentration, each extract is used for skin prick tests until a definite positive wheal and flare response (compared with the diluent as a control) is obtained. Inhalation tests may safely commence with a 10-fold dilution of the concentration producing the skin response. If no response is seen to skin prick tests, intracutaneous tests are sometimes carried out with 0.02 ml of the dilutions, 0.001 through 0.01 mg/ml. Higher concentrations can be expected to produce nonspecific responses. The lowest concentration producing a definitely positive response should be chosen for the initial inhalation test.

The risk of inducing an undue immediate reaction can be further reduced if, for example, a 10-minute cumulative challenge is administered by degrees in approximately 2-fold increments (periods of ½, 1½, 3, and 5 minutes) at 10-minute intervals. Lung function can therefore be measured between each incremental dose, allowing unnecessary further exposure to be avoided if the significant response is already evident.

Control Studies

A major benefit of laboratory challenge tests is that control tests can be carried out under identical circumstances. The tests are thus single blind (providing any characteristic taste, odor, etc. is adequately disguised) which greatly diminishes the possible influence of supratentorial factors or even fraud. Since control of the challenge exposure usually involves an investigator other than the supervising physician, it is also possible to use a double-blind technique, though the inconvenience of this is rarely justified. It is important that the test subject appreciate the need for one or more control studies, and that he or she be fully aware that each individual challenge exposure could involve an inert control agent. The true nature of each test exposure should not be revealed until all tests are completed. In practice, there is some advantage in administering a control challenge for the first test. Otherwise, there is risk that a prolonged late reaction may be provoked before the investigator is able to record true baseline levels of lung function under nonoccupational conditions. A subsequent control test(s) can always be given at a later, random point in the series if necessary.

Monitoring Investigations

Immediate reactions may progress rapidly, and so the test subject must be closely observed during the initial 30 to 60 minutes after challenge exposure begins. The subject should be free to leave the exposure chamber whenever he or she wishes, and should do so immediately if unduly troublesome symptoms occur. Lung function should be measured every 5 to 15 minutes, a convenient and adequate protocol comprising 10-minute intervals for the 30 minutes preceding and the 90 minutes following challenge onset. Late responses develop and resolve much more slowly, and so subsequent measurements need only be carried out at hourly intervals while the subject remains awake. Should the subject wake during the night, it is worthwhile obtaining further measurements (particularly following a control challenge), since subsequent late reactions might not reach their peak until such a time. Close supervision should be provided throughout, and in most cases hospital admission will be necessary. Appropriate treatment must be readily available throughout.

Measurement of ventilatory function provides the most reliable evidence of changing levels of airways obstruction, though symptoms and auscultory signs should be recorded also. Frequency of measurement is more crucial than its degree of sophistication, and forced expiratory volume in one second (FEV_1) has proved to be the most satisfactory monitoring test. If a spirometer is not readily available at the hospital bedside, inhalation provocation tests should also be monitored with a portable PEF measuring device, so that readings can be continued throughout the waking hours of the 24 hour study period. Late reactions which are not manifest until the evening or night following challenge can thereby be identified.

A 15 to 20% decrement in FEV_1 from baseline (prechallenge) levels conventionally defines a positive immediate reaction assuming that no appreciable immediate decline is seen after control challenge. In the latter circumstances, FEV_1 measurements following antigen challenge should be less than 80 to 85% of both mean baseline measurements and corresponding control test measurements. This double requirement in defining a positive result should also apply to late reactions in order to allow for the confounding effect of circadian change, which is a common characteristic of asthma in general. Measurements of PEF show greater variance than those of FEV_1 and so declines of 20 to 25% are generally required to define an unequivocally positive response. With both FEV_1 and PEF, however, these defining percentages are arbitrarily chosen. They provide useful guidelines, but it should be recognized that variance also differs between individual subjects, and that in any one subject, statistically significant changes in lung function may occur after quite different (and often much lesser) percent changes. In practice, it is usually best to conduct a further antigen challenge test using a higher exposure dose whenever equivocal results are obtained, though in these circumstances a 2-fold increment is usually advisable. In a few subjects, the degree of reactivity to antigen challenge appears to be limited and increasing challenge exposures produce similar mild or equivocal responses. In these circumstances, a confident diagnosis requires that the response is shown to be reproducible after further single blind antigen and control challenges.

Two further monitoring investigations have been used, though neither is essential, since both tend to be less sensitive than 1 to 2 hourly measurements of FEV_1 or PEF. The generation of blood and sputum eosinophilia are frequent, though not invariable, accompaniments of asthmatic exacerbations, and so the documentation of either may occasionally prove useful when equivocal results are obtained from ventilatory function tests. The optimum period for demonstrating blood eosinophilia can vary between 6 and 24 hours after challenge exposure, and so we recommend that samples be drawn shortly before each morning challenge exposure and again after 6 to 8 hours and 24 hours. Blood eosinophilia is best demonstrated by absolute eosinophil counts but an automated total white count plus differential is less costly and often adequate. Late (but not immediate) asthmatic reactions also tend to increase nonspecific bronchial reactivity, though this is not easily detected if the reaction is mild. Increased methacholine or histamine reactivity following a series of antigen challenge tests may consequently provide further evidence of the test antigen's relevance.

Contraindications

Assuming informed consent is obtained, the only major contraindication to inhalation provocation tests in the laboratory is severely impaired lung function. When baseline FEV_1 exceeds 70% of the predicted level, the protocol outlined is acceptably safe. When baseline levels are in the range 50 to 70% of predicted, extra caution should be exercised. Sequential challenge exposures should involve no more than 2-fold increments, and closer medical supervision should be provided so that unequivocally positive responses can be reversed with medication at the earliest moment. When baseline levels are less than 40% of predicted, provocation tests can rarely be justified.

A lesser problem is the need for continuing medication. Effective levels will clearly exert a masking effect on a triggering stimulus, while discontinuing medication may in some cases lead to unacceptably poor ventilatory function. Occupational exposure should cease, and provocation tests should be postponed until maximum recovery has occurred. When this is achieved, medication should be slowly reduced under the monitoring surveillance of regular measurements of PEF to the minimum level compatible with reasonable comfort and adequate baseline lung function (FEV_1 more than 50% of predicted). Antigen and control challenges should then be carried out under identical conditions; identical timing of medications, chamber exposures, and monitoring tests being particularly crucial. In these circumstances, sequential increases in antigen challenge exposure can be expected to provoke a significant effect if the antigen is a truly relevant factor.

Illustrative Examples

Dust Challenge—Ampicillin and Related Antibiotics[11]. Occupational asthma due to airborne dusts of ampicillin, benzyl penicillin and the intermediate product 6-aminopenicillanic acid (6-APA) was first described in 1974. Extensive use of chamber inhalation tests on three affected workers selected from different sections of a production line manufacturing ampicillin from benzyl penicillin showed that each gave reproducible late asthmatic reactions to com-

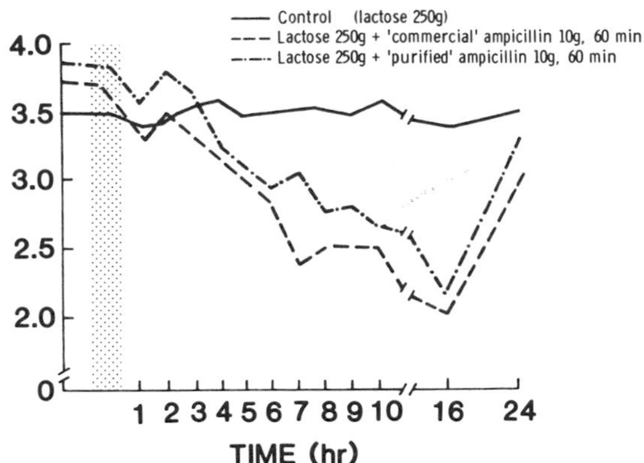

Fig. 6-4 Inhalation tests in a 39-year-old ampicillin worker, using "commercial" and "purified" samples of ampicillin. (From Davies RJ, Hendrick DJ, Pepys J: Asthma due to inhaled chemical agents: Ampicillin, benzyl penicillin, 6-aminopenicillenic acid and related substances. Clin Allergy 4:227, 1974.)

mercial samples of the particular antibiotic with which he worked. A second series of tests were then carried out to determine whether contaminants or the antibiotics themselves were responsible. In the ampicillin and benzyl penicillin workers, further challenges with purified samples provoked responses of undiminished severity (Fig. 6-4), whereas challenge (in the ampicillin worker) with a potent antigenic degradation product contaminating penicillins, benzyl penicilloic acid conjugated to polylysine, produced no response. The benzyl penicillin worker was also tested with commercial ampicillin (which differs structurally from benzyl penicillin only by a —NH_2 substitution for —H on the phenyl acetyl side chain), and a similar positive response was observed. When, however, both ampicillin and benzyl penicillin workers were tested with 6-aminopenicillanic acid (the antigenic configuration of the latter is markedly different from the two other penicillins, because of deletion of the phenyl acetyl side chain), little or no response was noted, irrespective of purification. These results identified the antibiotics themselves as the etiologic agents.

Tests in the 6-aminopenicillanic acid worker produced contrary results. Similar responses were observed to commercial samples of all three antibiotics, whereas little or no response was noted following challenge with purified samples (Fig. 6-5). A contaminant therefore appeared to be responsible, but tests involving benzl penicilloyl polylysine, 6-aminopenicillanic protein impurities and *Escherichia coli* amidase (used in the biologic degradation of benzyl penicillin) were negative.

Vapor Challenge—Toluene Diisocyanate (TDI). Commercially prepared TDI is a 4:1 mixture of two isomers, 2,4-TDI and 2,6-TDI. The 2,4 isomer is the most active chemically, and it is to 2,4-TDI only that current occupational exposure standards apply. TDI is used primarily for making polyurethane, and the more reactive 2,4-TDI is incorporated disproportionately in the foam produced. As a result, TDI exposure in polyurethane plants may predominantly involve unreacted 2,6-TDI; our recent measurements having shown proportions of up to 1:10, 2,4-TDI: 2,6-TDI (R. Rando, personal communication). It is consequently of some importance to investigate the re-

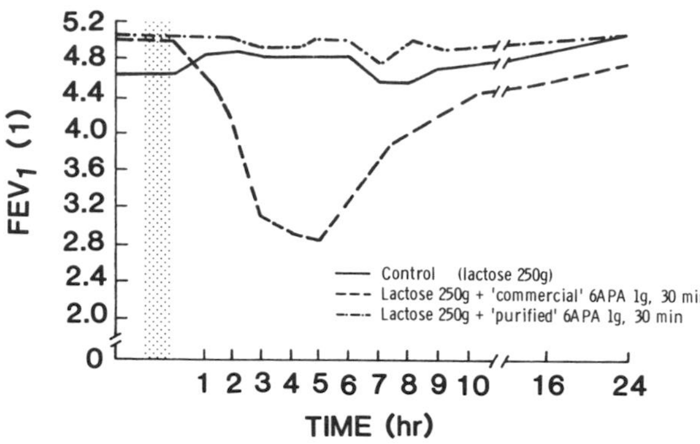

Fig. 6-5 Inhalation tests in a 26-year-old 6-APA worker, using "commercial" and "purified" samples of 6-APA. (From Davies RJ, Hendrick DJ, Pepys J: Asthma due to inhaled chemical agents: Ampicillin, benzyl penicillin, 6-aminopenicillenic acid and related substances. Clin Allergy 4:227, 1974.)

spective biologic potencies of these two isomers. Figure 6-6 shows the results of inhalation provocation tests that address this question in a worker exposed to TDI in its manufacture. His responses to the usual production mixture of TDI and pure 2,6-TDI were identical, providing preliminary evidence that the biologic affects of these two isomers are comparable. Further similar studies will be needed before current regulatory standards can be applied with equal confidence to all types of occupational exposure to TDI.

An additional question of possible importance to TDI exposure standards in the polyurethane industry, concerns concomitant exposure to respirable catalysts used in various foaming processes. The volatile tertiary amine, N-ethyl morpholine, for instance, may be used to produce polyester-based polyurethane. At present it is considered a mild respiratory irritant only, and workplace levels up to 5 ppm are permitted. It is not known whether it could

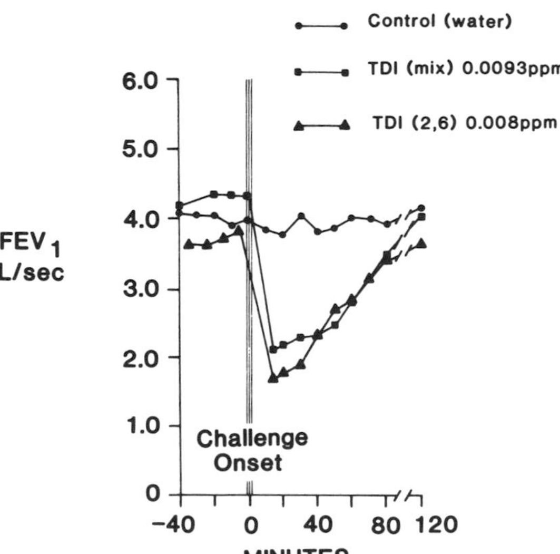

Fig. 6-6 Inhalation tests in a 41-year-old TDI worker, using the usual TDI isomer mix (80% 2,4-TDI: 20% 2,6-TDI) and pure 2,6-TDI.

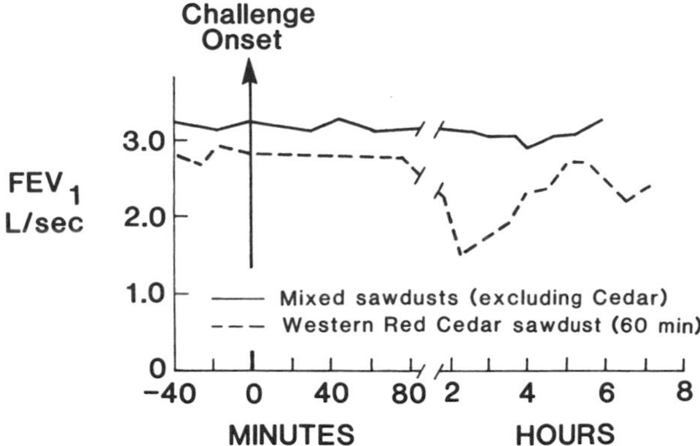

Fig. 6-7 Inhalation tests in a 54-year-old carpenter, using mixed sawdusts (excluding cedar) and western red cedar. (From Hendrick DJ, Jones RN, Weill H: Occupational lung disease. In Current Pulmonology. Vol 3, ed. Simmons DH. New York, Wiley, 1981. Reprinted by permission of John Wiley & Sons, Inc.)

augment the biologic effects of TDI when the two are inhaled together, but this does not seem to be an unreasonable consideration. The answer should be readily obtained from a series of inhalation provocation tests involving TDI sensitive polyurethane workers if challenges are carried out with TDI alone, N-ethyl morpholine alone, and the two together at known carefully controlled concentrations.

Dust Challenge—Wood Dusts[12]. Asthma in wood workers is a common occupational disorder, but different species have different antigenic potencies, and occasionally an occupation can be pursued without hazard simply by avoiding the particular species responsible for symptoms. Figure 6-7 illustrates the results of inhalation provocation tests in such a case, the carpenter in question having developed sensitivity to western red cedar alone.

Aerosol Challenge—Pigeon Antigen Solution[13]. This case illustrates the value of inhalation provocation tests when there are two possible etiologic agents in a worker's environment. The subject, a carpenter, related his increasing disability from asthma to occupational exposures to wood dust, but the history was not fully convincing (it did not suggest immediate type hypersensitivity) and it transpired he was also a pigeon fancier. Figure 6-8 shows the results of inhalation provocation tests which confirmed asthmatic (but not parenchymal) hypersensitivity to pigeon serum. With this evidence he gave up his birds and continued with his job. He recovered fully within six months, losing in addition a troublesome rhinitis and an intriguing hoarseness.

Conclusions

The techniques outlined, together with the illustrative examples, indicate how agents responsible for occupational asthma may be identified with a high degree of confidence. There are, however, limitations to their use which should be recognized. Inhalation provocation tests are time-consuming and potentially hazardous if not conducted responsibly, and not every worker is a suitable test subject. Results are not always easily interpreted, especially if tests are carried out many months after occupational exposure ceases (when hypersensitivity

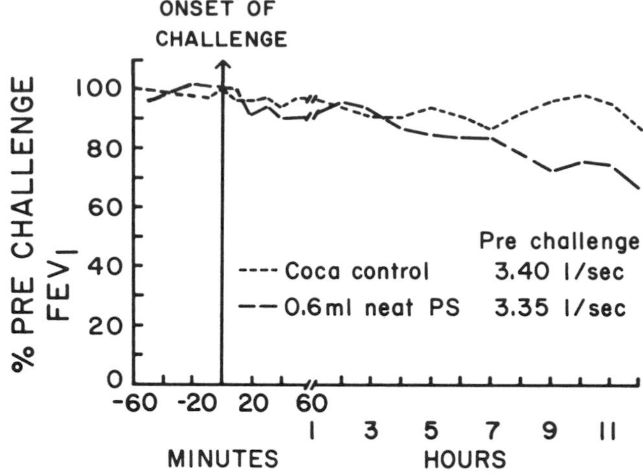

Fig. 6-8 Inhalation tests in a 37-year-old carpenter and pigeon fancier, using nebulized pigeon serum.

may have diminished or resolved), or if evidence of active asthma persists outside the workplace. In the latter circumstances, carefully conducted control studies are of crucial importance. Strict control of the challenge exposure is also of crucial importance, and the benefit of industrial hygiene measurements in both the workplace and the laboratory cannot be overstressed.

IMPLICATIONS

When investigations identify an agent as an inducer of occupational asthma, a number of implications should be recognized. The affected worker may feel obliged to seek redress and the investigating physician must be prepared to defend his or her diagnosis in the courts. The physician may also need to testify before regulatory bodies responsible for exposure standards in the workplace. Legislation for occupational lung disease is usually based on the results of epidemiologic studies that consider prevalence, incidence, and severity and their relationships with exposure to the inducing agent. For occupational asthma, legislated standards are not yet practical, since dose–response relationships vary greatly from individual to individual, and it is rarely economically feasible to limit exposure to levels that will prevent sensitization in all workers. Fortunately, the effects of occupational asthma are rarely life threatening, and in most cases symptoms regress if occupational exposure ceases promptly. In these circumstances, society must decide what prevalence is acceptable in the workforce at risk, with due regard to the economic viability of the production process involved.

Once an occupational asthma has been diagnosed, the worker should, ideally, avoid further exposure to the agent concerned. Otherwise there is a risk that asthma may persist, even when exposure to the initial inducing agent ceases. Duration of this exposure may be an important factor influencing outcome,[14] although some affected workers appear to be able to continue to work without undue difficulty providing continuing exposure is minimized (industrial hygiene is improved, the specific job is modified) and appropriate treatment is readily available. Important personal considerations are job satisfaction and the availability of alternative employment, and in certain cases these may outweigh the physician's concern over long-term risks. If the affected worker does choose to return to work this should be recognized as one further potential risk. Accidents can occur even in the best run factories, and the potential exists for spills or emissions involving massive exposures which could present a threat to life.

The choice of continuing employment should not, of course, lie with the affected worker alone, and at times it may be the employer who declines to permit continuing exposure. Not all employers are able (or willing) to relocate affected workers in sites of negligible exposure, and some jobs are lost as a result. Fear of this may understandably make the affected worker reluctant to report illness, both to the physician and to the employer. However, it is only when all involved parties are fully aware of the facts that the most appropriate form of management can be followed for the affected individual, and proper protective controls introduced for the other workers.

REFERENCES

1. Figley KD, Elrod RM: Endemic asthma due to castor bean dust. JAMA, 90:79, 1928.
2. Salvaggio JE, ed: Occupational and environmental respiratory disease. In: NIAID Task Force Report: Asthma and Other Allergic Diseases. Patterson R, Task Force Chairman. US Department of Health, Education and Welfare, NIH Publication 79-387, May 1979.
3. Davies RJ, Butcher BT, O'Neil CE, Salvaggio JE: The in vitro effect of toluene diisocyanate on lymphocyte cyclic adenosine monophosphate production by isoproterenol, prostaglandin and histamine—A possible mode of action. J Allergy Clin Immunol 60:223, 1977.
4. Carroll KB, Secombe CJ, Pepys J: Asthma due to non-occupational exposure to toluene (tolylene) diisocyanate. Clin Allergy 6:99, 1976.
5. Kumar P, Marier R, Leech SH: Hypersensitivity pneumonitis due to contamination of a car air conditioner. N Engl J Med 305:1531–1532, 1981.
6. Hammad Y, Corn M, Dharmarajan V: Environmental characterization. In: Occupational Lung Diseases, Research Approaches and Methods, eds. Weill H, Turner-Warwick M. New York, Marcel Dekker, 1981.
7. Karr RM, Lehrer SB, Butcher BT, Salvaggio JE: Coffee workers' asthma: A clinical appraisal using the radioallergosorbent test. J Allergy Clin Immunol 62:143, 1978.
8. Zeiss CR, Patterson R, Pruzansky JJ, et al: Trimellitic anhydride-induced airway syndromes. Clinical and immunologic studies. J Allergy Clin Immunol 60:96, 1977.
9. Nelson GO: Controlled Test Atmospheres, Principles and Techniques. Ann Arbor, MI, Ann Arbor Science, 1980.
10. Willeke K, ed: Generation of Aerosols and Facilities for Exposure Experiments. Ann Arbor, MI, Ann Arbor Science, 1980.
11. Davies RJ, Hendrick DJ, Pepys J: Asthma due to inhaled chemical agents: Ampicil-

lin, benzyl penicillin, 6-aminopenicillenic acid and related substances. Clin Allergy 4:227–247, 1974.
12. Hendrick DJ, Jones RN, Weill H: Occupational lung disease. In: Current Pulmonology, vol 3, ed. Simmons DH. New York, Wiley, 1981.
13. Hendrick DJ: Bird fancier's lung—Clinical, epidemiological and laboratory features. MD thesis, University of London, 1979.
14. Chan-Yeung M, Lam S, Koerner S. Clinical features and natural history of occupational asthma due to western red cedar (*Thuja plicata*). Am J Med 72:411, 1982.

7 Occupational Lung Disease in the Rural Environment

Guillermo A. doPico

Working in a rural environment has been long regarded as a healthy mode of life, yet clinical and epidemiologic observations indicate that farming, animal raising, and forestry are hazardous occupations. The risk extends to those involved in the processing, stocking, transporting, handling, and inspecting of agricultural, animal, and forestry products as well as to veterinarians. Technological advances, chemical and mechanical, are being applied ever more intensely in plant cultivation, animal raising, and forestry. The industrialization of rural occupations has resulted in new hazards that need to be recognized and prevented.

The hazards include exposure to a variety of agents that can cause lung disease by inhalation or by the circulation following dermal or intestinal absorption (Table 7-1). Some agents, e.g., neurotoxic chemicals, can cause respiratory failure by respiratory muscle paralysis without initial lung damage. Other inhaled agents cause cellular respiratory failure in other organs by interfering with oxygen transport or disrupting cellular enzymes.

Inhalation injury may result in airways reaction (bronchitis, asthma, and/or bronchiolitis) or in parenchymal reaction (alveolitis and/or pulmonary edema), which may be acute or chronic, reversible or irreversible, progressive, stable, or regressive (Fig. 7-1). Some exposures lead to characteristic symptoms with an identifiable etiology, therapy, and prevention for example, silo fillers' disease. Other agents cause less specific morbidity patterns with ill-defined pathogenesis, e.g., chronic expectoration in nonsmoking dairy farmers.

Table 7-1. Occupational Hazards in Rural Environment

Physical	Heat, cold, solar radiation, medication, lightning Man–machine interactions: accidents, vibration, noise Fatigue, effort, posture
Organic dusts (noninfectious)	Vegetable origin: grains, hay, pollen, cotton, wood Animal dander: hair, feathers, skin Fungi and bacteria antigens and toxins Insects and mites antigens
Chemicals	Pesticides (see Table 5-4) Fertilizers Antibiotics in animal feed
Toxic gases	From liquid manure: H_2S, NH_3, CH_4, CO_2 From vegetable matter: NO_2, CO_2 From gasoline-powered machines: CO
Oxygen deprivation	In sealed silos Animal confinement units Manure and septic tanks Drowning in silage, grain
Infectious agents	Animal related: viral, bacterial, parasitic, rickettsial Fungi: *Histoplasma, Blastomyces, Cryptococcus, Coccidioides, Sporotrichum*
Carcinogens	Aflatoxin: liver and lung cancer? Bovine leukosarcoma virus? leukemia? Pesticides?
Inorganic dusts	Silicates, asbestos, other natural fibers, silica Mt. St. Helen's ash (hazard?)
Psychological stresses	

The incidence of farm accident-related deaths is second only to that in the construction industry. There are 2000 deaths per year from accidents and 200,000 disabling injuries[1] including rib fractures, lung contusions, flail chests, and acute respiratory distress syndromes requiring intensive medical care. The

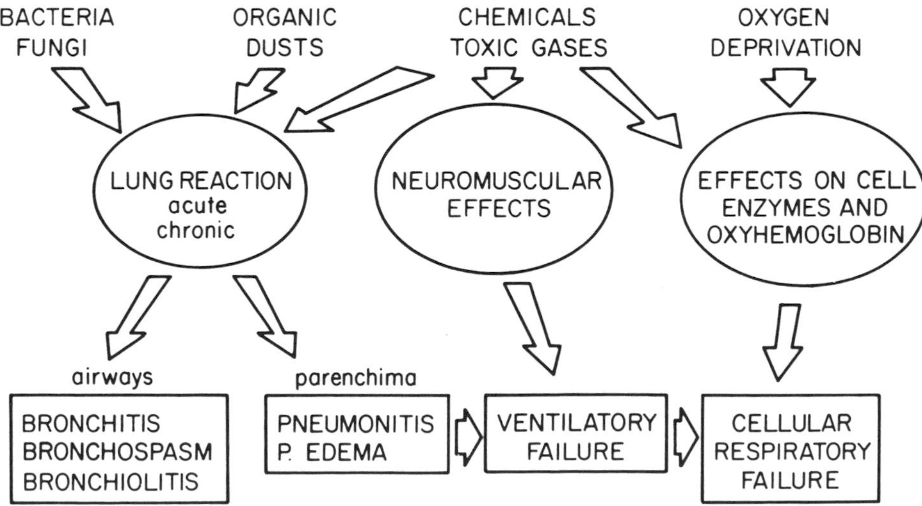

Fig. 7-1 Health effects of rural environmental hazards.

causes of farm accidents are multiple: fatigue, working under pressure, weather, illness, inexperience, poor equipment, insufficient awareness of risks and safety measures, and carelessness.

The population at risk is diverse and disperse. In the United States an estimated 12 million people live and work on over 3 million farms.[2] There is, in addition, a large population exposed to unprocessed agricultural, animal, and forestry products who may suffer from the same diseases as farmers. In rural communities environmental contamination by farming products may show health effects. Others at risk are government employees such as grain inspectors, researchers, buyers, gardeners, game keepers, river and forest keepers, veterinarians, and persons involved in building, supply, and servicing of farm operations.

EPIDEMIOLOGIC ASPECTS

Farmers, according to Wan and Wright,[3] have the highest prevalence of disabling respiratory diseases of any occupational group in the United States (22 per 100,000). The age-adjusted respiratory death rate for 1968–1972 in Vermont, primarily a rural state, was appreciably higher than the comparable 1970 United States rates for the white population. The male respiratory death rate was excessive in all categories (cancer, emphysema, pneumonia, influenza, and bronchitis).[4] Among Vermont dairy farmers, smokers had more respiratory symptoms than nonsmokers, and farmers reported chronic sputum production and dyspnea with greater frequency (25 and 40%) than non-mineral industry workers.[5]

In California 3 million farm laborers are employed by commercial farms involved in high output, energy-intensive agriculture. In this population, the mortality rate from respiratory disease in the farm laborer group (employees) tripled the rate of the management group.[6] Pneumonia was the predominant cause. Working and living conditions, climate, nutrition, and the increased use of chemicals may contribute to the rising death rate.

Among doctors, firefighters, farmers, and petrochemical workers in Ontario, Canada, farmers had the lowest FEV_1/FVC ratios, the highest prevalence of asthma and the second highest prevalence of chronic bronchitis.[7] Warren[8] found that 55% of Manitoba cattle farmers had cough and dyspnea related to moldy crop handling. One hour after exposure to moldy crop 9% of the farmers had fever and symptoms consistent with farmers' lung disease; 18% had attacks of wheezing with shortness of breath consistent with occupational asthma, 19% of the nonsmokers had chronic bronchitis, and 24% of the farmers had abnormal FEV_1/FVC ratio.

A group of petrochemical workers and farmers from a rural medical practice in the United Kingdom had a comparable frequency of chronic cough and expectoration and dyspnea. One third of the farmers had symptoms when handling hay.[9] In Switzerland among 500 asthma clinic patients, farmers had the highest mortality and worst pulmonary functions.[10]

In developed countries the respiratory diseases of importance for farmers are farmers' lung disease, asthma due to grain dust, silo fillers' disease, chronic bronchitis, and swine confinement exposure disease.

ORGANIC DUST-INDUCED DISEASES

Hypersensitivity Pneumonitis

Hypersensitivity pneumonitis or allergic alveolitis is a diffuse fibrosing interstitial inflammatory disease of the lung due to an allergic reaction to inhaled organic dusts. Diagnosis can be made by the combination of appropriate clinical, physiologic, radiographic, pathologic, and immunologic features, following a specific exposure to organic dusts derived from fungal, bacterial, or serum protein sources (Table 7-2). No single clinical feature or laboratory test is diagnostic of the disease. There is a wide variety of agents that can induce hypersensitivity pneumonitis in workers handling agricultural, animal, or forestry products in a wide variety of occupational settings (Table 7-2). One of the most common and extensively studied hypersensitivity pneumonitis is farmers' lung disease.

Farmers' Lung Disease

Farmers' lung disease is a hypersensitivity pneumonitis induced by the inhalation of moldy hay, fodder, and grain, moldy shredding or threshing dusts, and moldy vegetable dusts.[11] The exposures occur during forking out moldy bales of hay, threshing poor quality grains, or sweeping out closed barns that

Table 7-2. Hypersensitivity Pneumonitides Due to Organic Dusts In Agriculture and Related Industries

Disease/Occupation	Exposure/Material	Specific Antigen
Farmer's lung	Moldy hay, grain	*Micropolyspora faeni*
		Thermoactinomyces sp.
Bagassosis	Moldy sugar cane	*Thermoactinomyces* sp.
Malt workers	Moldy sprouting barley	*Aspergillus clavatus*
Wood workers	Moldy maple logs	*Cryptostoma corticale*
	Moldy logs	*Alternaria* sp., *Rhizopus* sp.
		Saccharomonospora viridis
	Moldy redwood sawdust	*Graphium* sp.,
		Aureo basidium sp.
Suberosis	Moldy cork	*Penicillium frequentans*
Mushroom workers	Mushroom compost	*Actinomycetes*
	Mushroom spores	*Pleurotus florida*
Bird breeders	Bird droppings	Avian proteins
pigeons, parakeets,	Dander	Feathers
chicken, turkeys	Feathers	
Rodent handlers	Urine, dander	Rodent protein
Cheese washers	Moldy cheeses	*Penicillium casei*
Vineyard sprayers	$CuSO_4$, hydrated lime	Unknown

may have contained moldy corn bedding. Improper storage of crops harvested in rainy weather in closed barns and silos will undergo self-heating, which favors the growth of thermophilic actinomycetes. These bacteria proliferate rapidly at 40–60°C. The hay gradually dries and the bale becomes discolored, dry, friable, and extremely dusty in one or two weeks. When a farmer breaks open these dry bales in the confines of a cow shed, the spore concentration may reach 1.6×10^9 spores/m^3 [12] and a man doing light work in this environment may retain an estimated 7.5×10^5 spores/min in his lungs.[13] The most abundant microorganisms found in moldy hay dusts are *Micropolyspora faeni* spores, the principal cause of farmers' lung disease in Britain[14,15] and in Wisconsin.[16] Elsewhere, other microorganisms have been incriminated, e.g., *Aspergillus* species in Finland.[17]

Epidemiology. Farmers' lung disease occurs in Europe and North America. Although true prevalence of the disease is unknown, in agricultural populations of the northern and midwestern states of the United States it is estimated to afflict 2 to 7 per 1000 farmers,[18] and in the United Kingdom 0 to 57 per 1000 farmers.[19,20] The high prevalence of 30/1000 farmers in Wyoming[21] is questionable, since positive serology occurs only in 5/1000. These prevalence rates are from survey studies that are difficult to compare and interpret because they utilized different criteria for identifying cases, epidemiologic designs, questionnaires, and sample selection. The methods and antigens for precipitin detection were not standardized in all surveys and in suspicious cases other confirmatory diagnostic features were not uniformly sought. Furthermore, the delayed symptoms of fever and dyspnea after exposure to agricultural dust, on which a prevalence rate for farmers' lung is based may not be due to allergic pneumonitis but to nonspecific febrile reactions without pneumonitis, e.g., grain fever.

Clinical Features. The *acute syndrome* is characterized by chills, fever up to 106°F, cough, dyspnea, myalgia, and malaise 3 to 8 hours after exposure to a variety of moldy farm dust (Table 7-3). Commonly fever, chills, and malaise would predominate and only when they subside and the farmer attempts to return to work, is dyspnea on mild exertion noticeable. At times, dyspnea and breathlessness are the striking initial symptoms.[22,23] The sputa are usually neither copious nor purulent, but hemoptysis occasionally occurs. Frequently the initial episode is not recognized by the farmer or his physician as farmers' lung disease and relapse often occurs on return to the same working environment.

Cyanosis may occur and classic inspiratory crackles are audible, usually not accompanied by wheezes or signs of consolidation. Provided further exposure is avoided, the acute symptoms usually subside spontaneously within 7 to 10 days but dyspnea may persist for months. Polymorphonuclear leukocytosis is frequently present. The usual radiographic features vary according to the duration and severity of the illness. The usual findings are generalized, diffuse, interstitial pneumonitis with fine nodular, reticular, or reticulonodular pattern with patchy areas of consolidation which may be confused with bacterial pneumonia.[22] A pattern resembling pulmonary edema can be seen in severe cases. The conglomerate densities tend to clear within a week or two, but the accentuation of the parenchymal markings may persist longer. A normal chest roent-

Table 7-3. Differential Characteristics of Acute Inhalation Diseases in Farmers

	Farmers' Lung	Silo Fillers' Dis.		Grain Fever	Mycotoxicosis	Grain Dust Asthma
Exposure	Moldy hay	Silo gas		Grain dust (large dose)	Moldy dust (large dose)	Grain dust
		Early	Late			
Onset after exposure	4–8 hours	Immediate or hours	Days or weeks	Immediate or hours	During or hours	Immediate or hours
Symptoms	Dyspnea, fever, chills, cough myalgias	Dyspnea cough	Dyspnea cough	Fever, chills myalgias	Fever, chills myalgias	Wheezing, chest tightness, dyspnea, cough
Radiologic findings	Diffuse, nodular; patchy consolidation	Pulmonary edema	Miliary pattern	Normal	Normal or reticulonodular	Normal
Function tests				(w/o asthma)		
VC	↓	↓	↓	0	0 or ↓	↓
RV/TLC	0	0	↑	0	—	↑
FEV_1/FVC	0	0	0	0	0	↓
$\dot{V}_{max\ 50}$	0 or ↓	?	↓	0	0 or ↓	↓
R_{aw}	0	0	0	0	0	↑
SG_{aw}	0	0	↓	0	0	↓
CL	↓	↓	↓	0	0 or ↓	0
DLco	↓	↓	↓	0	0 or ↓	0
Skin tests	Irritant effect	Not done		− or +	?	− or +
Bronchial challenge	Late, ↓DL, ↓VC, ↑WBC, fever	Not done		Late ↑WBC, fever, no Δ in DL	?	Immediate or late, ↓FEV_1, ↑R_{aw}, ↓$\dot{V}_{50}$
Etiologic agent	*M. faeni* *T. vulgaris*	Nitrous dioxide		?	Mycotoxins? Endotoxins? Proteases?	Grains, mites, insects, fungi
Pathologic finding	Alveolitis Granulomas Fibrosis	Pulmonary edema	Bronchiolitis obliterans	?	Alveolitis or none?	?
BAL	↑% lymphs ↑T/B cells	?		?	↑% neutrophils	?

genogram does not exclude the diagnosis of farmers' lung. In two reported patients lung biopsies were positive when radiographic findings had returned to normal.[22]

Pulmonary function tests reveal loss of lung volumes, decreased compliance, reduced diffusing capacity for carbon monoxide, hypoxemia, and hyperventilation.[23] The FEV_1/FVC ratio and airways resistance are usually normal, but evidence of small airways dysfunction can be recognized.[24] Most of these abnormalities are reversible.

Chronic disease develops insidiously with dyspnea on exertion, malaise, weight loss, fatigue, and unproductive cough. The most striking symptom is the breathlessness on exertion. Chronic interstitial pneumonitis may develop following subclinical or mildly manifested symptoms or after recurrent overtly symptomatic exposures to moldy material. Some farmers reported being sick from fall until spring when stored forage is fed to animals, experiencing some relief during the summer months.[22,23] The chest radiographs are indistinguishable from idiopathic diffuse fibrosing alveolitis. Hilar adenopathy does not occur and pleural changes are rarely seen. Physiologically the most common pattern is restrictive, with reduced VC, DLco and lung compliance and increased RV/TLC ratio without airflow obstruction.[23] Others show airflow obstruction or a combined pattern, restrictive and obstructed.[22] In some cases of airflow obstruction, the compliance is high suggesting emphysema.[24]

Pathologic Features. The histologic changes depend upon the intensity of the antigenic exposure and the stage of the disease at the time of the biopsy. Alveolitis characterized by interstitial alveolar infiltrates consisting of lymphocytes, plasma cells, activated macrophages, and occasional polymorphonuclear eosinophils are uniformly present while intraalveolar granulomas are found in about 70% of the biopsies.[25] Absence of granulomas does not exclude the diagnosis of farmer's lung disease. Interstitial fibrosis is common but usually not severe and mild bronchiolitis obliterans was often present. Vasculitis is not a common feature,[25] but has been reported.[26]

In the chronic stages, the histologic changes may be undistinguishable from other pulmonary fibroses.

Although immunofluorescence studies in hypersensitivity pneumonitis continue to be unrewarding,[27] they have demonstrated actinomycetes antigen in the bronchiolar walls and IgG, IgA, and IgM and complement products in the granulomatous lesions.[28]

Immunologic Parameters. There is no single immunologic laboratory test diagnostic for the disease but serum precipitins to the offending antigen is deemed necessary to diagnosis. Serum precipitating antibodies to moldy hay or to thermoactinomyces can be easily detected by conventional Ouchterlony double immunodiffusion.[29] Although in Britain and the United States serum *M. faeni* antibodies have correlated with symptoms of farmers' lung,[29,30] it is now accepted that serum precipitins are not in themselves evidence of disease. In rural populations the prevalence of precipitins to *M. faeni* varies from 3 to 18%,[21,30,31] and to *Thermoactinomyces vulgaris* 0.8 to 11%. In urban populations and in grain handlers the prevalence of antibodies to these organisms is about 1 to 3%.[32,33] In both farmers and office workers[32,34] no discernible significant difference in radiologic or pulmonary function were found between those with precipitins and those without. Precipitins are present during the first year in nearly all cases of farmers' lung disease, but the incidence falls 50% during the second to fifth year after the exposure ceases.[35] The long-term presence of precipitins suggests continued exposure and their detection may be useful in evaluating preventive measures and clinical follow-up. The diagnostic usefulness of precipitin detection is impaired by the poor standardization of the available extracts of actinomycetes species.

There has been an intensive search for a laboratory test that will identify patients with farmers' lung disease rather than the asymptomatic, precipitin-positive farmer. None of the many tests or assays developed appear to discriminate between disease and mere sensitization without disease. New methods have improved the detection and quantitation of precipitating antibodies and have demonstrated the complexity of the *M. faeni* antigen. These and other tests for cell-mediated immunity, response to mitogens, serum complement levels, angiotensin converting enzyme, and intradermal skin tests have limited diagnostic precision for farmers' lung disease.[36] Of the more recent tests, the ELISA (enzyme-linked immunosorbent assay) is said to be a sensitive, specific, and quantitative test.[37] It correlated better with the clinical diagnosis than the Ouchterlony double immunodiffusion technique. However, although those with farmers' lung had significantly higher ELISA values, symptomatic farmers and controls also had detectable levels. Because of its greater sensitivity and quantitative value the ELISA[37] could be useful for early diagnosis or for recognition of continued exposure to the agent in prospective studies. The small number of negative ELISA with weakly positive precipitins may be due to classes of antibody other than IgG such as IgA or perhaps IgM.[38]

Serum levels of IgG, IgA, and IgM are elevated, but IgE levels are usually normal. Skin tests with actinomycetes preparation cause nonspecific reactions.

Course. Recovery from the acute episode occurs in most patients. However, continued subclinical reexposure to the antigen or numerous subacute episodes of pneumonitis can lead to interstitial fibrosis and disability and in some instances to chronic obstructive pulmonary disease.[39] Death rates of 9 to 17% attributable to chronic farmers' lung have been reported.[39,40] In a long-term (2 to 40 years) follow-up study of 92 patients, breathlessness and chronic bronchitis were reported by 20 and 28% of the patients.[39] Radiographically 39% had some evidence of interstitial changes. Evidence of airways obstruction by FEV_1/FVC ratios was present in 25%, abnormal DLco in 30%, and hypoxemia in 40% of the patients. More than 50% of nonsmokers had abnormal $\dot{V}_{max\ 50}$, and $\dot{V}_{max\ 75}$. These abnormalities were mild and most patients did well even if they had remained on the farm. The degree of pulmonary function impairment correlated with a history of five or more symptomatic recurrences and the persistence of precipitins but not with continuing farming or the duration of disease.[39]

Diagnosis. In most cases the characteristic clinical, physiologic, and radiologic findings and the presence of serum precipitins to moldy hay and thermoactinomycetes suffice to diagnose farmers' lung disease. Conclusive evidence of farmers' lung disease can be obtained by demonstrating the typical granulomatous alveolitis by transbronchial or open lung biopsy or by inducing the clinicophysiologic syndrome by bronchial provocation test. These tests, however, are invasive and not without risks and the success of the latter depends upon administering an adequate dose of the appropriate antigen, factors that are not always well defined. The analysis of bronchoalveolar lavage fluid eventually may prove helpful in establishing the diagnosis and the activity of the allergic alveolitis. In this disease, bronchoalveolar lavage fluid show an increased proportion of lymphocytes[41] and mast cells[42] with higher T/B cell ratios and high IgG and IgM levels.[41]

Pathogenesis. The detailed pathogenesis is unknown but a current hypothesis ascribes the activation of the alveolar macrophage a central role in the production of the inflammatory granuloma (Fig. 7-2). The initial inflammatory reactions to organic dust could be nonspecific activation of the alternative complement pathway as well as a nonspecific adjuvant effect with subsequent generation of chemotactic factors attracting neutrophils and also recruiting and activating macrophages. Enzymes released from macrophages can lead to more chemotactic products and cleavage of C3 resulting in further recruitment and activation of macrophages and inflammatory cells. Hydrolases and oxidases from macrophages and neutrophils could cause tissue damage. Immunologically specific events would be also operative. Antigens in organic dust cause B

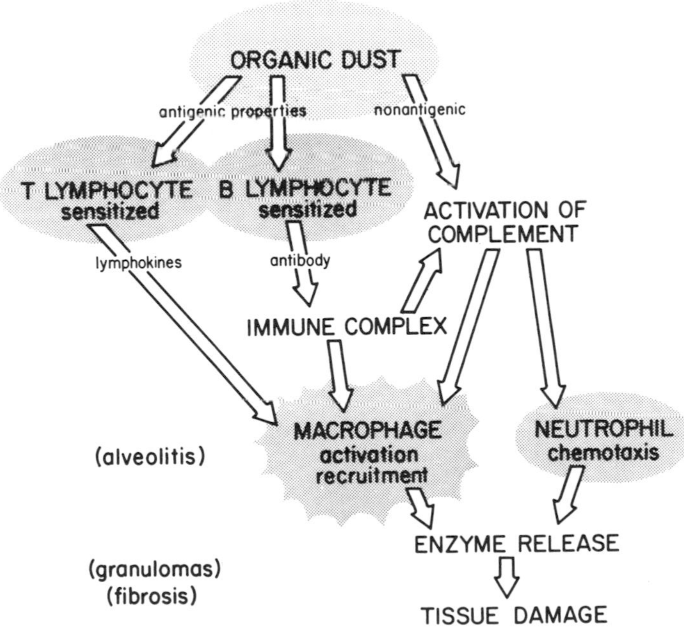

Fig. 7-2 Postulated events in the pathogenesis of farmers' lung disease.

lymphocytes and plasma cells to produce antibodies. Continued or recurrent inhalation of the antigen would result in immune complexes which activate macrophages when ingested. There is evidence that lymphokines from sensitized T cells produce further macrophage activation.

Prevention and Therapy. Avoidance of the antigen is the treatment of choice. In severe cases supplemental oxygen and prednisone may aid in symptomatic relief; 60–80 mg of prednisone daily for 7–10 days until the hypoxemia improves is justified. Long-term steroids are not advisable because they will hide the symptoms in the reexposed patients and do not necessarily prevent the development of lung lesions.

Before the farmer returns to his farm work, the moldy material must be thoroughly wetted down and totally removed by someone other than the victim. Adequate drying of hay and grain before bailing and storage is the most effective approach. In regions of high rainfall, equipment to dry the material is available but expensive. Face dust masks can be recommended but farmers seldom wear them. Masks tight enough to filter 1-μm spores impose too much airway resistance to air flow to be practical. It would seem reasonable to recommend that patients with recurrent episodes be urged to leave the farm, but the advice should take into consideration that farmers can continue to work without problems, without pulmonary function deterioration, or disabling disease and that for socioeconomic and psychological reasons, most farmers find it extremely difficult to discontinue farming. Mechanization of certain farm chores and assignment of dusty jobs to others are very effective measures in our experience.

Bird Breeders' Lung Disease

Hypersensitivity pneumonitis can result from exposure to dust from bird droppings and feathers containing avian proteins from pigeons, parakeets, parrots, turkeys, and chickens.

The reported prevalence of pigeon breeders' disease varied from 1 in 1000[44] to 21 in 100 breeders.[45] A history consistent with hypersensitivity pneumonitis has been found in 6% of 200 workers engaged in raising or processing turkeys.[46] After prolonged exposure to chickens 20% of 58 chicken farmers reported chest tightness and cough[47] and 69% of 200 turkey workers in Utah reported pulmonary symptoms, in 6% the history was consistent with allergic alveolitis, but none had restrictive lung disease.[46] The prevalence of respiratory symptoms associated with bird exposure in turkey raisers appears to be slightly higher than that observed in persons exposed to chickens or pigeons.[46]

As in farmers' lung disease the presence of precipitins to avian proteins or feathers is found in both those who have the clinical syndrome of hypersensitivity pneumonitis and a percentage of exposed but asymptomatic workers. Based on a case study of hypersensitivity to chicken feathers, Warren and Tse[48] suggested that precipitins in bronchial washings may offer a better diagnostic specificity than serum precipitins. The subject had serum precipitins to chicken serum, feathers, and droppings and positive immediate and late intradermal skin tests to chicken serum and feathers. Bronchial washing contained only weak precipitins against chicken serum but strong precipitins against feathers. Inhalation provocation studies were positive to chicken feather but not to chicken serum.

Mushroom Workers' Disease

Respiratory disease associated with the cultivation of mushroom was first described in 16 Puerto Rican mushroom farm workers in Pennsylvania in 1951.[49] Since then cases have been reported from Britain,[50–52] Canada,[53,54] and the United States.[55,56]

The disease appears to be relatively uncommon, considering the large-scale mushroom production in Europe and North America.

Mushroom cultivation involves the preparation of compost from wheat, straw, and horse manure inside the growing houses or outdoors. In high humidity conditions, the decomposing organic material can reach temperatures of 165°F in the interior of the piles so facilitating the massive growth of thermotolerant fungi and thermophilic actinomycetes, which appear as a grey film impregnating the compost. If grown outdoors, the compost is brought indoors. During the sowing of the spawn the compost is mechanically mixed giving rise to dust and steam rich in actinomycetes spores. Random air samples in a spawning shed in Britain yielded a count of 700×10^6 spores/m^3.[52] The growing mushrooms are picked periodically for several weeks until the nutrients of the compost have been exhausted. The spent compost is then removed.

The disease had been found associated with laying down of fresh compost,[49] spawning,[50,52] or when dumping spent compost.[55]

The etiologic agent responsible for the hypersensitivity pneumonitis in mushroom workers is unknown. The source of the antigen may be in the vegetable and animal-derived particles of the compost, in the fungi and bacteria dust or in the spores of the mushrooms themselves. Because the disease resembles farmers' lung disease, the precipitins to *M. faeni* and *T. vulgaris* were in a few patients,[50] the disease was originally attributed to these fungi, which are however seldom isolated from mushroom compost. The most common actinomycetes bacteria in the dust is *Streptomyces diastaticus*.[57] Precipitants to other fungi, bacteria, mushroom spores, mushroom extracts, pasteurized compost, untreated compost, and compost after spawning,[51,52,54] have been found but none are common to all affected workers. Precipitins to mushroom compost are also found in persons without contact with mushroom compost.[54]

Acute symptoms of hypersensitivity pneumonitis have been found associated with the inhalation of spores of *Pleurotus florida,* a dual skin reaction to prick tests with spore extracts and serum precipitins against the organism.[58]

Inhalation provocation test with antigens from mushroom or compost after spawning[52] or extracts of thermophiles isolated from a spawning shed[51] have been negative except in a patient that reacted to mushroom compost extract.

The characteristic respiratory febrile syndrome of hypersensitivity pneumonitis occurs usually 4 to 6 hours after exposure, after days or months of symptom-free work in the industry. Occasionally, however, the symptoms can develop within a few hours of the first exposure.[52] No diagnostic serologic tests exists.

Chest radiographs show diffuse finely nodular changes in the mid to lower lung fields which may become confluent and ill-defined opacities.

Characteristic is the loss of lung volumes, impaired diffusing capacity for CO and hypoxemia. Chronic interstitial pneumonitis has been described.[56]

Avoidance of the offending material should prevent the recurrence of the disease. Improved ventilation in spawning houses and respirators may help decrease sensitization of workers. Bilingual education of the workers in the health hazards of the profession and medical surveillance programs are advisable, since recurrent unreported episodes of allergic alveolitis may lead to chronic interstitial lung disease.

Bagassosis

Bagassosis is manifested as a hypersensitivity pneumonitis following exposure to dust from stored bagasse. Bagasse is the fibrous cellulose of sugar cane stalk after its juice has been extracted by crushing compression. Stored bagasse, like other vegetable material, heats spontaneously, becoming a media for growth of many different species of thermophilic fungi and bacteria. Particularly abundant is the etiologic agent of bagassosis, *Thermoactinomyces sacchari*.[59] Risk of bagassosis exists when there is exposure to dry and moldy bagasse during transportation of stalks, compression operations, shredding the bales at factories, milling bagasse to desired partical size, manufacturing operations turning bagasse for cattle, or poultry bedding. Bagasse has many possible uses including the manufacture of paper, particle boards, and fiber boards for containers or insulation. Bagassosis has been reported in the southern United States, Britain, India, the Philippines, Spain, Italy, and the West Indies. The incidence of bagassosis has markedly decreased since measures to prevent the growth of bacteria and fungi have been introduced. These preventive measures include the application of 1% propionic acid to mill fresh bagasse before bailing,[60] the use of Ritter system, i.e., continuous moisturing of large, loose mounds of bagasse; grinding and shredding operations in the open; exhaust ventilation; and enclosure of machinery when feasible. High efficiency respirators may be worn when needed and tolerable.

Malt Workers' Lung

The risk of inhaling spores of *Aspergillus clavatus* alleged to cause allergic alveolitis in malt workers[61,62] has been markedly reduced by the introduction of mechanical methods in distilleries and breweries. In Scotland it was estimated that 5% of the malt workers had symptoms attributable to environmental contaminants in the malting industry,[63] but confirmation of hypersensitivity pneumonitis was lacking. The *A. clavatus* in sputum and serum precipitins to *A. clavatus* are found in exposed workers regardless of whether they are symptomatic or not, but are not found in nonexposed workers.[62] The prick test with the *A. clavatus* causes a late reaction and the disease can be reproduced by bronchial challenge with *A. clavatus* spores.

Wood Workers' Hypersensitivity Pneumonitis

Wood workers' hypersensitivity pneumonitis can be prevented by spraying the logs during debarking with water containing detergent, the use of remote control operations, and the wearing of special respirators.[64] Monitoring of environmental spore concentrations or antigen concentration in the mill may prove to be useful in the future. Medical surveillance programs, including clinical and radiologic examinations, are desirable for early detection.

Cheese Washers' Lung

The hypersensitivity pneumonitis known as cheese washers' lung has been observed in Swiss cheese makers engaging in washing the molds off the surface of cheeses. Up to 10 to 15% of the workers were affected. Serum precipitins to *Penicillium casei* have been found in the sera of these patients.[44] These workers can also develop asthmatic symptoms and the association of asthma with pulmonary infiltrates makes the disease similar to allergic bronchopulmonary aspergillosis. Recently, cheese mites have been implicated in the etiology of the cheese washers' asthma.[65]

ASTHMA AND BRONCHITIS

The prevalence of occupational asthma in agricultural and forestry workers in the United States is unknown. Occupational asthma in rural environments has been ascribed to multiple agents: grain, wheat, oats, rye, barley, and grain dusts, flour, soybean, mexican bean, castor beans, coffee beans, antigens in particles of insects and mites (locusts, grain weevils, grain storage mites), fungi (spores of *Cladisporium, Verticillium*) mushroom spores, organophosphate insecticides, carbamates, animal dander, bird feathers, ammonia used as fertilizer, tobacco leaves, garlic dust, maiko, cotton, flax, hemp, sisal, and wood dusts.[66] In addition, farmers are in close contact with common environmental allergens, tree, grass and weed pollens, and basiodiospores.

The etiopathogenesis and diagnosis of occupational asthma are discussed in another chapter.

Airways disease in agricultural workers can be manifested by functional changes (airways obstruction, bronchial hyperactivity) and/or by respiratory symptoms such as cough, expectoration, wheezing, chest tightness, and dyspnea. The bronchial disease may be labeled as asthma or chronic bronchitis or acute bronchitis or simple bronchitis without airways obstruction when the clinicophysiologic syndrome fulfills established criteria, but in many cases the clinical manifestations cannot be clearly classified and may be called "asthmatic bronchitis'' ''chronic bronchitis with asthmatic component'' or reported as a symptom, for example, chronic productive cough or as a functional abnormality, FEV_1/FVC.

Grain Dust Asthma and Bronchitis

Ramazzini[67] described a bronchopathy in grain sifters in 1713. Asthma due to wheat,[68] grain smuts, grain molds,[69] grain mites,[70] grain dust,[71] durum wheat,[72] durum wheat dust,[72] and grain insects[72–74] have been described.

Grain dust is a complex mixture of materials derived from cereal grains as well as natural contaminants, for example, silica, fungi, bacteria, endotoxin, insects, mites, rat hair, pollen, and human additives (pesticides and their residues). The biologic potency of the dust is likely to vary with the grain and the type and concentration of the contaminants.

The prevalence of asthma, ''asthmatic'' symptoms, or acute bronchitis related to grain dust in farmers in the United States is unknown, but epidemiologic studies have shown a high prevalence of respiratory disorders among grain handlers in other occupations. A recent study[75] of a rural town and surrounding farming community of Manitoba Canada found that 40% of farmers engaged in harvesting and shoveling grain had shortness of breath during exposure to grain dust about an hour after work. They also found that symptoms of chronic cough, expectoration, and wheezing were more common in nonsmoking male farmers than in nonsmoking male nonfarmers.

Cross-sectional epidemiologic surveys[33,76–79] indicate a high prevalence of chronic bronchitis and asthma as well as conjunctival, laryngeal, nasal, and systemic (grain fever) symptoms in grain handlers. In addition, exposure to pesticides may provide acute neurologic, gastrointestinal, hepatic, and pulmonary symptoms and can cause chronic neurobehavioral effects.

Disease statistics of grain elevator operators may not apply to farmers since the patterns of exposure, and composition of the dust may be different in the various types of grain elevator and farm operations, but the respiratory problems resulting in exposure to grain dust appear to be identical. Farmers are usually exposed to grain dust while harvesting, transporting, storing, or feeding animals in open or closed environments. The grain elevator operator and longshoremen are exposed during loading and unloading of trucks, railroad cars, and ships, during grain distribution and transport within the elevator components, weighing, cleaning operations, equipment maintainance, and grain inspection. Federal and state grain inspectors are exposed while sampling and testing grain. Workers in feed, malt and flour mills, and food manufacture are also exposed to grain dust.

The total population at risk for the harmful effects of grain dust is unknown, but the number is certainly in the hundreds of thousands. In 1979, there were an estimated 13 million bushels of major grains produced in the United States requiring about 15,000 grain elevators, 250,000 grain elevator workers, 450,000 grain processors, and an unknown proportion of the 4 million farm operators.[80]

Clinical Features. The acute episodes are characterized by varying degrees of cough, expectoration, wheezing, and/or chest tightness, and dyspnea associated with conjunctivitis, blepharitis, rhinitis, pharyngitis, and laryngitis (Table 7-3). Cough and/or expectoration on exposure to grain dust has been reported in over 75% of smokers and in 50% of nonsmokers and wheezing and/or chest tightness in almost 60% of grain handlers.[76] In grain handlers the symptoms vary from once a day, to a few times a month. Wheezing and/or chest tightness and dyspnea tended to occur immediately or within 2 to 5 hours after starting to work, but in some workers wheezing was apparent in 2 hours after leaving work.[33] Smokers are more likely to have these complaints than nonsmokers. Durum wheat and barley dust were reported to be the most common inducers of symptoms, followed by spring wheat, rye, and oats dust. Less likely inducers of symptoms are corn, soy beans, and sunflower products.[33]

Exposure to grain dust can result in recurrent nocturnal asthma after a single exposure.[74]

Pulmonary Function Tests. Acute grain dust asthma is manifest as airways obstruction and is significantly reversed by bronchodilators or corticosteroids and/or avoidance of exposure. Chronic grain dust exposure has an adverse affect on the airways function of grain handlers of a similar magnitude to the effect of smoking, that can lead to chronic airways obstructive disease.[76] Severe cases, as described by Ramazzini[67] in 1713 lead to cor pulmonale.

Experimental exposure to 23–160 kg/m^3 of grain dust for 2 hours induced an immediate, significant fall in FEV_1, $\dot{V}_{max\,50}$ and $\dot{V}_{max\,75}$, marked increase in airways resistance, gas density dependence of pulmonary resistance, frequency dependence of resistance and compliance, and increased functional residual capacity but caused no change in static compliance or diffusing capacity.[71] Two or three hours after exposure, there was a persistence of frequency dependence of compliance, loss of gas density dependence of resistance and decrease in the magnitude of the resistance elevation so indicating the airways obstruction was predominantly central immediately after the exposure and predominantly peripheral at 2 to 3 hours after exposure.[71,81] The acute bronchoconstriction following a single exposure may persist for 36 to 48 hours[20] or recur daily.[74] Bronchial provocation challenges with grain dust are useful in identifying the occupational origin of the asthma. For identifying the etiologic agents, saline extracts of constituents of grain dust can be used. A negative reaction, however, should be interpreted with caution, as the antigen may not be soluble in saline. The type of reaction can be immediate, late, dual, or recurrent. Because asthmatic reactions are often late and not always detected by changes in FEV_1, the postchallenge period should extend for at least 24 hours and $\dot{V}_{max\,50}$, $\dot{V}_{max\,75}$, and airways resistance should also be measured.[72,82]

Chest radiographs are normal.

Immunologic Features. The skin test or serum levels of specific IgE is valuable in identifying potential etiologic agents from complex antigenic exposure and aids in selecting antigen for bronchial provocation tests. Farmers from Manitoba exposed to grain dust appeared to have a greater incidence of skin hypersensitivity to grain mites, grain dust, and grain molds than nonfarmers.[75]

In the northern United States, grain elevator workers and the population of the city where the elevators are located have a higher prevalence of airborne grain dust skin hypersensitivity than workers of a city not exposed to grain dust.[33,82] Sensitization to airborne grain dust is higher in atopic grain workers. Although symptoms on exposure to grain dust can develop in individuals with or without immediate skin hyperreactivity to airborne grain dust or other allergens present in grain dust as well as in atopic and nonatopic individuals, airways dysfunction is most likely to occur in allergic workers.[33,82] Actually, the allergic workers who develop severe asthma will likely leave the industry early in their employment.

Serum precipitins to fungi, airborne grain dust, and other contaminants of grain dust can be found in a small proportion of workers.[33] But the presence of these contaminants does not correlate with the presence of disease and has little diagnostic value.

Diagnosis. The diagnosis of occupational grain dust asthma is based on the following: a compatible history regardless of the length of employment, symptoms, physical and physiologic findings of airways obstruction brought on or aggravated by exposure to grain dust and relieved by its avoidance, and a negative chest radiograph. Bronchial provocation tests can identify the causative agents and confirm the occupational origin of the asthma.

Pathogenesis. The mechanism by which grain dust or grain dust constituents induce an acute or chronic bronchial reaction may be allergic, mechanical, or chemical. It is possible that all three mechanisms are responsible. Results from bronchial challenges[83,84] were interpreted as compatible with an allergic mechanism because of the type of response and its blockage by cromolyn. However, similar features occur with nonspecific or nonimmunologic mechanisms[85,86] and the direct stimulation of sensory irritant receptors.[87] We doubt that all grain dust-induced bronchial reactions are IgE- or allergic-mediated responses, but severe acute disabling and acute asthmatic reactions at low dust concentrations in sensitized individuals are probably allergic. We have hypothesized that the obstructive airways disease of grain handlers may be the result of recurrent mechanical or chemical irritation or of recurrent allergic inflammatory reactions with increased bronchomotor tone and nonspecific hyperreactivity. Grain particles may, by a nonallergic (predominantly) or allergic (less often) mechanism, activate rapidly adapting sensory (irritant) receptors and initiate a neuroreflex increase in bronchomotor tone. The sensitivity of these receptors may be heightened by bronchoepithelial damage caused by recurrent grain dust-induced chronic inflammatory changes.

Based on in vitro studies, complement activation by the alternate pathway has been implicated in the human reaction to grain dust.[88] In vivo, we have been unable to demonstrate serum complement activation either during the workshift exposure or during bronchial provocation challenges with wheat, barley, grain insects, mites, and grain dust extracts or airborne grain dust[71,82,33] in volunteer subjects. The lack of evidence of complement activation in the subjects' sera does not preclude the possibility of local activation of complement in the lung.

Prevention. Labor Canada adopted a TLV of 10 mg/m^3 of total grain dust to protect workers. No such standard exists in the United States where the nuisance dust standard of 15 mg/m^3 is used instead. Studies[33,89] show, however, that the respiratory effects can be found in workers exposed to dust levels below the current TLV. With current technology, it may not be possible to protect the health of all workers through dust control measures alone. Fungicide applications are unlikely to prevent the asthma or chronic bronchitis from occurring in the majority of the grain handlers, since fungi do not appear to be common etiologic agents. Although cromolyn inhalation has blocked experimentally induced grain asthma,[71,83] it is not recommended as an alternative to good dust control measures.

The reduction in exposure level can be accomplished by the following measures:

1. Efficient dust control using cyclones with dust bins for storage of dust, hooded conveyor belts, automation, and central vacuum systems.
2. Personal protection with airline respirators or enclosures can help while operating a machine, but they are not well tolerated when farmers perform hard labor with high minute ventilations because the mask adds a breathing resistance, becomes plugged up with dust quickly, and impairs proper vision and movement. An alternative is a cab on combine harvesters or a mechanism that provides a curtain of filtered air around the operator. These cabs and "air curtains" also somewhat restrict operator movement so some compromise between safety and comfort may be necessary. Exposure of drivers to airborne dust might also be decreased by harvesting across the wind and by design modifications to direct more dust away from the operator.
3. Preemployment identification of susceptible workers. This is a highly controversial issue because techniques to identify host susceptibility are inadequate. However, some individuals such as atopic workers with a history of asthma and nonspecific bronchial hyperreactivity can be advised of personal risk.
4. Periodic medical examinations to detect early sensitization and airways disease at a reversible stage is a worthwhile aim.

Insect and Mite Asthma

Exposure to pollen from trees, grasses, and weeds during the planting and harvesting season may cause rhinitis and asthma in farmers. However, in the Orkney Islands of the United Kingdom hay, grain dust, and house dust mites are more common inducers of rhinitis and asthma.[90] Farm dust asthma is related to occupational exposure; it is associated with a high mite count and causes a strongly positive immediate skin test reaction to mites and mite-specific serum IgE and a positive response bronchial provocation.[91,92] Common species of mites in grain dust are *Glysyphagus domesticus* and *G. destructor, Tyrophagus putrescens* and *Acaro siro,* and house dust *Dermatophagoides ptenrimissimus*.[90]

Laboratory workers who breed insects for research purposes may become sensitized and develop asthma. In locust breeders[93] occupational asthma develops more often and more quickly in atopic workers than in similarly exposed nonatopic workers. IgG and IgE antibody to locust antigens correlated significantly with degree of exposure and presence of disease. Bean sorters in Mexico were reported to develop asthma to a bean weevil called *Zabrotis subfasciatus*.[93]

Western Red Cedar Asthma

Red cedar asthma is a common type of occupational asthma in certain regions of North America, e.g., British Columbia. This type of asthma is not seen in loggers but in workers exposed to the red cedar wood dust in saw mills, carpentry, or wood carving. The type of asthmatic reaction induced by red cedar is late or dual in over 90% of the cases.[94]

Chan-Yeung and associates[94] recently reported information on red cedar asthma of significant clinical and medicolegal importance. Only half of the patients with red cedar asthma recovered completely after exposure ended. The remaining continued to have recurrent asthma. The persistence of their asthma was the result of the previous occupational exposure, since none of the patients had asthma prior to employment and when challenged they showed specific reaction to red cedar extract. Early diagnosis and early removal from exposure were associated with recovery. On those who continued to work, lung function deteriorated and nonspecific bronchial hyperreactivity increased.

ORGANIC DUST TOXIC SYNDROMES

Grain Fever

Grain fever is a short-term flulike illness developing during or after occupational exposure to high concentrations of grain dust. In survey studies 6–32% of the grain handlers reported symptoms consistent with grain fever syndrome. Some workers have a single episode after their first exposure to grain dust, whereas others report hundreds of episodes in their work life. The frequency of grain fever has markedly decreased since dust control systems became mandatory. High concentrations of dust above 200 mg/m^3 have been found in Canadian country elevators[95] and in American terminal elevators.[96] Nowadays, such high dust concentrations should occur only when dust control systems are not operating adequately. The grain fever syndrome has been reproduced in humans under experimental conditions at concentrations ranging from 23 to 164 mg/m^3 of respirable dust.[71]

The syndrome is characterized by facial warmth, headache, malaise, myalgias, feverish sensation, and chills, developing during or after work; symptoms subside in a few hours or overnight, vary in intensity from mild to severe, and may or may not be associated with respiratory symptoms such as throat and tracheal burning sensation, chest tightness, dyspnea, cough, and expectoration. Hyperthermia was not consistently present on subjects complaining of feverish sensation, chills, or facial warmth after experimental exposure to grain dust[71] and was seldom found in symptomatic workers during or after a work shift.[33]

The physiologic and radiologic features of work-related grain fever are unknown. Experimentally induced grain fever syndrome was associated with diffuse airways obstruction without evidence of parenchymal reaction[71] leukocytosis, ranging from 11,700 to 24,300 leukocytes/mm^3 with a left shift and no detectable evidence of activation of complement in the subject's sera. Although the symptoms subsided in a few hours or overnight, in 6 of the 12 subjects leukocytosis and/or airways obstruction persisted longer than 24 hours.[71]

Grain dust contains a wide variety of organic constituents, e.g., grain fungi, bacteria,[97] and endotoxins[88] that can be potentially responsible for the grain fever syndrome. Because grain fever clinically resembles hypersensitivity pneumonitis, it has been hypothesized to be a Type III allergic reaction[98] to fungi contained in the grain dust. However, physiologic or radiologic evidence of pneumonitis with grain fever has not been demonstrated. Also, grain fever, unlike hypersensitivity pneumonitis caused by inhalation of organic dust or materials, tends not to recur unless the exposure to grain dust is again massive and has not been found to be related to the presence of precipitins or immediate skin hypersensitivity to grain dust, or fungi.[33,71,76,83] Like the extracts of organisms associated with hypersensitivity pneumonitis, airborne grain dust also activates complement by the alternate pathway in in vitro studies.[88] In vivo experiments have not demonstrated activation of complement following bronchial provocation challenge with grain dust.[71,83] The fact that grain fever occurs on exposure to high concentrations of grain dust in subjects not previously exposed to grain dust implies that grain fever is a nonallergic reaction to grain dust not requiring prior sensitization.[20] Like other febrile reactions to inhaled vegetable dusts,[99,100] such as mill fever or mycotoxicosis, grain fever may be caused by the host response to bacterial or fungal endotoxins contained in the inhaled grain dust.

Grain fever subsides spontaneously. Prevention of future episodes by dust control measures should be instituted. No apparent residuals are found. Since it resembles infectious illnesses and hypersensitivity pneumonitis, chest radiograph and pulmonary function tests are required for differential diagnosis if the symptoms persist and the patient seeks medical attention.

Mycotoxicosis

Pulmonary mycotoxicosis[100] or atypical farmers' lung appears to be a distinct pathologic entity characterized by an acute inflammatory reaction to components of dust from moldy haylage, oats, ear corn, and shelled corn. In the pathogenesis of this disease, mycotoxins,[100] microbial proteinases, and activation of complement may be involved. In contrast to farmers' lung, there appear to be no host factors involved as several persons simultaneously exposed to heavy moldy dust concentrations will develop the same symptoms without preceding allergic sensitization. In this respect it resembles grain fever syndrome. The exposure occurs when farmers remove the extremely moldy top layer of silage prior to feeding livestock or when cleaning silos prior to storing new silage. The clinical presentation is similar to hypersensitivity pneumonitis with delayed onset of chills, fever, cough, dyspnea, myalgias, and arthralgias. Some cases show radiographic and histologic evidence of interstitial pneumonitis, impaired DLco and hypoxemia. There are no serum precipitins and no recurrences with reexposure to low concentrations. Five varieties of fungi were cultured from lung biopsy material.[100] Preliminary observations have shown that the predominant cells on bronchoalveolar lavage are neutrophils rather than lymphocytes.[36]

Green Tobacco Sickness

Green tobacco sickness is a self-limiting, short illness characterized by nausea, vomiting, dizziness, and prostration associated, in approximately 50% of the cases, with breathlessness and dry cough. The prevalence is high; 91% of field croppers studied in North Carolina[101] and 88% of Indian tobacco workers[102] developed this syndrome. Symptoms may start one hour after starting to work and may last for six hours. Criteria for diagnosis should include the characteristic symptoms, recurrence of the illness on repeated harvesting exposures, and the self-limiting nature of the illness. This illness resembles both organophosphate insecticide poisoning and heat exhaustion. The etiology is not clear, but nicotine dermal absorption is suspect. A threefold increase in the urine nicotine levels were observed in workers with symptoms.[102]

CHEMICALS AND TOXIC GASES

Farmers are exposed to an array of chemicals that may affect exposed skin (contact dermatitis) or exposed mucosa or may cause respiratory problems by inhalation, ingestion or dermal absorption. The chemicals can be natural or synthetic products used to improve or protect the quality and quantity of the production (Table 7-4) or may be natural by-products of chemical decomposition of organic material such as nitrous dioxide in silos and H_2S, NH_3, CO, CO_2, and methane in animal confinement units previously described.

Some chemicals do not cause lung disease per se but qualify as respiratory occupational hazards, since they may cause neuromuscular respiratory failure by their central nervous system or neurotoxic effects, e.g., tetanus from dinitrophenol poisoning.

Pesticides

Pesticides are defined as substances or a mixture of substances intended for preventing, destroying, repelling, or mitigating any insects, rodents, nematodes, fungi, or weeds or any other form of life declared to be pests; and substances intended for use as plant regulators, defoliants, or desiccants. Fumigants are substances that produce gas, smoke, or fumes used to destroy insects, bacteria, and rodents. As of 1979 there were 1400 active pesticide ingredients in 50,000 different formulations registered with the Environmental Protection Agency. In 1975 it was estimated that four billion pounds of pesticides were used worldwide, one billion of these in the United States.[103]

In the United States agriculture is the largest user of pesticides and fumigants for rodent and insect control, food storage (especially for grain), soil treatment, and control of pests on imported and exported food. Pesticides are also used for public health purposes in malaria control, forestry, highway right-of-ways, industries such as wood products, paper, paint, cotton, hemp, cosmetics, water, food processing, pest control, and homes and gardens.

The World Health Organization recorded 500,000 occupational and nonoccupational poisonings a year with a 1% death rate. Occupational death from pesticides in the United States appears to be relatively uncommon, considering that of the 192 deaths from pesticide poisoning in 1971–1973, only 24 were occupational in origin. The danger of poisoning exists in the manufacture, formulation, and application of pesticides as well as during harvesting, transport, storage, and distribution of agricultural products by migrant farm workers, crop dusters, flaggers, loaders, truckers, railroad workers, longshoremen, and grain elevator operators. Numerous mass poisonings of harvest crews have been reported in California.[104] Pesticides and fertilizers are capable of inducing occupational lung disease (Table 7-4).

Paraquat Poisoning. Paraquat is a bipyridilium herbicide capable of causing severe pulmonary fibrosis when ingested. The pulmonary damage by paraquat ingestion appears to be dose related. Large doses will produce pulmonary edema, intermediate doses will induce pulmonary fibrosis, and small doses will cause subclinical lung changes.[105] During the initial phase there is

Table 7-4. Selected Pesticides and Fertilizers Capable of Inducing Occupational Lung Disease

Type	Compound	Effect[a]
Insecticides	Chlorinated hydrocarbons (e.g., endrin)	P. edema
	Organo phosphates (e.g., malathion)	Bronchospasm P. edema P. failure
	Carbamates (e.g., sevin)	P. failure
Rodenticides	Sodium fluoroacetate	Arrythmias
	Strychnine	Tetanus failure
	Warfarin	P. hemorrhage
Fungicides	Formaldehydes, phenols	Irritation, asthma P. edema
	Compounds with arsenic	Lung cancer
	"Bordeaux mixture" with copper	Interstitial pneumonitis
Herbicides	Bipyridyls: paraquat	P. fibrosis, edema
	Sodium chlorate	Methemoglobin
Fumigants	Methyl bromide	P. edema
	Carbon disulfide	P. edema
Fertilizers	Anhydrous ammonia	Respiratory irritation

[a] P. = pulmonary.

destruction of alveolar epithelium followed by alveolar edema, hemorrhage, and extrusion of macrophages. Subsequent proliferation of fibroblasts lead to diffuse fibrosis.[106] Medial hypertrophy of pulmonary arteries with organized thrombi, have been described in human and experimental animal paraquat poisoning.[107]

Workers involved in normal agricultural use of paraquat do not develop adverse health effects.[108–110] Agricultural spray equipment is not designed to generate respirable spray particles. Therefore, the majority of the inhaled droplets are too large, 200 μm, to reach the alveolar spaces and are deposited in the upper airways. Persons overexposed to paraquat spray mists may develop temporary signs and symptoms of localized irritation of the upper respiratory tract or skin, but there were no substantiated cases of pulmonary fibrosis or systemic poisoning resulting from inhalation exposure.

Heavy smokers of paraquat-contaminated marijuana may experience cough, hemoptysis, and mouth irritation.[111] Severe systemic and pulmonary poisoning, however, can result from dermal absorption associated with extensive occupational exposures, preexisting cutaneous lesions, and poor hygiene.[107] In a fatal case, the worker had used a leaky spray reservoir on his shoulder resulting in a burnt ulcerated skin area, and subsequent dyspnea, cyanosis, respiratory failure, and death.[107] Bilateral fine nodular opacities were seen in the chest radiograph.

More recently[112] evidence of interstitial lung disease was reported in workers with chronic 3 to 5 years seasonal dermal exposure to paraquat. One symptomatic nonsmoker had restrictive disease with decreased vital capacity, TLC, DL, Pa_{O_2}, but normal FEV_1; an interstitial pattern on chest radiograph; diffusely positive gallium-67 scan suggestive of active alveolitis, and an open lung biopsy showed marked interstitial fibrosis. Two asymptomatic workers had radiographic evidence of interstitial lung disease by gallium-67 scan, and a decline in P_{O_2} during exercise.

The diagnosis depends on the physician's awareness that occupation paraquat poisoning can occur from dermal absorption. Gastrointestinal symptoms are followed by signs of renal and liver toxicity and rapidly progressive interstitial lung disease. There may be areas of erythema, abrasions, and ulcerations on the skin, mouth, or pharynx. Plasma paraquat levels within the first 24 hours may be helpful in assessing severity and prognosis.[105,113] Patients whose plasma concentrations do not exceed 2.0, 0.6, 0.3, 0.16 and 0.1 mg/liter at 4, 6, 10, 16, and 24 hours, respectively, are likely to survive.

Treatment should start soon as possible to decrease the accumulation of paraquat in the pneumocytes, emphasizing the removal or inactivation of paraquat. Gastric lavage and suspensions of clay are, obviously, not helpful in poisoning by dermal absorption. Instead, diuresis, hemodyalisis, or hemoperfusion should be used until paraquat is not detected in blood or dialysates. Corticosteroids have been used. Oxygen therapy should be used cautiously since paraquat generates superoxide anion, and would sensitize the lungs to O_2 at atmospheric pressure.[106] Pretreatment with clofibrate was reported to protect rat lungs from paraquat poisoning but has not been studied in humans.[114]

Organophosphate Compounds. Organophosphate compounds, for example, malathion, can be absorbed through the gastrointestinal tract, the skin, and the respiratory tract. Severe poisoning usually occurs by nonoccupational ingestion. Severe intoxication and death from occupational exposures are rare and occur by inhalation and dermal absorption during spraying or harvesting contaminated crops. It can occur also by ingestion, for example, drinking water from contaminated cupped hands. Organophosphate pesticides cause acetylcholinesterase inhibition, which results in increased cholinergic activity. Decreased erythrocyte cholinesterase (RBC-ChE) and/or plasma pseudocholinesterase activity are considered reliable indicators of exposure, the level of inhibition correlating with the severity of the clinical manifestation.[103] Normal cholinesterase activity, however, does not exclude exposure to the pesticide because regeneration of the enzyme and reversibility of the inhibition may occur rapidly. Reduction in enzyme activities between 50 and 90% of baseline are unlikely to be manifested clinically. It is recommended, however, that workers exhibiting RBC-ChE inhibition to 60% of baseline be removed from their jobs until recovery to 75% of baseline. Immediate evaluation of work practices should be undertaken when any worker's RBC-ChE is reduced to 70% of baseline.[115]

Mild poisoning causes headache, fatigue, dizziness, blurred vision, excessive sweating, nausea, vomiting, diarrhea, cramps, and salivation. These symptoms are nonspecific and can be confused with heat exhaustion and infectious disease. In moderate to severe poisoning, in addition to the above symptoms, the patient will complain of inability to walk, weakness, chest tightness, and will exhibit miosis and muscle twitching. RBC-ChE activity of 10–40% of baseline will be found. These symptoms can be mistaken for pneumonia, myocardial infarction, and encephalitis. Severe poisoning is associated with RBC-ChE activity of less than 10%. Convulsions, unconciousness, hemorrhagic pulmonary edema, flaccid paralysis, respiratory failure, and death are seen at this level.

The diagnosis is based on the definite history of exposure to organophosphate six hours or less before the onset of the symptoms of diffuse parasympathetic stimulation. A ChE below 50% of preexposure level or below a normal range confirms the diagnosis.

Treatment, in severe cases, should start immediately before laboratory confirmation of significant cholinesterase inhibition. Actually, the lack of normal response (dry mouth, tachycardia, flushed skin, midriasis) to a larger than normal dose of atropine (2–4 mg intravenously) supports the diagnosis of anticholinesterase poisoning. Atropine therapy should be carefully monitored because it may induce ventricular fibrillation in the cyanotic patient. In moderate to severe cases and particularly in those with signs of respiratory muscle weakness, pralidoxine chloride (2-PAM) should be administered (1 g intravenously at a rate slower than 500 mg/min but preferably over 15 to 30 minutes). The dose may be doubled in severe intoxications. PAM is most effective when given within 24 hours after poisoning. Atropine is antagonistic to the muscurinic effects and PAM accelerates the regeneration of ChE and reverts this muscle weakness. Morphine, aminophylline, and phenothiazines are contraindicated.[116] The airways should be kept open and ventilatory support given if necessary. Further absorption should be prevented by washing the skin and/or lavaging the stomach. The disease is reversible without sequelae.

The National Institute for Occupational Safety and Health recommended limits for malathion, parathion, and methoparathion are 15 mg/m^3, 0.05 mg/m^3, and 0.2 mg/m^3, respectively.

Proper clothing to reduce skin contact and engineering controls and/or suitable respirators to reduce chemical inhalation will help prevent poisoning. Well-designed tractor enclosures with temperature controls protect workers well. Handling of pesticide concentrates should be done with rubber gloves.[103] Medical personnel washing the intoxicated patients or veterinarian attending animals should wear rubber gloves and respirators if necessary. Ingestion should be reduced by avoiding contamination of foodstuffs, their containers, cigarettes, and washing before eating.

Carbamates. Carbamates are reversible cholinesterase inhibitors which, like the organic phosphates, can cause chest tightness and muscle weakness, but there are clinical and therapeutic differences. Atropine and ventilatory support are indicated, but PAM should not be used. ChE activity is not reliable for diagnosis because cholinesterase reactivates rapidly after carbamate poisoning. 1-Naphthol will be increased in urine samples.[117]

Dinitrophenol. The herbicide dinitrophenol can cause malaise, headache, dyspnea, sweating, thirst, hypothermia, dyspnea, respiratory failure, and death.[118] Dinitrophenols cause uncoupling of oxidative phosphorylation in the mitochondria of body cells.

Chlorinated Hydrocarbons. Most of the chlorinated hydrocarbon pesticides do not affect the lung. Endrin has been reported to cause pulmonary edema treated with ventilatory assistance and PEEP.[119]

Animal Confinement Related Diseases

The recent industrial approach to livestock production includes the raising of large numbers of animals in relatively small enclosed spaces with minimum labor. The buildings are equipped with mechanized systems for ventilation, feeding, watering, and manure removal. Many potential respiratory hazards for the animals and for the people working in these buildings have been recognized.[120,121] The animal wastes in the slated/floor pit systems which undergo an aerobic digestion within the pit for several months and are usually pumped out in liquid form for land application. Toxic volatile products from the organic matter fermentation include ammonia (NH_3), hydrogen sulfide (H_2S), methane, and CO_2 and carbon monoxide from hydrocarbon-burning heating units and can be found inside the confinment buildings at levels exceeding the threshold limit value (TLV).[120,122]

Fatal or near-fatal accidental exposures to toxic levels of these gases in man[123,124] and in animals[122] have been reported. Recently the subacute and chronic effects of swine confinements systems exposure have been studied.[120,121] Another potential hazard found in livestock confinment units is the high levels of aerosolized particles,[120] a high percentage of which is of respirable size. The major component of this dust is probably grain dust, but also it contains dried fecal material, dander, hair particles, bacteria, and endotoxin. Dust particles may absorb NH_3 and H_2S.[125]

The population at risk is large. In Iowa alone approximately 84,000 workers and 468 veterinarians are exposed to some degree to swine confinment systems. The total United States population exposed to swine, beef or dairy cattle, and poultry confinment systems is roughly estimated at 700,000.[120]

Epidemiologic studies have concentrated on the health hazards for men and animals in swine confinment systems because they are more numerous than beef cattle or poultry confinment systems and because more case studies have been reported for swine raisers.

Clinical Manifestations. ***Acute Pulmonary Reaction.*** Farm workers and veterinarians develop the acute respiratory symptoms within a few minutes to three hours of exposure to a swine confinment building atmosphere.[120] Cough, expectoration, chest tightness, wheezing and shortness of breath, rhinorrhea, scratchy throat, and eye irritation usually improve after 24 to 48 hours of nonexposure. The prevalence of acute pulmonary symptoms show positive correlation with the number of swine raised and with smoking, but no correlation with age, number of hours worked per week, or the type of building.

Delayed Reaction. Delayed symptoms 4 to 6 hours after exposure manifest as a flulike illness with fever, myalgias, headaches, cough, and chest tightness. These episodes resemble grain fever syndrome or allergic alveolitis.

Chemical gases particulate matter and bacterial endotoxin may be involved in the etiopathogenesis of the acute respiratory and systemic symptoms.

Acute Toxic Reactions. Near-fatal and fatal exposures to high concentrations of toxic gases from the decomposition of manure have been reported. Rapid buildup of ammonia, hydrogen sulfide, and carbon dioxide to acute toxic levels and rapid depletion of oxygen within minutes or a few hours can occur when (1) there is failure of the ventilation system, or (2) storage pit manure is agitated before being pumped out, even if the ventilation is operative.[123] Under condition (1), ambient concentration of CO_2 may increase to 15% and oxygen concentration may decline to 10% in 6 to 8 hours.[122] During condition (2), the toxic levels of above 500 ppm may be reached instantly or in few minutes. Workers are also in danger when entering manure pits or septic tanks for maintainance or to rescue victims of the toxic gases without the proper protective equipment.[122,124]

In these ambient situations sudden death can occur from asphyxia due to ambient hypoxia when large amounts of methane and carbon dioxide are present. In addition, carbon monoxide inhalation can produce high levels of carboxyhemoglobin and tissue hypoxia. In Iowa most of the eight deaths and six near-deaths associated with exposure to toxic gases in swine confinment operations investigated by Donham and coworkers[120] were ascribed to hydrogen sulfide exposure. Recently, three deaths and one near-death from exposure to gases in a liquid manure storage tank in Utah were ascribed to H_2S.[124]

Reenactment of the circumstances leading to the death of an Iowa farmer and his two sons and the Utah farmers and two of his rescuers revealed levels of hydrogen sulfide above 400 ppm. NIOSH recommends a maximum exposure to hydrogen sulfide of 10 ppm over a 10-minute period with immediate evacuation at 50 ppm.[126] The Utah victims had heart blood sulfide ion levels of 5, 3.6, and 0.8 mg/liter, whereas control blood levels did not exceed 0.05 mg/liter and in random autopsy cases levels did not exceed 0.4 mg/liter.[124]

A low concentration (10–50 ppm) of H_2S can induce numerous complaints such as eye and throat burning, headache, anorexia, dizziness, dyspnea, cough, sleep disturbances, and nausea; with higher doses, >150 ppm, the characteristic warning signal of the rotten egg odor is obliterated due to olfactory nerve fatigue. Keratoconjuctivitis, palpebral edema, arm cramps, hypertension, bronchitis, and hemorrhagic pulmonary edema may develop. Levels above 300 ppm and particularly at levels above 1000 ppm unconsciousness, convulsions, and sudden death occur.[126] Hydrogen sulfide has an adverse effect on the respiratory system by several mechanisms. It affects the cellular respiration through inhibition of cytochrome oxidases and affects ventilatory control by its toxic effect on the brain. It also directly irritates the airways and causes edema due to formation of an alkali sulfide. Although H_2S alone can cause fatal or near-fatal respiratory reactions, the role of other toxic gases, ammonia, methane, and carbon dioxide, and the resulting hypoxia cannot be minimized.

Ammonia can also reach toxic levels in swine confinement buildings. Ammonia is usually sufficiently irritating to the eyes and nose to repel the worker from the area. If immediate withdrawal is not possible, cough, glottal edema, bronchospasm, pulmonary edema, and pneumonia may follow. Mild exposures can produce headaches, salivation, burning of the throat, anosmia, perspiration, nausea, vomiting, and substernal pain.[117]

Prevention. Measures that will reduce the risk of exposure to toxic gases from liquid manure systems should include improvements in engineering designs, improvement in ventilation, development of building standards, and safety precautions such as evacuation of animals and workers from confinement houses during manure agitation, and education of farmers and rescue workers in the hazards of livestock of confinement spaces. Workers should not rely on the detection of rotten egg odor. Workers who must enter a closed space or tank containing liquid manure gases should wear a self-contained breathing apparatus with full face operated on pressure demand or other positive pressure mode. An observer capable of rapidly retrieving the person in the tank using the safety line should remain outside the tank. A frequent tragedy is that rescuers may collapse as fast as the original victim.

Therapy for H_2S poisoning consists of prompt removal from exposure without endangering the rescuer's life, oxygen and cardiopulmonary resuscitation, followed by mechanical ventilation if necessary. Nitrites may accelerate recovery by inducing methemoglobin that inactivates sulfides, thus protecting the cytochrome oxidases and aerobic cellular respiration. Methemoglobin can also impair oxygen transport. The respiratory reaction to hydrogen sulfide may resolve completely without sequelae.[124]

Silo Fillers' Disease (Nitrogen Dioxide Poisoning)

Nitrogen dioxide poisoning (NO_2) has been recognized as a toxic substance since 1914. However, it was not considered a hazard to farmers until 1949 when lethal concentrations of NO_2 were found in freshly filled silos. Although the majority of the symptomatic exposures are mild and self-limiting, some are sufficiently severe to cause pulmonary edema and/or bronchiolitis obliterans. Unfortunately, even though most patients recover without sequelae, almost one third fail to survive the initial episode of pulmonary edema or bronchiolitis.[127] This is particularly unfortunate since the disease and the exposure are preventable.

The incidence of silo fillers' disease is difficult to assess, and the true scope of the problem is probably underestimated. We found a 4% incidence of symptomatic exposure among 2000 randomly selected farmer operators. These suggest that there were over 6700 potentially dangerous exposures to NO_2 among 164,000 farmers in Wisconsin.[127]

NO_2 and its dimer, nitrogen tetraoxide, derived from plant nitrates form a yellow or reddish-brown gas at the top of the silo that emits an odor similar to household bleach. It begins to form within a few hours after the silo has been filled and reaches a peak concentration 1 to 5 days later and dangerous amounts persist for about 10 days.

Occasionally, NO_2, which is heavier than air, may concentrate at or near the silage surface or in depressions for several months if the silo has remained unopened and is tightly sealed. The farmer or the silo repairman is in danger of NO_2 poisoning when entering the silo within this period of time without adequate precautions. Current farming practices of filling up the silo in stages throughout the summer and fall creates the potential of poisoning several times during the season.

Larger amounts of NO_2 are likely to be produced when the vegetable or plants stored are high in nitrates. Larger nitrate concentrations in plants are found when the soils have been heavily nitrated by fertilizers, by drought, and by immaturity of the plants. Concomitant with NO_2 formation, CO_2, ammonia butyric acid, and free amines are produced and the oxygen concentration decreases. The current threshold limit value for NO_2 in industry is 5 ppm and >50 ppm is considered dangerous, even for short periods. Unfortunately, concentrations of NO_2 capable of inducing serious pulmonary injury (50–150 ppm) may be only mild irritants to the eyes and airways, thereby allowing a persistent individual to damage the lungs seriously before being forced out of a silo or work area. Silo concentrations as high as 4000 ppm have been measured.[128]

Acute experimental exposures in man to 1.6–2 ppm of NO_2 for 15 minutes resulted in an increase in airway resistance in normal subjects and in persons with chronic bronchitis.[129,130] Experimental exposure to 0.11 ppm of NO_2 for one hour increases the airways response of asthmatics to a bronchoconstricting agent.[131]

NO_2 inhalation, whether from agricultural or industrial sources, exerts the same deleterious effect upon the pulmonary tissue. Unlike most water-soluble irritant gases, which mainly affect the exposed airway mucosa, NO_2 hydrolyzes more slowly and is capable of reaching the bronchioles and alveoli. At these locations NO_2 undergoes almost complete hydrolysis to nitrous and nitric acids, resulting in a profound chemical pneumonitis and pulmonary edema. The clinical presentation depends on the concentration of NO_2 inhaled and the duration of exposure.

Clinical Manifestations. Mild exposures to NO_2 result in upper airway and occular irritation, cough, dyspnea, fatigue, cyanosis, vomiting, vertigo, somnolence, and even loss of consciousness. Although the symptoms may persist for one or two weeks, the likely result is complete recovery. More severe exposures, however, can result in death from bronchiolar spasm, laryngeal spasm, reflex respiratory arrest, or simple asphyxia. Alternatively minimal symptoms occur during exposure with progression to severe pulmonary edema several hours later. These patients will have severe dyspnea with hypoxemia, hyperventilation, and impaired pulmonary diffusing capacity.[132,133] Serious hemoglobin O_2 desaturation occurs due to impaired lung function and the formation of methemoglobin. The patient may also have severe metabolic acidosis caused by both the dissolution of NO_2 in body fluids to form nitrous and nitric acid and lactic acidosis secondary to tissue hypoxemia. Systemic hypotension from the direct vasodilatory effect of nitrates has been observed clinically[134] and experimentally.[135]

Chest radiographs show the characteristic pattern of noncardiac pulmonary edema.

The gross appearance of the lungs in fatal cases shows hemorrhagic pulmonary edema with fluid in the airways and patches of pneumonia. Microscopically there is edema and extensive damage of the epithelium of the small bronchi and bronchioles with generalized infiltration of the alveolar walls with lymphocytes, numerous macrophages in the alveolar spaces, and bronchiolitis obliterans in various stages of organization.

With appropriate therapy most patients survive pulmonary edema and symptoms improve, but bronchiolitis obliterans with recurrence of dyspnea and cough may develop 10 to 31 days after exposure. However, with appropriate supportive therapy and corticosteroids, the majority of patients have also survived this later manifestation.

Bronchiolitis may follow pulmonary edema or present as the initial manifestation of exposure.[127] The radiographs inhibit a miliary or fine nodular patterns. Lung biopsy at this stage will show bronchiolitis obliterans. During the delayed acute stage, frequency dependence of compliance, hypoxemia during exercise with normal elastic recoil and airways resistance have been found.[136] Regardless of the stage after acute accidental exposures, pulmonary function generally improved without any permanent disability. In some instances, there may be a mild degree of pulmonary dysfunction probably due to bronchiolitis obliterans manifested as mild hyperinflation,[133] abnormal $\dot{V}_{max\ 50}$, $\dot{V}_{max\ 75}$ or FEF_{25-75}, increased respiratory resistance,[137] and airways obstruction.[132]

Diagnosis. As with other occupational lung diseases, the diagnosis of silo fillers' disease depends on obtaining an adequate medical history. It is important to recognize that during exposure, the symptoms may be mild, becoming severe only after the exposure has ceased. In the case of bronchiolitis obliterans, this may occur several days or weeks later. In the latter disease, other causes (e.g., virus or miliary tuberculosis) have to be considered in the differential diagnosis. Careful clinical history should also allow the distinction between silo-fillers' disease and farmers' lung disease, both of which may result from exposures in the silo. Silo-fillers' disease occurs in freshly filled silos during harvesting season, whereas farmers' lung disease results from exposure to moldy, stored silage or foliage.

Treatment. As with other acute chemical intoxications, the initial step should be the removal of the patient from the source of exposure without endangering the health of the rescuers. Oxygen, bronchodilators, and ventilatory support should be provided if required. Any patient with significant exposures to NO_2 should be observed in the hospital for 48 hours and followed closely for an additional six weeks after discharge. If a patient has hypotension and shock, it should be remembered that it is usually due to a direct effect of nitrites on the blood vessels and not due to hypovolemia. Hence, volume expanders should be given cautiously and vasopressor drugs may be necessary to correct the normovolemic shock.

Corticosteroids should be started immediately in the presence of respiratory embarrassment due to pulmonary edema and to bronchiolitis. An unfavorable response to the premature cessation of corticosteroid therapy has been reported by us and others,[127,138] thus it is prudent to continue the therapy for a minimum of eight weeks.

Cyanosis or methemoglobinemia usually disappears within 24 to 72 hours after exposure. No therapy is required unless the concentration exceeds 30%. If therapy is indicated, methylene blue, 1–2 mg/kg body weight, given intravenously over a five-minute period at 1% solution is the treatment of choice. The total dose may be repeated as necessary, but should not exceed 7 mg/kg. The toxic effects of this therapy include dyspnea, precordial pain, restlessness, apprehension, a sense of oppression, and tremors.

Prevention. NO_2-induced lung disease is preventable by appropriate engineering modifications, application of safety standards, and workers' education. Gas tight or control environment silos do not require manual leveling of silage, but these are more expensive than the standard upright silos and not widely accepted.

Preventive Advice for Farmers.

1. Keep out of silos during the two-week danger period.
2. Close all doors before putting in silage.
3. Go up outside ladder to level of silage.
4. Remove doors down to silage if silo is not completely full.
5. Check fresh silage on steps of shoot; stains indicate the presence of NO_2. If unstained for two days, the concentration is probably not dangerously high.
6. Effect entry into silo only with complete O_2 support system.
7. Ventilate by opening the cover flaps and blowing for 24 to 48 hours before entering.

8. Never enter the silo alone or without a lifeline for rescue during the danger period.

It is important for farmers to remember that when the surface of the silage is convex they are more likely to encounter higher gas concentrations immediately on exposure than when it is concave, but when they descend into a central cavity, there may be higher concentrations than at the entry level.

INFECTIOUS DISEASES

Currently in the United States the direct effect of agricultural exposure to infectious agents on humans is probably less important than the potential of these agents for introducing a variety of toxins and antigens. Detailed descriptions of these diseases do not belong in this review, but salient features of each disease will be mentioned.

Zoonosis

A zoonosis is a disease agent transmitted naturally between man and other animals. The World Health Organization recognizes over 150 zoonoses. Those zoonoses that affect the respiratory tract and are acquired during on-farm or agricultural activities tend to produce subclinical or mild infections in man and are less common than strictly human infections. Since the farmer may not seek medical attention or the disease may go unrecognized as a zoonosis, the prevalence is not well-documented. In the healthier and more technologically developed countries in the world, classic zoonoses have come under control and only rarely do these diseases affect man or animal. Schnurrenberger[139] classed the zoonotic agents as high, medium, or low in terms of their hypothetical importance as agricultural respiratory agents of infection. Based on clinic or epidemiologic evidence 35 zoonoses were identified as causing respiratory involvement. Since disease occurrence depends on interactive factors involving host, agent, and environment, a disease of high importance under certain conditions may be of minimal concern in most agricultural settings, for example, leptospirosis, listeriosis, and mycobacterium avium infection. In endemic areas a high-risk hazard rating has been given to (1) brucellosis, (2) chlamydiosis, (3) hydatidosis, (4) Newcastle disease, (5) tularemia, (6) *Pasteurella multocida* infection, (7) Q fever, (8) salmonellosis, (9) South American hemorrhagic fever, and (10) North Asian tick typhus. The first eight of these are prevalent in the United States. One of these, hydatidosis, is transmitted to man by ingestion of the parasite but can cause pulmonary disease. Certain animal vaccines have caused disease in humans, for example, cholera.

The arena virus which causes South American hemorrhagic fever is a high-risk hazard in endemic areas of Argentina and Bolivia, but in the United States the risk is low. The disease is probably acquired by inhalation of dust contaminated with rodent urine. The reservoir is the musmusculus present in or near every farm. The clinical manifestation may vary from mild influenzalike to fatal hemorrhagic or neurologic symptoms. North Asian tick typhus has been reported from Japan west to Czechoslovakia, but risk is low in the United States.

Q Fever. *Coxiella burnetti* infection is endemic in the United States where up to 60% of thc cattle and sheep serve as main reservoirs. The agent becomes airborne from milk, urine, feces, and uterine contents of their hosts and can be isolated from the vicinity of infected animals. Its clinical features are similar to brucellosis and influenza with pneumonic infiltrates. A fourfold increase in complement-fixing antibody titers confirm the diagnosis. Those at risk of infection are farmers, veterinarians and slaughterhouse workers. Prevention is difficult since infected animals are healthy and productive.

Brucellosis. In the United States brucellosis is uncommon because of controlled slaughter and the population at risk is mostly limited to pig slaughterers and pigmeat processors exposed to *Brucella suis*. In the United Kingdom dairy farmers, cattle breeders, abattoir workers, and veterinarians are exposed to *B. abortus*-contaminated urine, feces, placentas, and aborted calves. In the Mediterranean countries, goats and sheep are infested with *B. mellitensis*. Interestingly, severe illness can also ensue in man from conjunctival or nasal exposure to droplets of the vaccine from Strain 19.

Chlamydiosis. The common reservoir of chlamydia in the United States is avian psittarines, but pigeons and turkeys can also be host. Several outbreaks of psittacosis have been reported in turkey farms and processing plants. The risk of infection is low in parakeet breeders, pigeon fanciers, railroad and zoo workers, and veterinarians, but is high in turkey slaughterers.[140,141] Q fever, brucellosis, and chlamydiosis in dairy farmers have to be differentiated from influenza, bacterial, and allergic pneumonitis. Occupational exposure, health of the animals, and a fourfold increase in complement fixing antibodies titers can aid in the diagnosis.

Leptospirosis. *Leptospira* bacteria contaminate urine and are sensitive to drying, so they do not represent a serious hazard for airborne transmission in dust except in dairy operations where droplets of urine may reach the milker's eyes or nasal cavity.

Listeriosis. *Listeria* bacteria usually causes meningitis or genital tract infection, but also may cause pneumonia. The organism may be found in man, animals (sheep and fowl), and the environment. In some instances, airborne infection results from exposure to contaminated straw and feces from lambing in calving pens.

Mycobacterium avium Intracellulary Complex. Current poultry husbandry practices in the United States have markedly reduced the prevalence of *M. avium* in poultry, unless poor management practices exist.

Pasteurella multocida is transmitted by insect bites can cause empyema, pneumonia, sinusitis, and pulmonary abscesses in rural workers.

Tularemia is transmitted by ticks and deer flys; rabbits are a major reservoir (*Francisella tularensis*). Pneumonia can result from inhalation of dried tick feces and blood in western sheep raisers and shearers, and of dust from haystacks infested by rodents in agricultural workers.[142,143]

Hydatidosis. In the United States ecchinococcosis affecting lung and liver can be found among the low socioeconomic groups of people of western states, who live in close contact with dogs or sheep.

The farm is an echo system in which man and animals live together, sharing the same environment and often the same hazards. If the environment is not suitable for the one it is also probably not suitable for the other. Proper farming techniques and animal disease controlled contribute at the same time to an increase in income of the farm, and improve the health and social conditions of farm workers.

Pulmonary Mycosis

The fungi causing pulmonary mycoses in the United States are mostly soil inhabitants and endemic in certain regions. Histoplasmosis and blastomycosis are found predominantly in the Mississippi Valley area and coccidioidomycosis in the semiarid southwest of the United States.

The growth of *Histoplasma capsulatum, Cryptococcus neoformans,* and probably blastomycosis is enhanced by nutrients from bird droppings. Hence, microepidemics of histoplasmosis, for example, can be found among workers or farmers disturbing blackbird and chicken roosting sites, during the demolition or bulldozing of buildings, or clearing of fields heavily contaminated with bird feces.[144,145] Farm workers are at risk of cryptococcosis when working in chicken roosting areas, barns, and stables. Acute blastomycosis is also prevalent in farm workers, farmers, and in other workers in contact with soil and wooded areas. Road construction workers in the southwest of the United States are exposed to dust containing Coccidioides immitis but cases of coccidiomycosis can occur outside the endemic areas from transported contaminated materials, e.g., cotton.[146]

The prevention of these mycoses is partially accomplished by avoiding unnecessary work in suspicious sites, for example, blackbird roosting sites. Respirators and protective clothes will also reduce exposure. Soils suspected of contamination with *H. capsulatum* should be treated with a 3% solution of formalin before being disturbed.[145] The state of California has established guidelines to help prevent coccidioidomycosis.[147]

POTENTIAL CARCINOGENS

Aflatoxins are metabolic products of fungi that grow on peanuts, grains, and other foods commodities. High levels are found particularly in crops grown in the southwest and southern United States. Aflatoxin has been found to produce hepatic and pulmonary carcinomas by ingestion, intratracheal, or intraperitoneal injection in animals.[148] Interesting, aflatoxin is a million times more carcinogenic than saccharine and much more potent than other well-known carcinogens such as benzidine.[149] Ingestion of high or large amounts of aflatoxin contaminated food can result in death of animals and humans. However, the acute lethal toxic effects should be of little concern to farmers, truckers, grain handlers, and processors because their level of exposure to aflatoxin contaminated dust would not even approach the LD_{50} given for monkeys.[148] A greater concern should be the extreme carcinogenicity of aflatoxin B_1 rather than its acute toxic effects. Although the carcinogenic potential of aflatoxin ingestion has been clearly demonstrated in fish and animals, the quality and quantity of data relating aflatoxin inhalation to human cancers is inadequate. Hence, currently available information does not conclusively establish aflatoxin as a human carcinogen. The International Agency for Research on Cancer (IARC) however, considers aflatoxin a probable carcinogen to humans.

It has been suggested that suitable dust control measures be used to prevent exposure of workers to aflatoxin-contaminated commodities.

The aflatoxin B_1 found in the lung tissue of a chemical engineer who died of bronchiolar carcinoma or pulmonary adenomatosis did not prove a cause–effect relationship since the levels of aflatoxin in lungs of people without carcinoma are unknown. Nevertheless, a colleague who also worked in a contaminated peanut meal sterilization plant died of the same disease a few months later.[150]

There are pesticides that are known or suspected as animal carcinogens, and some pesticides which are not carcinogens may have a carcinogenic contaminant.[151] There is no evidence of pesticide-related cancer in humans. The role of these chemicals exposure in the higher incidence of certain neoplasms in farmers, for example, stomach cancer, leukemia, prostate cancer, multiple myeloma, need to be investigated. Epidemiologic studies have detected associations between cattle raising or corn production and leukemia, multiple myeloma, and poultry production.[152]

INORGANIC DUST PNEUMOCONIOSIS

Pneumoconiosis due to inorganic dust such as silica and silicates do not appear to be a significant hazard for agricultural workers. However, some controversial data suggest that in certain regions and under certain occupational exposures, silicosis may occur. Dunner et al.[153] reported radiographic changes compatible with silicosis in dock workers exposed to grain. Silicosis was found in 13% of tractor drivers working on sandy soils of tree farms in Russia.[154] Silicate pneumoconiosis was found in seven farm workers from central California exposed to clay and micas used in pesticide sprays.[155] Only 5 to 10% of the particles were silicon dioxide and silicate cristobalite. Pneumoconiosis has been reported in horses from the Monterey peninsula of California. Those caring for the horses, however, did not show evidence of pneumoconiosis.[156] Calcified pleural plaques, chronic fibrosing pleuritis and pleural mesotheliomas are endemic among peasants of certain rural regions of Turkey where the soil is rich in asbestos fibers (see chapters 3 and 4 for further discussion).[157]

REFERENCES

1. National Safety Council: Farm Safety Rev 35:12, 1977.
2. Banks VJ, Kalhacher JV: Farm income recipients and their families: A socioeconomic profile. Rural Development Research Report No. 30, pp 1–10. Washington DC, USDA Economics Research Service, 1981.
3. Wan TTH, Wright A: Occupational differentials in chronic disability. J Occup Med 15:493, 1973.
4. Vital Statistics of Vermont. 1973 Annual Report. Burlington, VT, The State of Vermont Department of Health, 1973.
5. Babbott FL Jr, Gump DW, Sylwester DL, et al: Respiratory symptoms and lung function in a sample of Vermont dairymen and industrial workers. Am J Public Health 70(3):241–245, March 1980.
6. Carlson ML, Petersen GR: Mortality of California agricultural workers. J Occup Med 20:30–32, 1978.
7. Lefcoe NM, Wonnacott TH: Chronic respiratory disease in four occupational groups. Arch Environ Health 29:143–146, 1974.
8. Warren CP: Respiratory disorders in Manitoba cattle farmers. Can Med Assoc J 125(1):41–46, July 1, 1981.
9. Stuart-Harris CH, Hanley T: Chronic Bronchitis, Emphysema, and Cor Pulmonale. Bristol, England, John Wright, 1957, pp 214–228.
10. Bartschi R, Rogli J: Chronic bronchitis in a rural area and its prognosis. Respiration 26:231–238. 1969.
11. Rankin J, Dickie HA, Kobayashi M, Stahmann MA: Pathogenesis of farmer's lung. J Lab Clin Med 60:1008, 1962.
12. Lacey J, Dutkiewicz J: Isolation of actinomycetes and fungi from mouldy hay using a sedimentation chamber. J Appl Bacteriol 41:315, 1976.
13. Lacey J, Lacey ME: Spore concentrations in the air of farm buildings. Trans Br Mycol Soc 47:547, 1964.
14. Pepys J, Jenkins PA, Festenstein GN, et al: Farmer's lung: Thermophilic actinomycetes as a source of "farmer's lung hay" antigen. Lancet ii:607, 1963.
15. Morgan DC, Smyth JT, Lister RW, Pethybridge, RJ: Chest symptoms and farmer's lung: A community survey. Br J Ind Med 30:256, 1973.
16. Flaherty DK, Barboriak JJ, Emmanuel D, et al: Multilaboratory comparison of three immunodiffusion methods used for the detection of precipitating antibodies in hypersensitivity pneumonitis. J Lab Clin Med 84:298, 1974.
17. Katila ML, Mäntijärvi RA: The diagnostic value of antibodies to the traditional antigens associated with farmer's lung in Finland. Clin Allergy 8(6):581–587, Nov 1978.
18. Gruchow HW, Hoffmann RG, Marx JJ Jr, et al: Precipitating antibodies to farmer's lung antigens in a Wisconsin farming population. Am Rev Respir Dis 124(4):411–415, Oct 1981.
19. Morgan DC, Smyth JT, Lister RW, et al: Chest symptoms in farming communities with special reference to farmer's lung. Br J Ind Med 32(3):228–234, Aug 1975.
20. Grant IW, Blyth W, Wardrop VE, et al: Prevalence of farmer's lung in Scotland: A pilot survey. Br Med J 1:530, 1972.
21. Madsen D, Klock LE, Wenzel FJ, et al: The prevalence of farmer's lung in an agricultural population. Am Rev Respir Dis 113(2):171–174, Feb 1976.
22. Dickie HA, Raulin J: Farmer's lung: An acute granulomatous interstitial pneumonitis occurring in agricultural workers. JAMA 167:1069, 1958.

23. Rankin J, Jaeschke WH, Callies QC, Dickie HA: Farmer's lung: Physiopathologic features of the acute interstitial granulomatous pneumonitis of agricultural workers. Ann Intern Med 57:606, 1962.
24. Warren CPW, Tse KS, Cherniack RM: Mechanical properties of the lung in intrinsic allergic alveolitis. Thorax 33:315–321, 1978.
25. Reyes CN, Emanuel DA, Roberts RC, et al: The histopathology of farmer's lung (60 consecutive cases). Am J Clin Pathol 66:460–461, 1976.
26. Seal RME, Hapke EJ, Thomas GO, et al: The pathology of the acute and chronic stages of farmers' lung. Thorax 23:469–489, 1968.
27. Salvaggio JE, Karr RM: Hypersensitivity pneumonitis: State of the art. Chest 75(2 Suppl):270–274, Feb 1979.
28. Wenzel FJ, Emanuel DA, Gray RL: Immunofluorescent studies in patients with farmer's lung. J Allergy Clin Immunol 48:224, 1971.
29. Flaherty DK, Murray HD, Reed CE: Cross reactions to antigens causing hypersensitivity pneumonitis. J Allergy Clin Immunol 53:329, 1974.
30. Pepys J, Jenkins PA: Precipitin (FLH) test in farmer's lung. Thorax 20:21, 1965.
31. Roberts RC, Wenzel FJ, Emanuel DA: Precipitating antibodies in a midwest dairy farming population toward the antigens associated with farmer's lung disease. J Allergy Clin Immunol 57:518–524, 1976.
32. doPico GA, Reddan WG, Chmelik F, et al: The value of precipitating antibodies in the detection of hypersensitivity pneumonitis. Am Rev Respir Dis 113:451–455, 1976.
33. doPico GA, Rankin J, Flaherty D: Medical health surveillance of grain handlers. Final Report on HEW/CDC/NIOSH Contract No. 210-76-0175, 1980.
34. Marx JJ, Flaherty DK: Activation of the complement sequence by extracts of bacteria and fungi associated with hypersensitivity pneumonitis. J Allergy Clin Immunol 57:328–334, 1976.
35. Fitzgerald GR, Barniville G, Black J, et al: Paraquat poisoning in agricultural workers. Ir Med J 71(10):336–342, 21 July 1978.
36. Jones A: Farmer's lung: An overview and prospectus. Annu Am Conf Gov Ind Hyg 2:171–182, 1982.
37. Bamdad S: Enzyme-linked immunosorvent assay (ELISA) for IgG antibodies in farmer's lung disease. Clin Allergy 10(2):161–171, Mar 1980.
38. Patterson R, Roberts M, Roberts RC, et al: Antibodies of different immunoglobulin classes against antigens causing farmer's lung. Am Rev Respir Dis 114:315–324, 1976.
39. Braun SR, doPico GA, Tsiatis A, et al: Farmer's lung disease: Long-term clinical and physiologic outcome. Am Rev Respir Dis 119(2):185–191, Feb 1979.
40. Emanuel DA, Wenzel FJ, Bowerman CI, Lawton BR: Farmer's lung. Clinical pathologic and immunologic study of twenty-four patients. Am J Med 37:392–401, 1964.
41. Reynolds HY, Fulmer JD, Kazmierowski JA, et al: Analysis of cellular and protein content of bronchoalveolar lavage fluid from patients with idiopathic pulmonary fibrosis and chronic hypersensitivity pneumonitis. J Clin Invest 59:165–175, 1977.
42. Haslam PL, Dewar A, Butchers P, Turner-Warwick M: Mast cells in bronchoalveolar lavage fluids from patients with extrinsic allergic alveolitis. Am Rev Respir Dis, Pt II 125:51, 1982.
43. Salvaggio JE: Immunological mechanisms in pulmonary disease. Clin Allergy 9(6):659–668, Feb 1979.

44. Molina C: Broncho-pulmonary Immunopathology. Transl. J Pepys. Edinburgh, London, New York, Churchill Livingstone, 1976.
45. Christensen LT, Schmidt CD, Robbins L: Pigeon breeder's disease—A prevalence study and review. Clin Allergy 5:417–430, 1975.
46. Boyer RS, Klock LE, Schmidt CD, et al: Hypersensitivity lung disease in the turkey raising industry. Am Rev Respir Dis 109:630–635, 1974.
47. Elman AJ, Tebo T, Fink JN, Barboriak JJ: Reactions of poultry against chicken antigens. Arch Environ Health 17:98–100, 1968.
48. Warren CP, Tse KS: Extrinsic allergic alveolitis owing to hypersensitivity to chickens—Significance of sputum precipitins. Am Rev Respir Dis 109(6):630–635, June 1974.
49. Bringhurst LS, Byrne RN, Gershon-Cohen J: Respiratory disease of mushroom workers. JAMA 171:15–18, 1959.
50. Sakula A: Mushroom-worker's lung. Br Med J 3:708–710, 1967.
51. Jackson E, Welch KMA: Mushroom worker's lung. Thorax 25:25–30, 1970.
52. Stewart CJ: Mushroom worker's lung—Two outbreaks. Thorax 29:252–257, 1974.
53. Craig DB, Donevan RE: Mushroom-worker's lung. Can Med Assoc J 102:1289–1293, 1970.
54. Chan-Yeung M, Grzybowski S, Schonell Me: Mushroom worker's lung. Am Rev Respir Dis 105:819–822, 1972.
55. Lockey SD: Mushroom worker's pneumonitis. Ann Allergy 33:282–288, 1974.
56. Johnson WM, Kleyn JG: Respiratory disease in a mushroom worker. Occup Med 23:49–51, 1981.
57. Kleyn JG, Hohnson WM, Wetzler TF: Microbial aerosols and actinomycetes in etiological considerations of mushroom workers lungs. Appl Environ Microbiol 41:1454–1460, 1981.
58. Schulz KH, Felton G, Hansen B: Allergy to spores of *Pleurotus florida*. Lancet 29, 1974.
59. Lacey J: *Thermoactinomyces sacchari* sp. nov., a thermophilic actinomycete causing bagassosis. J Gen Microbiol 66:327–338, 1971.
60. Lehrer SB, Karr RM, Salvaggio JE: Extraction and analysis of coffee beans allergens. Clin Allergy 8:217–226, 1978.
61. Riddle HFV, Channell S, Blyth W, et al: Allergic alveolitis in a maltworker. Thorax 23:271–280, 1968.
62. Channel S, Blyth W, Lloyd M, et al: Allergic alveolitis in maltworkers. Q J Med 38:351–376, 1969.
63. Grant IWB, Blackadder ES, Greenberg M, Blyth W: Extrinsic allergic alveolitis in Scottish maltworkers. Br Med J 1:490–493, 1976.
64. Emanuel DA, Wenzel FJ, Lawton BR: Pneumonitis due to *Cryptostroma corticale* (maple bark disease). N Engl J Med 274:1413–1418, 1966.
65. Renaud J, Pétavy AF, Duriez-Vauchelle T, et al: Analyse antigénique des acariens due from et vue d'une étude de la maladie des fromagers. Rev Fr Mal Respir 7:441–447, 1979.
66. Parker WR: Occupational asthma. In: Occupational Lung Disorders, London, Butterworth, 1982, Chap 12, pp 416–422.
67. Ramazzini, B: Demorbis Artificum Diatriba, 1713. Transl. W. Cave Wright. Chicago, IL, University of Chicago Press, 1940.
68. Cohen VL, Osgood H: Disability due to inhalation of grain dusts. J Allergy 24:193, 1953.

69. Darke CS, Knowleden J, Lacey J, Ward M: Respiratory disease of workers harvesting grain. Thorax 31:294, 1976.
70. Cuthbert OD, Brostoff J, Wraith DG, Brighton WD: "Barn allergy": Asthma and rhinitis due to storage mites. Clin Allergy 9(3):229–236, May 1979.
71. doPico GA, Flaherty D, Bhansali P, Charaje N: Grain fever syndrome induced by inhalation of airborne grain dust. J Allergy Clin Immunol 69:435–443, 1982.
72. doPico GA, Jacobs S, Flaherty D, Rankin J: Pulmonary reaction to durum wheat—A constituent of grain dust. Chest 81:55–61, 1981.
73. Lunn JA, Hughes DTD: Pulmonary hypersensitivity of the grain weevil. Br J Ind Med 24:158, 1968.
74. Davies RJ, Green M, Schofield N: Recurrent nocturnal asthma after exposure to grain dust. Am Rev Respir Dis 114:1011, 1976.
75. Warren CPW, Holford-Stretens V, Wong C, Manfreda J: Respiratory disorders in grain farmers. In: Occupational Lung Disease, eds. Gee JBL, Morgan WKC, Brooks SM. New York, Raven Press, 1984, pp 191.
76. doPico GA, Reddan WG, Tsiatis A, et al: Pulmonary reaction to grain dust and its constituents. Chest 80:56–60, 1980.
77. doPico GA, Reddan WG, Flaherty D, et al: Respiratory abnormalities among grain handlers. A clinical, physiologic and immunologic study. Am Rev Respir Dis 115, 115:915–927, 1977.
78. Broder I, Mintz S, Hutcheon M, et al: Comparison of respiratory variables in grain elevator workers and civic outside workers of Thunder Bay, Canada. Am Rev Respir Dis 119:193–204, 1979.
79. Chan-Yeung M, Schulzer M, MacLean L, et al: Epidemiologic health survey of grain elevator workers in British Columbia. Am Rev Respir Dis 121:329–338, 1980.
80. Department of Labor, OSHA: Hazards in grain handling facilities. Fed Regist 45:10732–10737, 1980.
81. doPico GA, Bhansali P, Dempsey J: Site of airways constriction induced by grain dust exposure. In: Occupational Lung Disease, eds. Gee JBL, Morgan WKC, Brooks SM. New York, Raven Press, 1984, pp 194.
82. doPico GA, Flaherty D, Reed C, Rankin J: Pulmonary and systemic reaction to grain dust. American Academy of Allergy, Annual Meeting, San Francisco, CA, March 9, 1981 (abstract).
83. Chan-Yeung M, Wong R, MacLean L: Respiratory abnormalities among grain elevator workers. Chest 75:461–467, 1979.
84. Warren P, Cherniack RM, Tse KS: Hypersensitivity reactions to grain dust. J Allergy Clin Immunol 53:139–149, 1974.
85. Pepys J, Hutchcroft BJ: Bronchial provocation tests in etiologic diagnosis and analysis of asthma. Am Rev Respir Dis 112:829–859, 1975.
86. Breslin B, Pepys J: Effect of sodium cromoglycate on asthmatic reactions to environmental temperature changes. Clin Allergy 5:325–329, 1975.
87. Boushey HA, Holzman MJ, Sheller JR, Nadel JA: Bronchial hyperreactivity. Am Rev Respir Dis, 121:389–413, 1980.
88. Olenchock SA, Mull J, Major P: Conversion of C_3 and consumption of hemolytic complement by extracts of airborne grain dust. Chest 1977.
89. Chan-Yeung M, Schulzer M, MacLean L, et al: A follow-up study of the grain elevator workers in the port of Vancouver. Arch Environ Health 36:75–81, 1980.
90. Cuthbert OD: The incidence and causative factors of atopic asthma and rhinitis in an Orkney farming community. Clin Allergy 11(3):217–225, May 1981.

91. Ingram CG, Jeffrey IG, Symington IS, Cuthbert OD: Bronchial provocation studies in farmers allergic to storage mites. Lancet 2(8156–8157):1330–1332, Dec 22–29 1979.
92. Cuthbert OD, Brighton WD, Jeffrey IG, McNeil HB: Serial IgE levels in allergic farmers related to the mite content of their hay. Clin Allergy 10(5):601–607, Sep 1980.
93. Burge PS, Edge G, O'Brien IM, et al: Occupational asthma in a research centre breeding locusts. Clin Allergy 10(4):355–363, July 1980.
94. Chan-Yeung M, Lam S, Koener S: Clinical features and natural history of occupational asthma due to western red cedar (*Thuja plicata*). Am J Med 72:411–415, 1982.
95. Williams N, Skoulas A, Merriman JE: Exposure to grain dust. I. Survey of the effects. J Occup Med 6:319–321, 1964.
96. Occupational Safety and Health Administration (OSHA) Citation. OSHA area office files. Milwaukee WI and Minneapolis MN, May 1974.
97. Lacey J: The microflora of grain dust. In: Occupational Pulmonary Disease. Focus on Grain Dust and Health. eds. Dosman J, Cotton D. New York, Academic Press, 1980, pp 417–440.
98. Becklake MR: Grain dust and health: State of the art. In: Occupational Pulmonary Disease. Focus on Grain Dust and Health, eds. Dosman J, Cotton D. New York, Academic Press, 1980, p 189.
99. Pernis B, Vigliani EC, Cavagna C, Finulli M: The role of bacterial endotoxins in occupational disease caused by inhalated vegetable dusts. Br J Ind Med 18:120–129, 1961.
100. Emanuel DA, Wenzel FJ, Lawton BR: Pulmonary mycotoxicosis. Chest 67:293–297, 1975.
101. Gehlbach SH, Williams WA, Perry LD, Woodall JS. Green-tobacco sickness. An illness of tobacco harvesters. JAMA 229(14):1880–1883. Sept 30, 1974.
102. Ghosh SK, Parikh JR, Gokani VN, et al: Studies on occupational health problems during agricultural operation of Indian tobacco workers: A preliminary survey report. J Occup Med 21(1):45–47, 1979.
103. Moses M: Pesticides. In: Public Health and Preventive Medicine, 11th ed. ed. Last JM. New York, Appleton-Century-Crofts, 1980, pp 731–750.
104. Kahn E: Pesticide related illness in California farm workers. J Occup Med 18:693–696, 1976.
105. Higenbottam T, Crome P, Parkinson C, Nunn J: Further clinical observations of the pulmonary effects of paraquat ingestion. Thorax 34(2):161–165, Apr 1979.
106. Rebello G, Mason JK: Pulmonary histological appearances in fatal paraquat poisoning. Histopathology 2(1):53–66, Jan 1978.
107. Levin PJ, Klaff LJ, Rose AG, Ferguson AD: Pulmonary effects of contact exposure to paraquat: A clinical and experimental study. Thorax 34(2):150–160, Apr 1979.
108. Swann AA: Exposure of spray operators to paraquat. Br J Ind Med 26:322–329, 1969.
109. Howard JK, Sabapathy NN, Whitehead PA: A study of the health of Malaysian plantation workers with particular reference to paraquat spraymen. Br J Ind Med 38(2):110–116, May 1981.
110. Ford JE: A review of the findings of potential health effect, associated with agricultural use of paraquat. Annu Am Conf Gov Ind Hyg 2:87–92, 1982.

111. Dasta JF: Paraquat poisoning: A review. Am J Hosp Pharm 35(11):1368–1372, 1978.
112. Keogh BA, Schoenberger, Price DL, Crystal R: Dermal exposure to paraquat as an occupational cause of interstitial lung disease. Am Rev Respir Dis 125:82 part II, 1982.
113. Proudfoot AT, Stewart MS, Levitt T, Widdop B: Paraquat poisoning: Significance of plasma-paraquat concentrations. Lancet 1(8138):330–332, Aug 18, 1979.
114. Frank L, Neriishi K, Sio R, Pascual D: Clofibrate pre-treatment and protection form paraquat-induced lung disease damage and lethality. Am Rev Respir Dis, Pt II 125:231, 1982.
115. Criteria for recommended standard, occupational exposure to malathion. NIOSH 76-205. National Institute of Occupational Safety and Health, US Department of Health, Education and Welfare. Washington, DC, US Printing Office, 1976.
116. Milby TA: Prevention and management of organophosphate poisoning. JAMA 216:2131–33, 1971.
117. US Dept of Health, Education and Welfare. Occupational Diseases—A Guide to Their Recognition. DHEW (NIOSH) Publication 77–181, 1977.
118. Bidstrup PL, Payne DJH: Poisoning by dinitro-ortho-cresol, report of eight fatal cases occurring in Great Britain. Br Med J 2:16–19, 1951.
119. Jedeikin R, Kaplan R, Shapira A, et al: The successful use of "high level" PEEP in near-fatal Endrin poisoning. Crit Care Med 7(4):168–170, Apr 1979.
120. Donham KJ, Rubino M, Thedell TD, Kammermeyer J: Potential health hazards to agricultural workers in swine confinement buildings. J Occup Med 19(6):383–387, June 1977.
121. Donham KJ, Gustafson KE: Human occupational hazards from swine confinement. Annu Am Conf Gov Ind Hyg 2:137–142, 1982.
122. Muehling AJ: Swine Housing and Waste Management: A Research Review. Cooperative Extension Service, University of Illinois, 1969, pp 65–78.
123. Morse DL, Woodbury MA, Rentmeester K, Farmer D: Death caused by fermenting manure. JAMA 245(1):63–64, Sept 2, 1981.
124. Osbern LN, Crapo RO: Dung lung: A report of toxic exposure to liquid manure. Ann Intern Med 95(3):312–314, 1981.
125. Curtis SE, Drummond JG, Grunloh DS, et al: Relative and quantitative aspects of aerial bacteria and dust in swine houses. J Anim Sci 41:1512–1219, 1975.
126. Criteria for a recommended standard-occupational exposure to hydrogen sulfide. NIOSH No. 77-158, National Institute for Occupational Safety and Health, US Dept of Health, Education, and Welfare. Washington, DC, US Government Printing Office, 1977.
127. Horvath E, doPico G, Barbee R, Dickie H: Nitrogen dioxide-induced pulmonary disease: Five new cases and a review of the literature. J Occup Med 20(2):103–110. Feb 1978.
128. Dowell AR, Kilburn KH, Pratt PC: Short-term exposure to nitrogen dioxide. Arch Intern Med 128:74–80, 1971.
129. Von Nieding G, Krekeler H, Wagner M, Koppenhagen K: Studies of the acute effects of NO_2 on lung function: Influence on diffusion, perfusion and ventilation in the lungs. Int Arch Arbeitsmed 31:61–72, 1973.
130. Von Nieding G, Krekeler H: Protective action of atropine, maclastine and orciprenaline on provocation tests with NO_2 in health subjects and patients with chronic non-specific bronchitis. Int Arch Arbeitsmed 29:55–63, 1971.

131. Orehek J, Massari JP, Gayland P, et al: Effect of short-term, low level NO_2 exposure on bronchial sensitivity of asthmatic patients. J Clin Invest 57(2)301–307, Feb 1976.
132. Jones GR, Proudfoot AT, Hall JI: Pulmonary effects of acute exposure to nitrous fumes. Thorax 28:61–65, 1973.
133. Moskowitz RL, Lyons HA, Cottle HR: Silo-filler's disease: Clinical physiologic and pathologic study of a patient. Am J Med 36:457–462, 1964.
134. Greenbaum R, Bay J, Hargreaves MD, et al: Effects of higher oxides of nitrogen in the anaesthetized dog. Br J Anaesth 39:393–404, 1967.
135. Clutton-Brock J: Two cases of poisoning by contamination of nitrous oxide with higher oxides of nitrogen during anaesthesia. Br J Anaesth 39:388–392, 1967.
136. Fleming GM, Chester EH, Montenegro HD: Dysfunction of small airways following pulmonary injury due to nitrogen dioxide. Chest 75:720–721, 1979.
137. Becklake MR, Goldman JI, Bosman AR, Freed CC: The long-term effects of exposure to nitrous fumes. Am Rev Tuberc 76:398–409, 1957.
138. Morrissey W, Gould I, Carrington C, Gaensler E: Silo filler's disease. Respiration 32(1):81–92, 1975.
139. Schnurrenberger PR: Agricultural respiratory hazards—Occupational zoonoses. Annu Am Conf Gov Ind Hyg 2:145–154, 1982.
140. Dickerson MS, Bilderback WR, Pessarra LW: Ornithosis (chlamydiosis) outbreaks in Texas. Texas Med J 72:57–61, 1976.
141. Leachman RD, Yow EM: The epidemiology of psittacosis and report of a turkey-borne outbreak. Arch Intern Med 1958.
142. Jellison WL, Kohls GM: Tularemia in sheep and in sheep industry workers in western United States. Public Health Monogr 28, 1955.
143. Stuart BM, Fullen RL: Tularemic pneumonia: Review of American literature and report of additional cases. Am J Med Sci 210:223, 1945.
144. Di Salvo AF, Johnson WM: Histoplasmosis in South Carolina: Support for the microfocus concept. Am J Epidemiol 109:480–492, 1979.
145. Storch G, Birrford JG, George RB, et al: Acute histoplasmosis. Description of an outbreak in northern Louisiana. Chest 77:38–42, 1980.
146. Gehlbach SH, Hamilton JD, Conant NF: Coccidioidiomycosis. An occupational disease in cotton mill workers. Arch Intern Med 131:254–255, 1973.
147. Schmelzer LL, Tabershaw IR: Exposure factors in occupational coccidioidiomycosis. Am J Public Health, 58:107–113, 1968.
148. Shotwell DL, Burg WR: Aflatoxin in corn: Potential hazard to agricultural workers. Annu Am Conf Gov Ind Hyg 2:69–83, 1982.
149. McCann J, Ames BN: Detection of carcinogens as mutagens in the salmonella/microsome test: Assay of 300 chemicals: Discussion. Proc Natl Acad Sci USA 73:950–954, 1976.
150. Dvorackova I: Aflatoxin inhalation and alveolar cell carcinoma. Br Med J 1(6011):691, 1976.
151. Criteria for a recommended standard-occupational exposure during the manufacture and formulation of pesticides. NIOSH No. 78-174. National Institute for Occupational Safety and Health, US Dept. of HEW, 1978.
152. Burmeister LF: Cancer mortality on Iowa farmers, 1971–1978. J Natl Cancer Inst 66:461–464, 1981.
153. Dunner L, Herman R, Bagnall DJ: Pneumoconiosis in dockers with grain and seeds. Br J Radiol 19:506, 1946.

154. Dynnik VI, Khizhniakova LN, Baranenko AA, et al: Silicosis in tractor drivers working on sandy soils on tree farms. Gig Tr Prof Zabol 12:26–28, 1981.
155. Sherwin RP, Barman ML, Abraham JL: Silicate pneumoconiosis of farm workers. Lab Invest 40:576–582, 1979.
156. Schwartz LW, Knight HD, Whittig LD, et al: Silicate pneumoconiosis and pulmonary fibrosis from the Monterey-Carmel peninsula. Chest 80(Suppl):82–85, 1981.
157. Baris YI, Artvinlim M, Sahin AD: Environmental mesothelioma in Turkey. Ann NY Acad Sci 330:423–432, 1979.

8 Beryllium-Induced Lung Disease: Immunologic Mechanisms and Diagnostic Approaches

Ronald P. Daniele

Beryllium has found wide application in new technologies and modern industry because of its important physical properties, including light weight, high melting point, high strength : weight ratio, and excellent alloying properties. It is currently used in the manufacture of such diverse products as thermal coatings, nuclear reactors, rocket heat shields, brakes, x-ray tubes, and dental plates. The inhalation of particles or aerosols of beryllium metal, beryllium oxide, or beryllium salts may cause either an acute or a chronic lung disease called berylliosis.[1] Besides absorption from the upper respiratory tract, beryllium compounds can also gain access and cause injury to the host by direct contact with the eye or exposed areas of the skin.

The acute form of the disease is a toxic and dose-related injury to the lung. This involves a pneumonitis associated with pulmonary edema and bronchiolitis; irritative injury of the upper airways may also occur. The acute form of the disease is rarely seen today because in the early 1950s it was perceived that acute and chronic diseases could be caused by beryllium oxides used as phosphors in the production of fluorescent lamps. The elimination of this type of use and tighter controls over the contamination in the environment have substantially reduced the risk of acute beryllium pulmonary disease.

In contrast to acute disease, chronic berylliosis is a multisystem disorder; it may progress from acute injury but usually occurs without antecedent events. One to 25 years may intervene between exposure and occurrence of clinical symptoms, and then it is usually a progressive illness with intervals of remission. The chronic form involves a granulomatous interstitial pneumonitis that may progress to fibrosis. The acute form is a toxic pneumonitis, whereas the chronic disease is an inflammatory reaction in the lung, which has many of the characteristics of hypersensitivity lung disease (see below). This chapter will focus on the chronic form of disease, emphasizing immunopathogenetic events.

HISTOPATHOLOGIC FEATURES

An important pathologic feature of berylliosis is that it is a multisystem disorder. This is explained by the fact that once beryllium compounds or metals gain access via the lung or skin, they bind to tissue and blood proteins and are distributed widely throughout the body, including the spleen, liver, and kidney. The histopathologic hallmark in affected tissues is the noncaseating epithelioid granuloma.[1,2] In the lung, which has been most extensively studied and where histopathologic features predominate, there is usually a mononuclear cell infiltration of the alveolar walls. The cell types comprise mainly histiocytes, lymphocytes, and a variable number of plasma cells. The cellular infiltration is usually associated with granulomas diffusely scattered throughout the interstitial, peribronchial, and perivascular areas. These granulomas are indistinguishable from those of sarcoidosis and hypersensitivity pneumonitis and consist of epithelioid cells and giant cells surrounded by lymphocytes and fibroblasts. In earlier descriptions of the granulomas in berylliosis, some emphasis was placed on the asteroid bodies or cholesterol crystals that may be present within giant cells. These cell inclusions, however, are not specific for berylliosis. The surrounding airway epithelium may be hyperplastic, and characteristically there are large collections of mononuclear cells in the airways. Within the granulomas and the adjacent alveolar walls, there is a variable amount of fibroblast activity, as demonstrated by stainable collagen. It is believed that, as the inflammatory lesions mature, interstitial fibrosis supervenes. Similar to sarcoidosis, interstitial fibrosis may progress to destructive changes of the alveolar walls and ducts resulting in honeycombing of the lung. Interestingly, in the chronic form there appears to be little relationship between the clinical severity of pulmonary disease and the amount and duration of exposure to beryllium.

Similar to saroidosis, granulomatous lesions can be found in extrapulmonary sites, including abdominal lymph nodes, spleen, liver, bone marrow, kidneys, and adrenals. Granulomas may also occur in myocardium, skeletal muscle, and bone. The skin may also be involved in berylliosis, but this usually results from direct contact and may precede the pulmonary lesions.

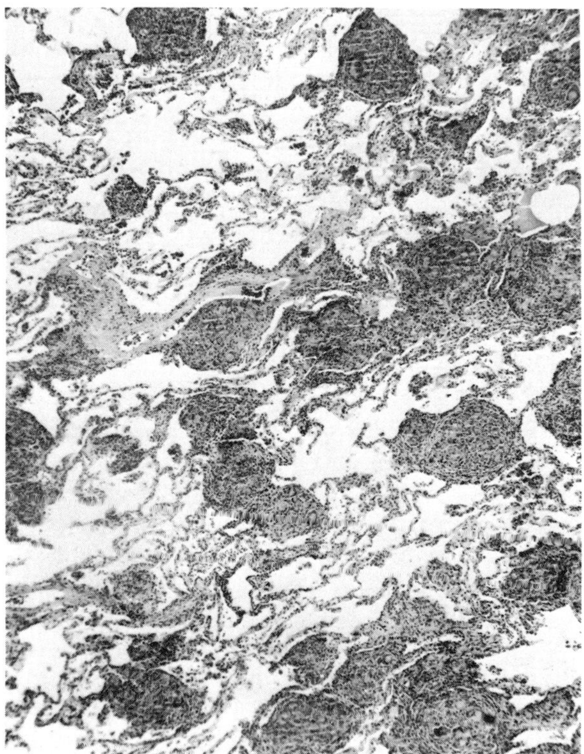

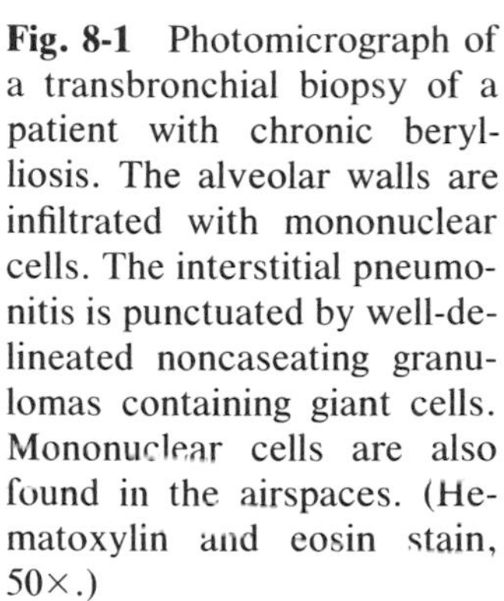

Fig. 8-1 Photomicrograph of a transbronchial biopsy of a patient with chronic berylliosis. The alveolar walls are infiltrated with mononuclear cells. The interstitial pneumonitis is punctuated by well-delineated noncaseating granulomas containing giant cells. Mononuclear cells are also found in the airspaces. (Hematoxylin and eosin stain, 50×.)

Key histopathologic features in chronic berylliosis, which may render some clues as to pathogenesis, include the following (see Fig. 8-1):

1. A mononuclear infiltrate in the alveolar walls.
2. Infiltrates may coalesce into well-defined granulomas containing epithelioid cells, giant cells, and macrophages in various states of activation.

These stereotypic changes also occur in diseases such as hypersensitivity pneumonitis and sarcoidosis, which are believed to be primarily immunologic in pathogenesis.

CLINICAL FEATURES

The initial and most conspicuous symptom is dyspnea on exertion. There may also be a dry, nonproductive cough precipitated by exertion or occurring spontaneously, sometimes during sleep. The onset of symptoms is usually gradual and may be accompanied by anorexia, fatigue, malaise, and weight loss. These symptoms may also be associated with physical findings of low-grade fever, tachycardia, tachypnea, and central cyanosis. In more advanced and severe cases, findings of digital clubbing or right heart failure (cor pulmonale) may be prominent.

Roentgenographic findings usually consist of a diffuse interstitial infiltrate.[3] This process may be seen as a fine granularity involving both lungs, the so-called ground glass appearance. It may also appear as a reticular nodular infiltrate involving both lungs. Hilar lymph nodes are often enlarged in patients with chronic berylliosis, but the degree of enlargement is seldom as great as that found in sarcoidosis. These roentgenographic findings may resemble those of sarcoidosis (Stages II and III). However, unlike sarcoidosis, hilar adenopathy is not seen in the absence of parenchymal infiltrates (i.e., Stage I). A late chest roentgenographic finding, and one which augurs a poor prognosis, is the presence of honeycombing or a coarse reticular pattern.

Pulmonary function abnormalities are predictable from the pathologic changes noted above.[4] The lungs are stiff and there is a decrease in pulmonary compliance. This results in a reduction in static lung volumes (vital capacity, total lung capacity), but the ratio of forced expiratory volume in one second to vital capacity usually remains normal. A decrease in the effective gas exchanging area results in a reduction in diffusing capacity. This may be an early finding. Hypoxemia is caused by mismatching of ventilation to perfusion and results from disruption and reduction in the gas exchanging units. Characteristically, hypoxemia becomes worse with exercise.

Laboratory abnormalities include hyperuricemia and hypercalcuria/hypercalcemia. It was once thought that serum angiotensin-converting enzyme activity was relatively specific for sarcoidosis; however, recent studies have shown that both angiotensin-converting enzyme and serum lysozyme may be significantly elevated in patients with chronic berylliosis as well as sarcoidosis.[5] Beryllium may also be detected in the urine of patients with chronic berylliosis.[6] However, the identification of beryllium in the urine indicates that there has been previous exposure to beryllium, but not the presence of active pulmonary disease.

It is clear that in berylliosis there are clinical, roentgenographic, and laboratory findings that are strikingly similar to sarcoidosis. As mentioned, however, isolated bilateral hilar adenopathy is rarely seen in chronic berylliosis. Moreover, uveitis and erythema nodosum are seen in sarcoidosis but not berylliosis. More important, the natural history and response to steroid therapy differ in these two diseases. Two thirds of the patients with sarcoidosis improve or resolve spontaneously, and for those patients who receive steroid therapy, there are dramatic short-term improvements in roentgenographic findings, pulmonary function, and clinical abnormalities. Chronic berylliosis frequently progresses relentlessly to fibrosis, and the response to steroids is less conspicuous.

DIAGNOSIS

The diagnosis of chronic berylliosis is based on a history of exposure to beryllium, clinical and histologic abnormalities compatible with the disease, and an elevated concentration of beryllium in lung or other tissues. The beryllium content of lung or affected tissues is usually determined by emission spectroscopy or laser probe techniques. However, to obtain sufficient amounts of tissue for this analysis, lung tissue must be obtained by open lung biopsy or thoracotomy and intrathoracic lymph nodes by mediastinoscopy. Recent analytic studies of lung tissue have defined borderline levels of beryllium in tissue upon which diagnosis can be made with confidence.[7] Lung tissue and mediastinal nodes from known cases of beryllium disease and sarcoidosis and from normal controls were analyzed.[7] It was found that 0.02 μg of beryllium per gram dry tissue represented a level that separated patients with known beryllium disease from controls. These studies showed further that, although beryllium disease is never present in the absence of beryllium in tissue, measurable levels of beryllium may be found in normal lung tissue or lymph nodes. Even after an invasive biopsy procedure and analysis of the tissue, the diagnosis may still be in doubt because of the similarity of this disease to other granulomatous diseases, especially sarcoidosis, and the fact that beryllium may be detected in the lungs of exposed individuals who do not have disease. These considerations have led investigators to seek more specific tests of beryllium exposure and disease (e.g., immunologic assays).

IMMUNOLOGIC ASPECTS OF CHRONIC BERYLLIOSIS

Because of the similarities, immunologic aspects of chronic berylliosis will be compared to sarcoidosis. In patients with chronic berylliosis, there may be a lymphopenia in peripheral blood that is reflected mainly by a reduction in circulating T cells.[8] However, unlike patients with sarcoidosis, peripheral blood lymphocytes from patients with chronic beryllium disease do not appear to have impaired responses to polyclonal mitogens such as phytohemagglutinin.[9] Similar to sarcoidosis, there is hyperreactivity of the B cell system as evidenced by an increase in the circulating immunoglobulins (IgA and IgG).[10]

Perhaps the most significant immunologic feature of chronic berylliosis is the evidence of hypersensitivity to beryllium that may be detected by beryllium patch test[11] or in vitro response of lymphocytes to beryllium compounds.[12] For the patch test, a solution of beryllium sulfate or beryllium nitrate is applied to the skin and elicits an erythematous reaction within 48 to 72 hours in sensitized individuals. This skin reaction progresses over several weeks to skin granulomas. Unfortunately, the beryllium patch test has been abandoned because (1) false negative reactions can occur, (2) introduction of beryllium into the skin will sensitize an unaffected individual, and (3) some reports indicate that the patch test may worsen existing disease.

Similarly, in sensitized individuals, the in vitro culture of lymphocytes with soluble beryllium salts, beryllium fluoride, or beryllium sulfate, elicits a blastogenic response of blood lymphocytes and the liberation of certain lymphokines, such as macrophage migration inhibition factor.[13] However, a positive patch test or an in vitro lymphocyte proliferation test does not indicate disease, but merely that an individual has been exposed and sensitized to beryllium compounds. Some investigators have found that in patients with disease there is a good correlation between clinical severity of chronic disease and the degree of the proliferative response by sensitized lymphocytes.

Such a test provides one means of distinguishing patients with sarcoidosis from those with chronic berylliosis. Patients with sarcoidosis will not exhibit a positive patch test or respond to beryllium compounds in vitro. Furthermore, patients with chronic berylliosis fail to respond to the Kveim-Siltzbach skin test.

These relatively specific immunologic responses in affected individuals coupled with the pathologic features of a mononuclear interstitial pneumonitis with granulomas lend some support to the hypothesis that this disease is caused by a delayed hypersensitivity reaction to beryllium compounds. Additional evidence for a primary immunologic basis for this disease is the low prevalence rate among exposed individuals, the prolonged latent period after exposure, and the response to steroids. Evidence for the presence of a *specific cellular immune* reaction, especially in the lungs, comes from recent studies of the local immune abnormalities.

LOCAL IMMUNE REACTIONS IN THE LUNG

A relatively new approach to study diffuse interstitial lung diseases has been the application of segmental bronchoalveolar lavage. Bronchoalveolar lavage fluid recovered from patients with sarcoidosis and hypersensitivity pneumonitis has been evaluated by several laboratories.[14,15] These disorders are characterized by increased numbers of lymphocytes in lavage fluid but the degree of lymphocytosis is usually greater in hypersensitivity pneumonitis than in sarcoidosis.

Immunologic studies of lung lymphocytes in chronic berylliosis appear more informative with respect to pathogenesis.[8] The most conspicuous abnormality was the recovery of cells by a standardized lavage in patients with chronic berylliosis; the total number of cells recovered was nearly seven times that of normal subjects and twice the number of cells recovered in patients with sarcoidosis. Moreover, lymphocytes were the predominant cell type in lavage fluid, equaling 60–80% of the total cells (Fig. 8-2). This pattern is similar to that found in hypersensitivity pneumonitis. Furthermore, the majority of these cells appear to be activated as demonstrated by various membrane markers of T cell activation. These include the capacity to form rosettes at 37°C (stable or active rosettes) as well as the expression of distinct differentiation markers, such as DR framework antigens (manuscript in preparation). When lymphocytes from the lung and peripheral blood were incubated with soluble beryllium salts, the degree of proliferation was dose dependent with the highest response occurring at 10^{-4} M of beryllium sulfate and beryllium fluoride (Fig. 8-3).[8] The peak response for bronchoalveolar lymphocytes that were stimulated with beryllium occurred after 3 days in culture, whereas the peak response for peripheral blood lymphocytes occurred 5 to 7 days in culture. The response of blood lymphocytes to antigenic stimuli usually occurs 5 to 7 days after stimulation.

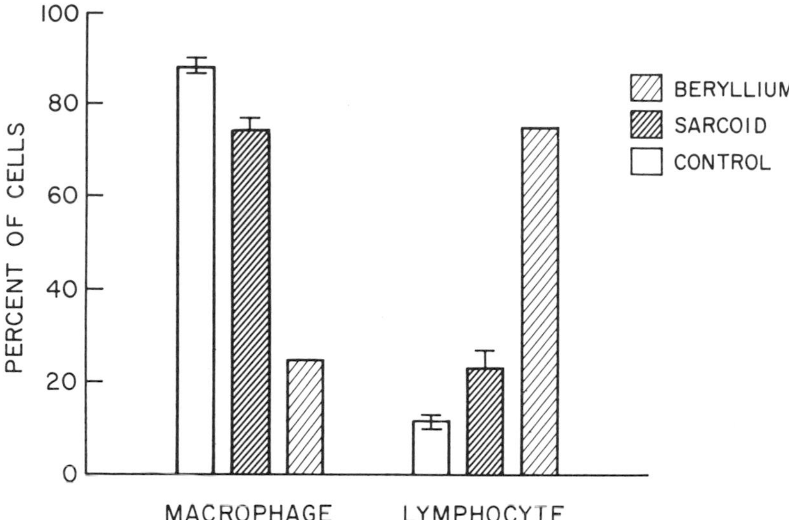

Fig. 8-2 Proportions of cell types in bronchoalveolar lavage fluid in patients with chronic berylliosis (n = 2), sarcoidosis (n = 22), and age-matched controls (n = 25). The proportions of lymphocytes in sarcoidosis and chronic berylliosis are increased in comparison to controls, but is greater in berylliosis. The lymphocytosis in lavage fluid is similar to that found in hypersensitivity pneumonitis.

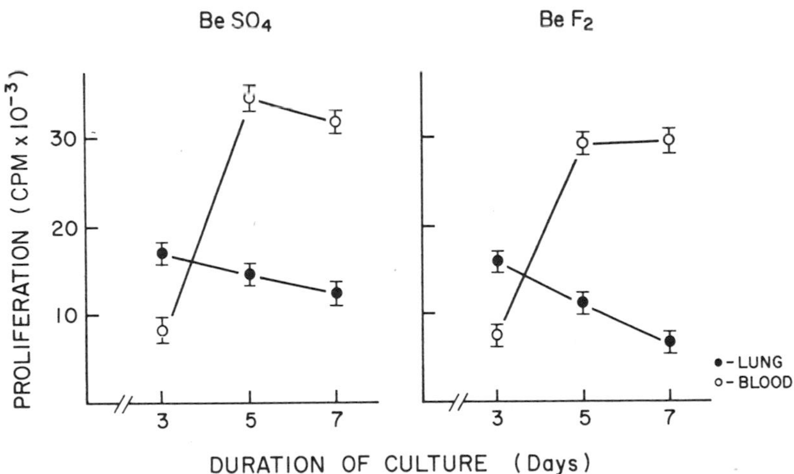

Fig. 8-3 The time course for the response of lymphocytes in bronchoalveolar lavage fluid (●) and those in peripheral blood (○) to doses of beryllium salts producing optimal proliferation; for both $BeSO_4$ and BeF_2, the concentration was 10^{-4} M.

The fact that lung lymphocytes responded with a peak response after 3 days indicates that a large number of antigen specific lymphocytes were present within the lung and bronchoalveolar airspaces. It is also of interest that the magnitude of the peak lung lymphocyte response to beryllium after 3 days in culture was more than double that of comparable numbers of peripheral blood lymphocytes, indicating that the proportion of lymphocytes in lavage fluid that were sensitive to beryllium was greater than in blood. Taken together, these observations are consistent with the idea that there is an immunologically mediated response in the lungs of these patients. Evidence for the specificity of this immune response is that beryllium salts are not mitogens nor do they stimulate lymphocyte proliferation in unsensitized individuals or in patients with active sarcoidosis (unpublished).

Similar findings have also been observed in patients with hypersensitivity pneumonitis that is provoked by exposure to antigens in pigeon serum and droppings.[16,17] The similarity in pathologic findings, lung lavage, results, and immunologic abnormalities suggests that chronic berylliosis may be a type of hypersensitivity pneumonitis exhibiting predominantly a cell-mediated immune response in the lungs. A question not yet answered is whether a positive response of lung lymphocytes to beryllium salts necessarily indicates the presence of active pulmonary disease.

Besides extending our understanding about pathogenesis, studies of lung cells obtained by bronchoalveolar lavage may have a practical and valuable application in replacing open lung biopsy as the definitive approach for establishing the diagnosis of chronic berylliosis.

CURRENT THOUGHTS ON IMMUNOPATHOGENESIS

The histopathologic hallmark of chronic berylliosis is an interstitial pneumonitis consisting of mononuclear cells. This infiltrate is composed of lymphocytes, monocytes, and macrophages in various states of activation. In general, that analysis of the cell types recovered by lavage in these patients reflects the type of cells found in the interstitial infiltrates of the biopsy specimens (Ref. 8 and unpublished findings). While the studies of lavage fluid reveal that these cells are made up almost entirely of T cells, it remains to be established whether the interstitial cell infiltrates are similarly composed of T cells. Similar to what has been proposed for sarcoidosis,[18] these histopathologic features coupled with the immunologic studies at both systemic and lung level suggest the following immunopathogenic sequence of events:

The initial event is the deposition of antigens in the lung. By as yet poorly understood mechanisms antigens are presented to the local immune apparatus of the lung with lymphocyte recruitment. The ability of beryllium to bind to tissue and blood proteins permits beryllium antigen to be distributed widely throughout the body. Beryllium is an element and thus acts as a hapten. When coupled with host proteins, the hapten carrier complex is recognized by the immune system as a foreign antigen and generates a cellular immune response.

The development of chronic disease in selected hosts indicates that the antigen persists at sites of granulomatous involvement. One mechanism that might explain the persistence of antigens at such sites as the lung comes from studies showing that alveolar macrophages are able to incorporate beryllium into the polyphagosome.[19] Persistence of the antigen and chronic stimulation of the immune system may lead to activation and proliferation of T cells and the liberation of lymphokines, which figure importantly in the recruitment, activation, and localization of mononuclear phagocytes. The pulmonary recruitment and retention of monocytes from the blood may explain ensuing granuloma formation whereby monocytes progressively differentiate into macrophages, multinucleated giant cells, and epithelioid cells. This immunologic train of events may also explain the recruitment and stimulation of fibroblasts, leading to an increase in their numbers and the deposition of extracellular matrix proteins. The factors that determine the fate of granulomas and interstitial pneumonitis in a given patient remain obscure. It is likely that, given the low prevalence rate among exposed individuals, there are unique host factors which contribute to the initiation and perpetuation of this cell-mediated reaction after exposure to beryllium.

Besides their practical significance, further studies in chronic berylliosis may provide important clues in understanding immunopathogenic events in similar diseases, such as sarcoidosis, where the etiology remains obscure.

ACKNOWLEDGMENTS

This work was supported by the following grants from the National Heart, Lung and Blood Institute: Research Career Development Award HL-00210 and HL-30715.

REFERENCES

1. Frieman DG, Hardy HL: Beryllium disease. The relation of pulmonary pathology to clinical course and prognosis based on a study of 130 cases from the U.S. Beryllium Case Registry. Hum Pathol 1:25–44, 1970.
2. Jones Williams W: Beryllium disease—Pathology and diagnosis. J Soc Occup Med 27:93–96, 1977.
3. Weber AL, Stoeckle JD, Hardy HL: Roentgenologic patterns in long-standing beryllium disease. Am J Roentgenol 93:879–890, 1965.
4. Andrews JL, Kazemi H, Hardy HL: Patterns of lung dysfunction in chronic beryllium disease. Am Rev Respir Dis 100:791–800, 1969.
5. Lieberman J, Nosal A, Schleissner LA, Sastre-Foken A: Serum angiotensin-converting enzyme for diagnosis and therapeutic evaluation of sarcoidosis. Am Rev Respir Dis 120:329–335, 1979.
6. Lieben J, Dattoli JA, Vought VM: The significance of beryllium concentrations in urine. Arch Environ Med 12:331–334, 1966.
7. Sprince NL, Kazemi H, Hardy HL: Current (1975) problem of differentiating between beryllium disease and sarcoidosis. Ann NY Acad Sci 278:654–664, 1976.

8. Epstein PE, Dauber JH, Rossman MD, Daniele RP: Bronchoalveolar lavage in a patient with chronic berylliosis: evidence for hypersensitivity pneumonitis. Ann Intern Med 97:213–216, 1982.
9. Morison WL: Phytohaemagglutinin and transfer factor in the leucocyte migration inhibition test in patients with sarcoidosis. Thorax 31:87–90, 1976.
10. Resnick H, Roche M, Morgan WKC: Immunoglobulin concentration in berylliosis. Am Rev Respir Dis 101:504–510, 1970.
11. Curtis GH: The diagnosis of beryllium disease, with special reference to the patch test. Arch Ind Health 19:150–153, 1959.
12. Deodhar SD, Barna B, Van Ordstrand HS: A study of the immunological aspects of chronic berylliosis. Chest 63:309–313, 1973.
13. Marx JJ Jr, Burrell R: Delayed hypersensitivity to beryllium compounds. J Immunol 111:590–598, 1973.
14. Reynolds HY, Fulmer JD, Kazmierowski JA, et al: Analysis of cellular and protein content of bronchoalveolar lavage fluid from patients with idiopathic pulmonary fibrosis and chronic hypersensitivity pneumonitis. J Clin Invest 59:165–175, 1977.
15. Dauber JH, Rossman MD, Daniele RP: Bronchoalveolar cell populations in acute sarcoidosis: observations in smoking and nonsmoking patients. J Lab Clin Med 94:862–871, 1979.
16. Schuyler MR, Thigpen TP, Salvaggio JE: Local pulmonary immunity in pigeon breeder's disease: A case study. Ann Intern Med 88:355–358, 1978.
17. Moore VL, Pedersen GM, Hauser WC, Fink JN: A study of lung lavage materials in patients with hypersensitivity pneumonitis: In vitro response to mitogen and antigen in pigeon breeder's disease. J Allergy Clin Immunol 65:365–370, 1980.
18. Daniele RP, Dauber JH, Rossman MD: Immunologic abnormalities in sarcoidosis. Ann Intern Med 92:406–416, 1980.
19. Hart BA, Pittman DG: The uptake of beryllium by the alveolar macrophage. J Reticuloendothel Soc 27:49–58, 1980.

9 Cellular and Humoral Mechanisms in Byssinosis

Ragnar Rylander

BACKGROUND

A characteristic respiratory ailment has long been known to exist among workers handling cotton and flax. Ramazzini[1] described symptoms of cough and asthma among dressers of flax and hemp. The term byssinosis (from the Egyptian word bysan meaning small fibers) was introduced during the nineteenth century. Based on epidemiologic studies of the disease among Lancashire cotton mill workers,[2] Schilling classified the symptomatology (see Table 9-1) and the prevalence of the disease at various work sites within cotton mills. Byssinosis has not only been observed among workers in cotton and flax mills but also in those handling soft hemp and sisal. Reviews of the present state of the art were presented at a recent international conference.[3]

The original definition of byssinosis refers to a subjective feeling of chest tightness. This symptom usually occurs for the first time on a Monday following a weekend break, but in severe cases, after long-term exposure, it may occur on any day of the week. Measures of respiratory function have demonstrated that the function decreases over the working shift. These changes are most often described as a loss in forced expiratory volume in one second (FEV_1). The subjective chest tightness and respiratory changes may, however, occur independently.

After long-term exposure, lung function may be impaired before the shift as well, particularly among smokers. Histopathologic examinations of tissue

Table 9-1. Symptomatic Classification of Byssinosis According to Schilling et al. (1963)

Grade 0:	No symptoms
Grade 1/2:	Occasional chest tightness or cough on the first day of the work week
Grade 1:	Chest tightness and/or shortness of breath on every first day of the work week
Grade 2:	Chest tightness and/or shortness of breath on the first and other days of the work week
Grade 3:	Grade 2 symptoms accompanied by evidence of permanent loss of lung function.

from cotton workers show mucus gland hypertrophy—chronic bronchitis—but no excess of emphysema and no fibrosis.[4]

A further effect associated with exposure to cotton dust is mill fever. This is characterized by an increase in body temperature, a feeling of dryness in the throat, and sometimes joint pains. The fever appears after several hours at work, peaks in the afternoon or evening, and disappears by the following day. After repeated exposure a tolerance develops and the fever then only appears on a return to work after a long absence such as annual holidays or a long sick leave. Mill fever closely resembles the fever seen in humidifier disease, and chest tightness has also been reported in episodes of humidifier fever.[5]

It is evident from the foregoing discussion that exposure to cotton and flax dust causes a series of symptoms distinctly different from those found in other pulmonary diseases. The chest tightness is different from the symptoms in an asthmatic attack. It is characterized by the development of tolerance during the work week and is not found among cotton mill workers working 7 days per week.[6]

Airway function decreases slowly, the maximum decrease occurring 4 to 6 hours after the initiation of exposure. This development of respiratory function impairment resembles certain types of occupational asthma, but in contrast to this disease, it is characterized by the development of tolerance over the work week.

The chronic bronchitis found among cotton workers is indistinguishable from that caused by tobacco smoke, for example, but emphysema is not present.

The question of whether byssinosis is a permanent, disabling disease and if the changes deteriorate over the years after the cessation of exposure, is dealt with in Chapters 10 and 11. It is noteworthy, however, that studies on mortality in cohorts of workers from cotton and flax mills, have not detected an excess in general mortality or mortality from respiratory disease.[7,8] Slightly elevated death rates from renal disease and heart disease have been found, but it is difficult to assess the importance of these observations without further analysis.

What then is the pathogenesis of this curious assembly of symptoms? In the following sections we review the cellular and humoral mechanisms which have been suggested to play a role in byssinosis. The etiologic agent(s) for the disease will not be reviewed, although reference will occasionally be made to bacterial endotoxins, in view of the accumulating evidence for a major role of these substances in the pathogenesis of byssinosis.[9]

HUMORAL REACTIONS

Histamine Release

Because bronchoconstriction is encountered in byssinosis, a good deal of attention was devoted in the early research to the possibility that cotton dust caused the liberation of histamine. Studies demonstrated, however, that the histamine content in the dust itself was insufficient to provoke bronchoconstriction. A direct or indirect influence of chemical compounds in the cotton dust on mast cells was then suggested as a possible mechanisms.

Although much effort has gone into studies of histamine release, no convincing evidence for its importance as a primary pathogenic mechanism for byssinosis has been produced. It is true that cotton dust is positive in in vitro test systems where the histamine release is measured in terms of contractions of an ileum preparation. However, in vitro experiments with chopped lung tissue from guinea pigs, rats, cats, sheep, and pigs have not produced evidence of histamine release after incubation with extracts of cotton flax or hemp dusts. The Monday phenomenon could be explained by a buildup of histamine in the mast cells over the exposure-free weekend and a rapid depletion on Mondays. Difficult to explain, however, is the gradual onset of the bronchoconstriction over the working day as well as the difference in the subjective feeling of chest tightness in byssinosis and the "air hunger" present in asthma or after a histamine provocation.

Although it is quite possible that histamine liberation takes place at some stage during the different reactions involved in the development of byssinosis, it is unlikely that it represents a major mechanism responsible for the initiation of the disease.

Antigen–Antibody Reactions

The observation that the development of typical symptoms of byssinosis requires a certain exposure period, ranging from a few to several years of employment, suggested the hypothesis that an antigen–antibody reaction was involved in the pathogenesis.

Massoud and Taylor[10] reported the presence of specific antibodies against cotton dust extract in the serum of byssinotic subjects. In a later report, the antigen was identified as tetrahydroxyflavone, but the reaction after inhalation of this compound did not mimic that seen after challenge with cotton dust extract. Kutz et al.[11] demonstrated that aqueous extracts of cardroom cotton dust contained polyphenolic tannins that precipitated globulins in a pseudoimmune fashion. No precipitating antibodies were detected to any of the antigens tested.

Rylander et al.[12] measured antibody activity against a major antigenic component in cotton and flax dust—gram-negative bacteria—in the serum and nasal secretions of cotton mill workers. Samples were taken from cotton mill workers and the activity was evaluated using the ELISA technique. No difference in IgG, IgM, and IgA antibody activity could be found between cotton mill workers and control subjects not exposed to cotton dust, nor were any differences found over the work shift among workers with or without symptoms. In a study of 13 cotton workers, IgE serum antibody activity was measured using the radioallergosorbent technique. No indications were found of increased antibody levels in this population, nor was any relation found to the FEV_1 decrements over a Monday work shift. Radioallergosorbent antibody values before and after the shift were similar.[13]

Evidence exists, however, that atopy is more common among persons showing an FEV_1 decline over the work shift in cotton seed oil mills than among persons without such changes.[14] This may be interpreted to mean that persons with increased immunologic responses may be more prone to develop byssinosis. The mechanism through which this takes place could, however, be a different immunologic response mechanism than antibodies for instance cell-initiated responses. It is plausible that such cell responses could be partly mediated through the presence of antibodies. Walker and Beasky[15] have demonstrated that the platelet aggregation caused by endotoxin, a substance always present in cotton dust, is modified in the presence of antibodies to the polysaccharide portion of the endotoxin.

Complement Activation

The direct or indirect activation of complement will cause the appearance of factors C3a and C5a, the latter rapidly transformed to C5 desArg. These components are active in the first phase of inflammation and also cause bronchoconstriction. Several researchers have considered that complement activation might be the cause of the symptoms appearing after exposure to cotton dust.

Wilson et al.[16] demonstrated that extracts of cotton dust activated the alternative complement pathway in fresh normal human serum in vitro. The activation was dose dependent and highly related to the amount of endotoxin in the dust. It has also been shown, using in vitro models or i.v. injections, that endotoxins have the ability to activate complement via the alternative pathway.

In spite of this evidence for complement activation by cotton dust, the real-life situation may be more complex. Cochrane[17] evaluated the importance of the complement system in shock induced by endotoxin in rabbits and monkeys. Hypotension, thrombocytopenia, neutropenia, and death after an i.v. injection of two different endotoxins were not influenced by the decomplementation of the animals. Snella and Rylander[18] exposed guinea pigs to aerosols of endotoxin and found a dose-dependent increase in neutrophils in the airways. Decomplementation of the animals prior to the endotoxin exposure did not influence the response and no neutrophil increase was seen after inhalation of zymosan, a potent complement activator.

Although the experimental evidence cited above does not rule out a participation of complement in the development of byssinosis, it suggests that other factors, probably of regulatory capacity, are involved. The role of complement may then be to enhance a reaction, most likely initiated by cell systems rather than initiate the reaction by themselves.

CELL REACTIONS

The Macrophages

The primary defense cell of the lungs against inhaled agents is the pulmonary macrophage. Exposure to any kind of airborne dust, of a size small enough to penetrate down into the alveoli, will result in rapid phagocytosis of the particles by the macrophages.

In guinea pigs exposed to aqueous extracts of different cotton dusts, an increase in the number of macrophages took place within 24 hours after the exposure.[19] This increase is not dose dependent, contrary to the neutrophil response, and could well be due to alterations in the adherence characteristics of the macrophages, making more cells available for lavage.

These data suggest that cotton dust is phagocytosed and stimulates the activity of macrophages. These are secretory cells with a capacity to induce the excretion of lysosomal enzymes, chemotactic factors, prostaglandins, complement factors, platelet activating factor (PAF-acether), and others.

Prostaglandins are a group of unsaturated long-chain fatty acids which contain a cyclopentane ring and hydroxyl and keto groups. Fowler et al.[20] demonstrated that water-soluble compounds extracted from cotton bract, a major component of cotton dust, can induce rabbit macrophages to generate prostaglandins $F_{2\alpha}$ and E in vitro.

It has been suggested that prostaglandins of the E type are mediators of endotoxin fever,[21] although other data suggest that it is caused by endogenous pyrogen, also secreted by macrophages, particularly after endotoxin exposure. When exposed to zymosan, macrophages release prostaglandins with a maximum 1 to 2 hours after incubation.[22] Treatment of macrophages with endotoxin (1–100 μg/ml) was found to cause a dose-dependent accumulation of PGE_2 and $PGF_{2\alpha}$ in the culture medium with a maximum after 24 to 48 hours. Peritoneal macrophages from C3H/HeJ mice, which do not respond to endotoxin, do not release $PGF_{2\alpha}$ after incubation with endotoxin.[23]

These data show that prostaglandins can be released by macrophages, both by a general, nonspecific phagocytosis and by endotoxins present in cotton dust. It is thus conceivable that prostaglandin synthesis is independent of phagocytosis. If the prostaglandin response after pure phagocytosis in humans reacts according to the in vivo model, bronchoconstriction caused by cotton dust particles should appear more rapidly than actually occurs. The slow initiation by endotoxin is more applicable to the reactions observed after human exposure to cotton dust.

Thromboxane A_2 and prostacyclin are metabolic derivatives of prostaglandins, the former being a potent bronchoconstrictor and the latter a dilator. Both substances can be produced by macrophages after exposure to endotoxin in vitro.[24]

The concept that the alveolar macrophage generates substances that cause the observed reactions in byssinosis is at first appealing. Although macrophages can produce a variety of such agents, their products are less important than secretions from other kinds of cells which can be activated by macrophages. The specificity of the reaction to cotton dust and quantities produced are not defined.

The role of the macrophage is thus to act as a cellular "orchestra leader" tuning in other cell types, which are then responsible for the final pathologic effects. Of primary interest among such secondary cell reactions are those caused by neutrophils.

Neutrophil Responses

Neutrophil Migration. A major reaction following inhalation of cotton dust or aqueous extracts thereof, is neutrophil invasion of the airways. This has been shown to occur both in animal experiments and when humans are exposed to cotton dust.[9] The reaction is caused by the lipid A part of the endotoxin in the dust.[25] The response is seen in animals 1 to 2 hours after the cessation of exposure and reaches a peak 12 to 24 hours thereafter. After subchronic exposure over a period of several weeks, the response is diminished and, although still higher than in control animals, it is significantly lower than the acute response. This change in the magnitude of response after long-term exposure could be related to the clinical observation that an increased pulmonary response to cotton dust is observed as the exposure continues.

The neutrophils are recruited into the lung from the blood and the bone marrow pool. Migrating neutrophils are commonly accompanied by platelets when moving into areas of inflammation.[26] During this recruitment, the neutrophils become sticky and attach to the endothelial wall. In animal experiments it has been demonstrated that this causes an increase in the pulmonary capillary pressure.[27] Neutrophils are short-lived and readily secrete their intracellular enzymes and generate oxidizing substrates, for example, H_2O_2 and O_2^-. Neutrophils are also the major source of leukotrienes, which are powerful bronchoconstricting agents. Neutrophils also secrete platelet-activating factor (PAF-acether) which itself is a potent bronchoconstrictor and also induces platelets to secrete serotonin.[28]

It is therefore suggested that the neutrophil is a major effector cell in the development of byssinosis. Further studies on the pathogenesis of the disease should focus on the response of this cell to cotton dust.

Leukotrienes. As regards the pathogenesis of byssinosis, leukotrienes are particularly interesting in view of their potent bronchoconstrictor activity.

Leukotrienes are formed from arachidonic acid by the lipoxygenase pathway. Leukocytes are a major source of leukotrienes, although they may also be secreted by macrophages. Some leukotrienes are potent peripheral airway bronchoconstrictors whereas histamine and prostaglandin $F_{2\alpha}$ have little effect. The leukotriene LTC_4 administered as an aerosol is 100 times more potent than histamine in decreasing the air flow in lungs of monkeys and 3800 times more active than histamine in decreasing the air flow in the lungs of human volunteers. LTC_4, LTD_4, and LTE_4 also increase vascular permeability at much lower concentrations than histamine. LTB_4 may also stimulate the release of lysozymal enzymes from granules of neutrophils and eosinophils. Rouzer et al.[29] demonstrated that mouse pulmonary macrophages, challenged with zymosan, synthesized LTC series.

Platelet-Activating Factor. Bomski et al.[30] reported that the number of circulating platelets in cotton workers decreased over the working shift. The reduction was only found over the first day of the working week but not on Friday.

Platelets respond to platelet activation factor (PAF-acether) which is secreted by several cell types.[31] In early studies it was found to be secreted by IgE-sensitized basophils after stimulation with the specific antigen, although this reaction seems to be limited to rabbits. Several researchers have, however, shown that neutrophils secrete PAF-acether after stimulation with zymosan or ionophore. When incubated with gram-negative bacteria isolated from cotton, human neutrophils were found to induce platelets to release serotonin, presumably due to PAF-acether production.[32] Macrophages also secrete PAF-acether after stimulation with ionophore and probably endotoxin.

PAF-acether induces bronchoconstriction if platelets are present. It is one of the most potent bronchoconstrictors so far described and acts on guinea pigs at concentrations of 60 ng/kg, as compared to arachidonic acid at 0.2 mg/kg, serotonin at 5 μg/kg and histamine at 10–20 mg/kg.

PAF-acether secretion apparently influences the platelets selectively. Henson and Laudes[33] reported that PAF does not induce the coagulation cofactor, platelet factor 3, in rabbit platelets. Henson[26] has suggested that antibodies to platelets react with a surface determinant related to PAF-induced reactions, possibly a receptor. If PAF is an endogenous mediator of platelet and neutrophil reactions, and if modifications in the reaction chain can be induced by antibodies, this may constitute an explanation for the gradual development of subjective chest tightness among cotton workers. Further studies are needed, however, to explore these hypotheses.

PAF-acether could also act as an inhibitor of neutrophil activation and represent an inbuilt shutoff mechanism for the initial macrophage–neutrophil reaction initiated by cotton dust or endotoxin,[34] although contradictory data exist.[35]

PAF-acether also activates neutrophils via a specific receptor and induces a concentration-dependent chemotactic response and, at lower concentrations, a chemokinetic activation of neutrophils.[36] A possible mechanism for the neutrophil migration into the lung after cotton dust exposure could thus be PAF-acether secretion from macrophages but there are also other alveolar macrophage-derived chemotactic factors.

PERSPECTIVE

The foregoing information indicates some of the constellation of reactions at the cellular level, which can be induced by exposure to cotton dust or to endotoxin, one of the major toxic components therein. There is no shortage of possible mechanisms to explain both the major cell responses to such exposures—the invasion and activation of neutrophils—and the subsequent bronchoconstriction. More traditional bronchoconstrictors are, for example, histamine, in the absence of convincing evidence of an effect on mast cells, of diminishing interest. Instead, the focus is changing to new, more potent compounds released by cells known to be activated by cotton dust, such as macrophages, neutrophils, and platelets.

Several of the descriptions of the various mechanisms discussed in this review are based upon observations in vitro. Conceptually it would be hazardous to draw firm conclusions about the nature of reactions occurring on in vivo based solely upon in vitro experiments. In vitro observations do, however, provide the background information needed for appropriate in vivo experiments, both in animals and in humans.

Another aspect of the problem concerns why only certain persons react with byssinosis. Even under extreme exposure conditions, a large proportion of the workers are asymptomatic. What is the inherent defect, or hyperreactivity, that predisposes to the development of symptoms in certain individuals? Is it a hyperreactive cell response, or a lack of inhibitory factors that normally damp cellular reactions to dust exposure?

A model of the cellular events in byssinosis based upon the information reviewed here is presented in Fig. 9-1. In this scheme inhaled cotton dust

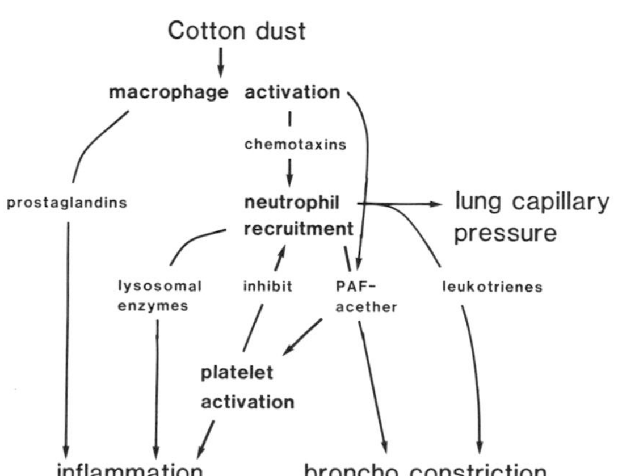

Fig. 9-1. Suggested mechanisms for various symptoms in byssinosis.

causes an activation of macrophages. These secrete chemotaxins and perhaps also PAF-acether, which mobilizes neutrophils into the lung tissue. During this process a physical clogging and secretion induced constriction of the pulmonary capillaries occur. The neutrophils in turn secrete leukotrienes, which induce bronchoconstriction, and PAF-acether, which activates platelets. Both neutrophils and platelets secrete products causing local inflammation. At the same time, a further leukocyte recruitment is arrested by the activated platelets.

It is evident that the above model is only a suggestion for further research. It suggests, however, how the present concepts of cell mediators can be applied in an attempt to explain the pathogenesis of an unusual disease syndrome of some practical importance. Only through a better understanding of the mechanisms behind the pathogenesis can the etiologic agent(s) of the disease be correctly identified and adequate measures undertaken to prevent its occurrence.

REFERENCES

1. Ramazzini B: De Morbis Artificum (1713). Transl. Wright WC, Disease of Workers. New York, Hafner, 1964.
2. Schilling RSF: Byssinosis in cotton and other textile workers. Lancet ii:261–265, 1956.
3. Weill H, ed: International Conference on Byssinosis. Chest 79(suppl):1S–136S, 1981.
4. Pratt PC: Comparative prevalence and severity of emphysema and bronchitis at autopsy in cotton mill workers vs controls. Chest 79:49S–53S, 1981.
5. Rylander R, Haglind P: Airborne endotoxins and humidifier disease. Clin Allergy 14(1): January, 1984.
6. Morgan PGM, Ong SG: First report of byssinosis in Hong Kong. J Ind Med 38:290–292, 1981.
7. Berry G, Molyneux MKB. A mortality study of workers in Lancashire cotton mills Chest 79:11S–15S, 1981.
8. Elwood PC, McAulay IR, Elwood JH: The flax industry in Northern Ireland twenty years on. Lancet 1112–1114, May 1982.
9. Rylander R: Bacterial toxins and etiology of byssinosis. Chest 79:34S–38S, 1981.
10. Massoud A, Taylor G: Byssinosis antibody to cotton antigens in normal subjects and in cotton card-room workers. Lancet ii:607–610, 1964.
11. Kutz SA, Mentnech SM, Olenchock SA, Major PC: Precipitation of serum protein by extracts of cotton dust and stems. Environ Res 22:476–484, 1980.
12. Rylander R, Wold A, Haglind P: Nasal antibodies against Gram-negative bacteria in cotton mill workers. Int Arch Allergy Appl Immunol 69:330–334, 1982.
13. Rylander R, Haglind P, Butcher BT: Reactions during workshift among cotton workers. Chest 84:403–407, 1983.
14. Jones RN, Butcher BT, Hammad YY, et al: Interaction of atopy and exposure to cotton dust in the bronchoconstrictor response. Br J Ind Med 37:141–146, 1980.
15. Walker RI, Beasky WJ: Evidence that antipolysaccharide antibodies alter platelet response to endotoxin in tolerant rabbits. Can J Microbiol 26:1241–1246, 1980.

16. Wilson MR, Schul A, Dry R, et al: Activation of the alternative complement pathway by extracts of cotton dust. Clin Allergy 10:303–308, 1980.
17. Cochrane CG: The pathogenesis of inflammatory injury produced by bacterial lipopolysaccharides. In: Advances in Immunopathology, eds. Weigle WO, LaJolla E. London, Arnold, 1982.
18. Snella M-C, Rylander R: Airway cell reactions after acute and subacute inhalation of bacterial lipopolysaccharide. Eur J Respir Dis 63:550–557, 1982.
19. Rylander R, Nordstrand A: Pulmonary cell reactions after exposure to cotton dust extract. Br J Ind Med 31:220–223, 1974.
20. Fowler SR, Ziprin RL, Elissalde MH Jr, Greenblatt GA: The etiology of byssinosis—Possible role of prostaglandin $F_{2\alpha}$ synthesis by alveolar macrophages. Am Ind Hyg Assoc J 42:445–448, 1981.
21. Rietschel ET, Schade U, Lüdertz O, et al: Prostaglandins in endotoxicosis. In: Microbiology, Schlessinger D. ed. Washington, DC, American Society of Microbiology, 1980, pp 66–72.
22. Weidemann MJ, Peskar BA, Wrogemann K, et al: Prostaglandin and thromboxane synthesis in a pure macrophage population and the inhibition by E-type prostaglandins, of chemiluminescence. FEBS Lett 89:136–139, 1978.
23. Wahl LM, Rosenstreich DL, Glode LM, et al: Defective prostaglandin synthesis by C3H/HeJ mouse macrophages stimulated with endotoxin preparations. Infect Immun 23:8–13, 1979.
24. Cook JA, Wise WC, Halushka PV: Thromboxane A_2 and prostacyclin production by lipopolysaccharide-stimulated peritoneal macrophages. J Reticuloendothel Soc 30:445–450, 1981.
25. Helander I: Acute pulmonary toxicity and pyrogenicity of inhaled lipid A. FEMS Microbiol Lett 13:283–287, 1982.
26. Henson PM: Platelet activating factor (PAF) as a mediator of neutrophil–platelet interactions in inflammation. In Russo-Marie F, Vargaftig BB, Beneviste (eds). Pharmacology of inflammation and allergy. INSERM Paris, Vol 100, pp 63–81, 1980.
27. Guntheroth WG, Kawabori I, Stevenson JG, Cholvin NR: Pulmonary vascular resistance and right ventricular function in canine endotoxin shock. Proc Soc Exp Biol Med 157:610–614, 1978.
28. Blumenthal KM, Rourke JJ, Wilder MS: Platelet activation by cultured mouse peritoneal macrophages. J Reticuloendothel Soc 27:247–257, 1980.
29. Rouzer CA, Scott WA, Hamill ALK, Cohn ZA: Synthesis of leukotriene C and other arachidonic acid metabolites by mouse pulmonary macrophages. J Exp Med 155:720–733, 1982.
30. Bomski H, Otawski J, Bomska H: Hämatologische und serologische Untersuchungen bei Byssinosis-gefährdeten Arbeitern. Int Arch Arbeitsmed 27:309–323, 1971.
31. Benveniste J, Jouvin E, Pirotzky E, et al: Platelet-activating factor (PAF-acether): Molecular aspects of its release and pharmacological action. Int Arch Allergy Appl Immunol 66:121–126, 1981.
32. Holt PG, Holt BJ, Beijer L, Rylander R: Platelet serotonin release by human polymorphonuclear leucocytes stimulated by cotton dust bacteria. Clin Exp Immunol 51:185–190, 1983.
33. Henson PM, Laudes RR: Activation of platelets by platelet activating factor (PAF) derived from IgE sensitized basophils. IV. PAF does not activate platelet factor (PF3). Br J Hematol 34:269, 1976.

34. O'Donnell MC, Siegel JN, Fiedel BA: Platelet activating factor: An inhibitor of neutrophil activation? Clin Exp Immunol 43:135–142, 1981.
35. O'Flaherty JT, Miller CH, Lewis JC, et al: Neutrophil response to platelet-activating factor. Inflammation 5:193–201, 1981.
36. Czarnetzki BM, Benveniste J: Effect of 1-*O*-octadenyl-2-*O*-acetyl-sn-glycero-3-phosphocholine (PAF-acether) on leucocytes. 1. Analysis of the in vitro migration of human neutrophils. Chem Phys Lipids 29:317–326, 1981.

10 Is Byssinosis Associated with Chronic Obstructive Lung Disease?

E. Neil Schachter
Gerald J. Beck

Extensive clinical and epidemiologic evidence now exists to document that chronic lung disease results from prolonged exposure to dust in the cotton textile industry. In this chapter we review some of the historical landmarks that have called attention to lung disease in textile workers and examine the cross-sectional and longitudinal studies that offer compelling evidence that an excess of respiratory symptoms and lung function impairment characterize this disease in older workers. Such findings have led medical and legislative organizations in the United Kingdom to establish dust standards in the cotton textile industry protecting workers from respiratory impairment and disability and to provide compensation for disabled workers. More recently, these concerns have also been recognized in the United States and have led to adoption of comprehensive cotton dust standards.

HISTORICAL BACKGROUND

In his lucid chapter on the "diseases of dressers of flax and hemp" from the landmark treatise on the "Diseases of Workers" Bernardini Ramazzini[1] noted in 1713 that "a foul and poisonous dust flies out from these materials, enters the mouth, then the throat and lungs, makes the workmen cough incessantly, and by degrees brings on asthmatic troubles." This characterization of disease associated with the processing of various natural vegetable fibers such as hemp, flax, and cotton foreshadowed the writings of a number of English physicians of the nineteenth century who wrote on diseases associated with cotton textile manufacture. Kay[2] in 1831 and later Leach[3] in 1863 were to call attention to excess respiratory disease in English towns engaged in the processing of cotton.

Leach, a factory surgeon described the disease as follows: "Cardroom operatives suffer from spasmodic cough, sore throat, expectoration of blood, pneumonia and confirmed asthma, with oppression of the chest." Although pneumonia and hemoptysis have not proven to be features of contemporary byssinosis, the other symptoms graphically portray what is seen today. The term byssinosis was first correctly used by a Belgian physician, Adrien Proust,[4] who in 1877 described various syndromes associated with the inhalation of cotton dust. Whereas data are not available to argue whether these early investigators distinguished acute and chronic components of this disease, it is clear that epidemiologists in Great Britain studying cotton textile workers in the period 1900–1930[5,6] documented both increased morbidity and mortality in these groups, suggesting the presence of a chronic disease. As a result of the continued findings of respiratory disease in cotton workers in the United Kingdom in the 1930s a compensation scheme was begun in 1941, based on the report of the Departmental Committee on Compensation for cardroom workers,[6] which was designed to help totally incapacitated men who had worked for at least 20 years in dusty rooms. A number of other authors have extensively documented these historical findings.[7–10]

In the United States, McKerrow and Schilling[11] reported respiratory findings in byssinotic workers in 1961. Nevertheless, despite extensive studies in the British literature and a growing number of studies in this country, acceptance of cotton textile worker's lung disease as either an acute or chronic respiratory occupational lung disease has been slow in developing in the United States. Only in the last ten years have standards been established in this country and an approach to compensation has yet to be formulated.

EPIDEMIOLOGIC CHARACTERIZATION

The characterization of byssinosis has been based primarily on chronic respiratory symptoms (e.g., cough, phlegm, or chest tightness) as well as symptom complexes (e.g., chronic bronchitis or Schilling's grades of byssinosis). Schilling's grading of byssinosis initially allowed the study of cotton textile workers to be established on a sound epidemiologic basis.[8,9] These grades of byssinosis suggest a progression of disease from a reversible "asthma-like" reaction to dust in the cotton mills on the first day of the work week (Grade 1) to one of irreversible airway obstruction (Grades 2 and 3). The findings of subjective symptoms of respiratory impairment have frequently been supplemented by objective evidence of lung function loss. The original grading included only Grades 1 and 2. Schilling later proposed Grade 3, which further described the chronic phase of the disease. This proposal was adopted by the 1962 Byssinosis Conference in England.

Chronic impairment of lung function in byssinosis has been characterized in terms of (1) the loss of respiratory function measured either as a percent of the predicted value for an individual (based on healthy nonsmokers), or as (2) the residual of a specific lung function defined as the observed value minus the predicted value. Various predicted values for nonsmokers have been developed (e.g., Schoenberg et al.[13]). In general, the lung function most commonly reported is the forced expiratory volume in one second (FEV_1), since many studies suggest that the chronic lung disease of cotton textile workers is primarily one characterized by airway obstruction. A second measure of irreversible lung function loss has been the annual rate of decline in lung function in workers as compared to control groups. Since an accelerated loss suggests a greater cumulative decrement, such measurements are of particular interest.

CROSS-SECTIONAL STUDIES

Cross-sectional studies beginning with those of Schilling et al.[8] have demonstrated increasing prevalences of byssinotic symptoms with increasing years of exposure in the industry. Table 10-1, adapted from Schilling's study, demonstrates increasing prevalences of byssinosis (all grades) with increased time worked in the mill, in particular for the higher grades of byssinosis. Increased prevalences of byssinosis in those workers with longer exposure were also reported by Molyneux and Tombleson[14] in Lancashire mills and by Schrag and Gullett[15] in cotton textile workers in the southern United States. Moreover, even among young workers with relatively few years in the cotton industry significant prevalences of advanced byssinosis exist.[16]

Cross-sectional data obtained from our Columbia, South Carolina study reported by Bouhuys and associates[17,18] have shown that other chronic respiratory symptoms and symptom complexes, such as wheeze or chronic bronchitis, are much more prevalent in older cotton textile workers than in control populations. Table 10-2 shows the prevalences of chronic bronchitis by sex and smok-

Table 10-1. Prevalence of Byssinosis by Length of Work History

	Byssinosis Grades			Total Byssinotic
Years Exposure	0	I	II	(I + II)
0–9	14 (67%)	4 (19%)	3 (14%)	7 (33%)
10–19	22 (47%)	18 (39%)	7 (15%)	25 (53%)
10–29	22 (35%)	22 (35%)	19 (30%)	41 (65%)
30+	17 (29%)	23 (39%)	19 (32%)	42 (71%)

Adapted from Schilling RSR, Hughes JPW, Dingwall-Fordyce I, et al: An epidemiological study of byssinosis among Lancashire cotton workers. Br J Ind Med 12:217–227, 1955.

Table 10-2. Prevalence of Chronic Bronchitis by Sex and Smoking Status in Three Populations of Whites Aged 45–74 Years

Sex	Smoking Status	Cotton Textile Workers Columbia, S.C. 1973	Controls[a] 1972–74	U.S. HANES[b] 1971–75
Men	Nonsmokers	7.7%	2.1%	1.0%[c]
	Smokers	36.6%	21.1%[d]	13.8%[c]
Women	Nonsmokers	12.3%	3.1%[c]	1.1%[c]
	Smokers	21.4%	7.6%	7.1%[c]

[a] Nontextile workers in Lebanon and Ansonia, Connecticut and Winnsboro, South Carolina.

[b] Based on the Health and Nutrition Examination Survey of NCHS to be representative of the U.S. noninstitutionalized population.

[c] Compared to cotton textile workers $p < .001$.

[d] Compared to cotton textile workers $p < 0.05$.

ing status in the population of cotton workers and in two control groups. The prevalences in the community controls are quite similar to those from the national data, and in all cases the cotton textile workers have more chronic bronchitis than do the controls, even when controlling for sex and smoking status.

Many of the cross-sectional studies make observations on lung function among cotton textile workers. A number of these studies document abnormal lung function related to work in the mill or presence of symptoms, particularly grades of byssinosis. As early as 1955[8] abnormal lung function in cotton workers with byssinosis was noted. This dysfunction increased with higher grades of byssinosis as well as with age. Lammers et al.,[19] studying English and Dutch workers, established that indirect maximum breathing capacity in workers with byssinosis was significantly lower than in those without byssinosis. Similar findings were reported for FEV_1 by Schrag and Gullett[15] in the United States. For example, in a group of 95 carders (67 asymptomatic and 28 with byssinosis symptoms), the mean (± 1 SD) FEV_1 was 3.0 ± 0.31 liters for those without byssinosis and 2.4 ± 0.4 liters for those with byssinosis. Similar (and also significant) differences were seen in this study in weavers and spinners. Zuskin et al.[20] studied two mills in the southern United States and found that 54% of all carders, 21% of the spinners, and 12% of a control group had FEV_1 less than 80% of predicted. In a larger study involving 10,133 workers at Burlington Industries, Imbus and Suh[21] found that in active workers with $<10\%$ across the shift change in FEV_1 and without byssinotic symptoms, FEV_1 was 86.4% of predicted on the average, whereas in those with byssinotic symptoms the mean FEV_1 was 81.1% of predicted; for workers with $\leq 10\%$ across-shift changes, those without byssinotic symptoms had FEV_1 of 82.2% of predicted on the average, while in those with byssinotic symptoms the figure dropped to 71.3%.

Further evidence of lung dysfunction among cotton textile workers has been documented in Sweden,[22] in winding room workers in England,[23] and in the United States by Merchant et al.[24] A study of 18 plants in the United States, sponsored by the American Textile Manufacturers Institute,[25] specifically concluded that there was chronic lung disease in cotton textile workers. The authors of this study state: "Evidence of a chronic or progressive effect, as indicated by simultaneous objective and subjective findings accompanied by a significant deficit in the predicted normal FEV_1, was present in 4.9% of carders and 0.6% of noncarders in our study."

When smoking is taken into consideration, cotton textile workers still have a greater than expected loss of lung function, as was shown for 646 active and retired workers from four mills in Columbia, South Carolina.[17] For instance, in lifetime nonsmokers aged 45 and over, the cotton textile workers had an average FEV_1 decrement of 0.28 liters more than controls for men ($p < 0.01$) and 0.19 liters more than controls for women ($p < 0.001$). Moreover, the pattern of lower lung function in cotton textile workers with byssinosis compared to those without byssinosis holds when workers were classified by their smoking status.[26] The independence of the cotton effect on lung function from the smoking factor can also be appreciated in Fig. 10-1 using the Columbia, South Carolina data. This is a plot of the cumulative distribution of FEV_1 expressed as a percent of predicted for nonsmoking cotton textile workers and controls. At

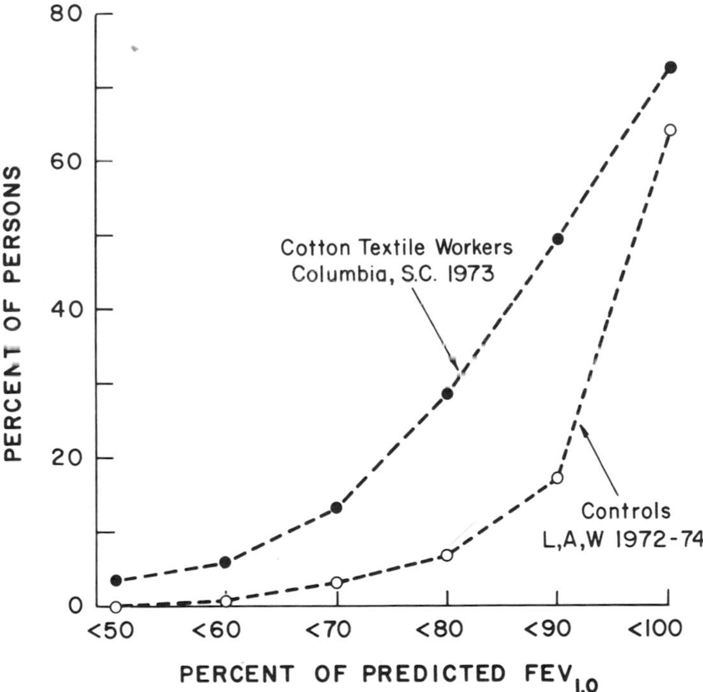

Fig. 10-1 Cumulative distribution of percent of predicted FEV_1 in nonsmoking cotton textile workers (n = 310) and controls (n = 553). L = Lebanon, Conn.; A = Ansonia, Conn.; W = Winsborough, S.C.

each level of FEV_1 the cotton workers have a greater number of individuals with that level (or worse) of lung function impairment. In general, at a given level there are at least three times as many impaired cotton workers as compared to controls. These cumulative distribution curves are significantly different ($p < 0.0001$) by the Kolmogorov-Smirnov test. More recently we have performed a two-way analysis of variance for each lung function measurement allowing separate effects for cotton dust exposure and smoking. For the forced vital capacity (FVC) and FEV_1 these two effects were separate and not significantly different in magnitude, except in women where the cotton effect was greater. For maximal expiratory flow rates at low lung volumes (MEF_{50} and MEF_{25}) the smoking effect was larger than the cotton effect. These differences may reflect different areas of major pathologic damage by these two agents. A further analysis related lung function loss to packyears of smoking and work in the textile mill. For example, for a man 45 years or older, the number of packyears smoked would have to be 56 in order to result in the same loss of FEV_1 as a cotton worker with an average of 35 years of work in the mill.

LONGITUDINAL STUDIES

In addition to confirming the results of the cross-sectional studies listed above, longitudinal studies reported in the last ten years have permitted us to examine the effect of cotton dust exposure on the rate of lung function loss in cotton textile workers as well as the incidence of new symptoms.

Fox et al.,[27] in a study of several thousand mill operatives examined in 1966–1968 and again in 1968–1970 showed an increase in the prevalence of byssinosis with years of exposure (3% for less than 5 years, 31% for more than 20 years). Regressions on the average percent predicted FEV_1 showed a decrease of 0.14% per year for cotton textile workers as compared to only 0.02% per year for controls. In a study by Berry et al.[28] cotton textile workers were examined every 6 months for up to 3 years. The FEV_1 declined at an average rate of 54 ml/year in cotton workers as compared to 32 ml/years for workers manufacturing artificial fibers. As in the Bouhuys et al.[17] study, the more recent Beck et al.[26] study found a separate cotton effect and smoking effect for FEV_1 loss. These effects were seen to be approximately equal in magnitude.

In a 10 month follow-up study performed by Merchant et al.[29] cotton textile workers had very large declines in FEV_1. These declines were related to job in the mill. Finally, in a recent study from Bombay by Kamat et al.[30] prevalences of both specific and nonspecific symptoms were associated with longer service in the cotton mills. In addition, mean annual decreases in FEV_1 were greater, in general, with increasing years worked in both symptomatic and asymptomatic individuals. Similarly, a trend of increasing yearly FEV_1 change was noted by dust exposure levels.

Thus all major longitudinal studies to date (including our own, discussed below) document an excessive loss of lung function over time resulting from exposure to cotton dust. Also, these lung function abnormalities have been related to an increased level of symptoms. These studies imply the development of progressive and chronic lung disease in cotton textile workers.

A PROSPECTIVE STUDY OF COTTON TEXTILE WORKERS IN COLUMBIA, SOUTH CAROLINA

Methods

In the review of other prospective studies given above, we have not included results from the most recent longitudinal study,[26] which is unique for two reasons. It is the only study of respiratory health among cotton textile workers that includes workers no longer working in the mills, and it is presently the only long-term prospective study of cotton textile workers in the United States. For these reasons it is worthwhile to summarize the major findings from this study separately and to give further results that provide evidence of chronic lung disease in cotton textile workers.

The cohort of active and retired cotton textile workers was from Columbia, South Carolina and worked in one of four mills there. These workers were first studied in 1973 and then again in 1979. The selection of the cohort of workers has been described in detail elsewhere[18] and included workers who had at least 3 years of work in the mills by 1955. Company personnel records and union membership lists were used to identify eligible workers. However, length of employment was not always available unless the person was actually contacted. Therefore, it was not possible to know the proportion of eligible persons who participated for the entire study. For a subgroup of the cohort (those working in the cardroom or weaveroom prior to 1946), a tabulation showed that 95% (152/160) of those workers still living in the Columbia area participated in the study. It is not surprising that many of the eligible workers had moved from the area or were not traceable (58% of the above subgroup) at the time of the first study in 1973. A concentrated effort, including word of mouth, was made to locate all eligible workers, and it was concluded that the total study group ($n = 692$) was representative of active and retired cotton textile workers who continue to live in the community. The analysis used the 646 whites aged 45 years or older in 1973. The average years worked in the mill by this group was 35 years.

The cross-sectional data were compared to a combined group of controls (whites, aged 45+) from three communities, two in Connecticut (Ansonia and Lebanon) and one in South Carolina (Winnsboro). These towns were combined because it was shown that they did not differ significantly in terms of lung function or most respiratory symptoms.[18,31] The overall response rates to the follow-up surveys in Columbia and Lebanon were about 60%. An in-depth analysis comparing those persons who were restudied and those who were not (but were still alive), using their cross-sectional data, showed no consistent (and only a few significant) differences in terms of demographic data, lung function, or respiratory symptoms.[32] That is, those followed up were not healthier or sicker than those not reseen.

Lung Function Impairment

Loss of lung function was measured over the 6 years of follow-up in the two cohorts.[26] The mean FEV_1 decline of 42 ml/year in male cotton textile workers was significantly larger ($p = 0.017$) than the 27 ml/year decline in male controls. The respective figures for females were 30 and 15 ml/year and were significantly different ($p < 0.001$). When classified by smoking status, the cotton textile workers had larger losses of FEV_1 (or residual FEV_1) than did controls in all groups except male ex-smokers. Examining the regression coefficients in a forward stepwise multiple regression of this data we showed that a significant ($p < 0.001$) loss of FEV_1 was attributable to smoking and to work in the mill simultaneously, and these losses were nearly identical: 23 ml/year for the mill effect and 26 ml/year for the cigarette effect.

Respiratory Symptoms

In this prospective study the incidence rates of seven respiratory symptoms or conditions (including byssinosis) over the 6 years follow-up in controls and cotton textile workers were reported. In all cases, for men and for women, the incidence rates were significantly higher ($p < 0.001$) in cotton textile workers than in controls. The rates in the cotton workers were always higher than controls, although not always significantly, even when classified into nonsmokers and smokers separately.

When cotton textile workers were divided by the presence or absence of byssinosis and compared to nonbyssinotic controls in terms of their annual decline in FEV_1 (ΔFEV_1/year) controls had consistently smaller rates of decline than did cotton workers. In particular, even cotton workers without byssinosis had larger annual declines than controls (see Table 10-3). These findings were, in general, similar when the subjects were classified by smoking status

Table 10-3. Mean Annual Loss of FEV_1 (ml/year) Over Follow-up in Controls and Cotton Textile Workers by Byssinosis Status and Sex

	Controls	Cotton Textile Workers	
	No Byssinosis	No Byssinosis	Byssinosis
Males	28	40	49[a]
(*n*)	(139)	(127)	(40)
Females	15	29[b]	36[b]
(*n*)	(132)	(165)	(51)

[a] Compared to controls $p = 0.06$.
[b] Compared to controls $p < 0.01$.

(e.g., smoker, nonsmoker, ex-smoker). These greater rates of losses in cotton workers are consistent with the previously mentioned lower levels of FEV_1 in workers with byssinosis.[26]

Respiratory Impairment

The degree of pulmonary impairment in a person can be quantitated by comparing their observed lung function to their predicted value (based on their age, sex, height, and weight and calculated assuming their being a nonsmoker with no respiratory symptoms). A person can be defined as having impaired lung function if their observed FEV_1 is less than 1.96 standard errors of their predicted FEV_1. Under this definition only 2½% of healthy nonsmokers would be expected to have impaired lung function. We have used this definition of pulmonary impairment to examine in the Columbia, S.C. cohort whether cotton textile workers have more lung dysfunction than expected and whether it is related to the presence (and degree) of byssinosis. Table 10-4 gives the percent of impaired controls and cotton textile workers. When cotton textile workers were classified by byssinosis grade the prevalence of impairment increased with increasing grades of byssinosis. For example, 28% of male cotton workers with Grades 0 or 1 byssinosis had impairment. By contrast 58% of male workers with Grade 3 had impairment.

Employment Status

This study was unique in that it followed cotton textile workers that were both active and retired. We thus had the opportunity to classify our workers by their work status at both points in our survey. When we compared those workers who were active at both exams (A-A) with those who had retired between the two surveys (A-R) we noted that the annual loss of FEV_1 was about twice as great in the retiring workers as compared to the active workers. This was true for both impaired and nonimpaired workers (e.g., see Table 10-5) for results on men. Most of the retiring workers were under 65. This suggests that often workers retire at an early age and that this retirement may be prompted by accelerating lung dysfunction or actual respiratory impairment.

Table 10-4. Percent of Controls and Cotton Textile Workers with Impairment[a] at Follow-up

Sex	Controls	Cotton Textile Workers
Male	11%	31%
(*n*)	(141)	(167)
Female	1%	15%
(*n*)	(136)	(216)

[a] Impaired = observed $FEV_1 <$ predicted $FEV_1 - 1.96$ SE.

Table 10-5. Mean Annual Loss of FEV_1 Over Follow-up in Male Cotton Textile Workers by Impairment Status

Impairment Status	Retirement Status	
	A-A[a]	A-R
Not Impaired[b]		
ΔFEV_1/year (ml/year)	22	53
(*n*)	(43)	(38)
Impaired		
ΔFEV_1/year (ml/year)	55	99
(*n*)	(8)	(6)

[a] See text for definition.

[b] Impaired = observed FEV_1 < predicted $FEV_1 - 1.96$ SE.

We have previously documented that accelerated lung function loss probably also occurs after workers have left the industry.[33]

SUMMARY

Numerous studies, both clinical and epidemiologic, have consistently documented an excess of respiratory symptoms and lung function impairment among cotton textile workers. This impairment is clearly distinct from that of other airway toxic agents such as cigarette smoke. Most recent longitudinal studies of cotton textile workers have shown accelerated lung function loss, an excess incidence of respiratory symptoms, and a high prevalence of lung function impairment. Our own studies would suggest that this chronic disease is responsible for early retirement and significant disability among cotton textile workers.

In England disability for chronic lung disease caused by cotton dust has been recognized and compensated for over 40 years. Recently, WHO[34] has acknowledged the worldwide distribution of this chronic occupational lung disease. In conclusion, there is convincing evidence that work in the cotton textile industry causes chronic lung disease in many cotton textile workers. Recognition of this occupational lung disease in the United States is important in implementing regulations for the prevention of further illness and for the compensation of disabled workers.

ACKNOWLEDGMENTS

We wish to thank L. Maunder and R. Schilling for valuable input on the analysis of the Columbia, South Carolina follow-up data. Technical assistance was provided by J. Petonito and D. Verlezza. We thank NCHS for making the HANES data available, which was analyzed under BRSG support from NIH.

Support for the cotton textile workers follow-up study came from Contract J-9-M-8-0168, U.S. Department of Labor. We also wish to thank Ms. Martha Krill for her typing and editorial assistance.

REFERENCES

1. Ramazzini B: Diseases in Workers (1713). Transl. from Latin, W Wright. Chicago, University of Chicago Press, 1940.
2. Kay JP: Observations and experiments concerning molecular irritation of the lungs as one source of tubercular consumptions and on spinners phthisis. North Engl Med Surg 1:348, 363, 1831.
3. Leach J: Surat cotton, as it bodily affects operatives in cotton mills. Lancet 2:648–649, 1863.
4. Proust AA: Traité d'hygiene publique et privee. Paris, Masson, 1877.
5. Collis EL: Report of the Inspector of Factory Workshops. London, Her Majesty's Stationers Office, 1909.
6. Hill AB: Industrial Health Board, Report No. 59. London, 1930.
7. Harris TR, Merchant JA, Kilburn KH, Hamilton JD: Byssinosis and respiratory diseases of cotton mill workers. J Occup Med 14:199–206, 1972.
8. Schilling RSR, Hughes JPW, Dingwall-Fordyce I, Gilson JC: An epidemiological study of byssinosis among Lancashire cotton workers. Br J Ind Med 12:217–227, 1955.
9. Schilling RSF: Byssinosis in cotton and other textile workers. Lancet 2:261–265, 319–324, 1956.
10. Schilling RSF: Epidemiological studies of chronic respiratory disease among cotton operatives. Yale J Biol Med 37:55–74, 1964.
11. McKerrow CB, Schilling RSF: A pilot inquiry into byssinosis in two cotton mills in the United States. JAMA 1977:850–853, 1961.
12. Bouhuys A, Gilson JC, Schilling RSF: Byssinosis in the textile industry: Research, prevention and control. Arch Environ Health 21:475–478, 1970.
13. Schoenberg JB, Beck GJ, Bouhuys A: Growth and decay of pulmonary function in healthy blacks and whites. Respir Physiol 33:367–393, 1978.
14. Molyneux MKB, Tombleson JBL: An epidemiological study of respiratory symptoms in Lancashire Mills. Br J Ind Med 27:225–234, 1963–66.
15. Schrag PE, Gullett AD: Byssinosis in cotton textile mills. Am Rev Respir Dis 101:497–503, 1970.
16. Mustafa KY, Bos W, Lakha AS: Byssinosis in Tanzanian textile workers. Lung 157:39–44, 1979.
17. Bouhuys A, Schoenberg JB, Beck GJ, Schilling RSF: Epidemiology of chronic lung disease in a cotton mill community. Lung 154:168–186, 1977.
18. Bouhuys A, Beck GJ, Schoenberg JB: Epidemiology of environmental lung disease. Yale J Biol Med 52:191–210, 1979.
19. Lammers B, Schilling RSF, Walford J, et al: A study of byssinosis, chronic respiratory symptoms, and ventilatory capacity in English and Dutch cotton workers, with special reference to atmospheric pollution. Br J Ind Med 21:124–134, 1964.
20. Zuskin E, Wolfson RL, Harpel G, et al: Byssinosis in carding and spinning workers. Arch Environ Health 19:666–673, 1969.
21. Imbus HR, Suh MW: Byssinosis: A study of 10,133 textile workers. Arch Environ Health 26:183–191, 1973.

22. Belin L, Bouhuys A, Hoekstra W, et al: Byssinosis in cardroom workers in Swedish cotton mills. Br J Ind Med 22:101–108, 1965.
23. Mekky S, Roach SA, Schilling RSF: Byssinosis among winders in the cotton industry. Br J Ind Med 24:123–132, 1967.
24. Merchant JA, Lumsden JC, Kilburn KH, et al: An industrial study of the biological effects of cotton dust and cigarette smoke exposure. J Occup Med 15:212–221, 1973.
25. Braun DC, Jurgiel JA, Kaschak MC, Babyak MA: Prevalence of respiratory signs and symptoms among U.S. cotton textile workers. J Occup Med 15:414–419, 1973.
26. Beck GJ, Schachter EN, Maunder LR, Schilling RSF: A prospective study of chronic lung disease in cotton textile workers. Ann Intern Med 97:645–651, 1982.
27. Fox AJ, Tombleson JBL, Watt A, Wilkie AG: A survey of respiratory disease in cotton operatives; Part 1: Symptoms and ventilation test results. Part II: Symptoms, dust estimations and the effect of smoking habit. Br J Ind Med 30:42–47, 48–53, 1973.
28. Berry G, McKerrow CB, Molyneux MKB, et al: A study of acute and chronic changes in ventilatory capacity or workers in Lancashire cotton mills. Br J Ind Med 50:25–36, 1973.
29. Merchant JA, Lumsden JC, Kilburn KH, et al: Intervention studies of cotton steaming to reduce biological effects of cotton dust. Br J Ind Med 31:261–274, 1974.
30. Kamat SR, Kamat GR, Salpeker VY, Lobo E: Distinguishing byssinosis from chronic obstructive pulmonary disease: Results of a prospective five-year study of cotton mill workers in India. Am Rev Respir Dis 124:31–40, 1981.
31. Bouhuys A, Beck GJ, Schoenberg JB: Priorities in prevention of chronic lung disease. Lung 156:129–148, 1979.
32. Beck GJ, Maunder LR, Schachter EN, Schilling RSF: Follow-up of active and retired cotton textile workers. Report to the U.S. Department of Labor. Springfield, Virginia: National Technical Information Service, Publication 82-240516.
33. Beck GJ, Schachter EN, Maunder LR, Bouhuys A: The relation of lung function to subsequent employment status and mortality in cotton textile workers. Chest 79S:26S–30S, 1981.
34. World Health Organization Task Group on Vegetable Dust: Environmental health criteria on vegetable dusts; dusts causing byssinosis. Geneva, WHO, 1981.

11 Chronic Effects of Cotton Dust Inhalation: A Fact?

Mario C. Battigelli

Exposure to the dust of cotton processing provokes respiratory effects of an acute nature, such as chest tightness, dyspnea, and related respiratory discomfort. These asthmalike effects are characteristically self-limiting, and have been clearly documented since the earliest reports in the literature (see Mareska and Heyman, 1845;[1] Collis, 1908;[2] Bokser and Ryabova, 1932;[3] Prausnitz, 1936[4]). Schilling described a typical case in the early 1950s by repeating a worker's own words, "I am a *dead horse on Mondays, but could fell a bull on Tuesday*."[5]

It is assumed by many that the evolution of an asthmalike effect into a less reversible and possibly chronic manifestation of respiratory functional injury is a consequence of exposure to cotton dust. This consequential relationship between cotton dust and chronic respiratory effects has no adequate or persuasive documentation in the literature. It is well known that numerous allegations claim a variety of morbid events in textile workers exposed to cotton dust, particularly in the literature of the nineteenth century. The U.S. Public Health Service observed in 1947 that pulmonary tuberculosis, hemoptysis, hypertension, fevers, headache, tonsillitis, intestinal disorders, radiologic abnormalities, cardiomegaly, lymphoadenitis of both cervical and axillary regions, among others, have been noted in textile workers by observers often not able to provide information on any reference population.[6] An additional drawback of these publications is that the intensity–duration of the exposure is generally not measured, or even estimated. From an extensive review of the literature (36 major reports were analyzed by the Public Health Service), Caminita et al.[6] stated that the textile population surveyed by the observers of different language is, in general, characterized by low income, inadequate diet, poor housing and insufficient sanitation. It is not difficult to understand that the neglect of these causative factors of ill health may have contributed to the facile assumption of a causality link between cotton dust exposure and chronic respiratory ailments. Moreover, the limited familiarity of older observers with the extent and frequency of chronic respiratory disorders in the general population readily explains the error of invoking an occupational etiology for common respiratory disorders occurring coincidentally in textile workers. Finally, the incomplete realization of the devastating effects of cigarette smoking has further contributed to the misinterpretation of cause and effect. For the accurate identification of etiologic factors of chronic disorders, an attentive and critical assessment of epidemiologic observations is needed. This requirement, however, is often omitted, even from recent publications. For instance, a series of reports, all based on a survey of textile workers in South Carolina, has epitomized the confusion existing on cause–effect relationship in this context.[7] The textile workers surveyed comprised a group of 645 individuals aged 45 and older and were obtained from a study implemented in 1973 in the community of Columbia, South Carolina. Workers were recruited from several cohorts and mill departments, identified by heterogeneous means. As the authors acknowledge in their earliest paper,[7] this sample was not adequately controlled, and the participants' response to the survey was poor.* The reference population was matched by race, age, and sex, but not for sampling techniques, or for geographic, ethnic, social, tenure, or economic factors. Now it is well known in the field of epidemiology that the failure to account for these discrepancies generates error in assessing the etiology of disorders with strong dependence on these social characteristics.[8]

Observations obtained outside the United States do not assist in solving the question of causality of cotton dust exposure in chronic respiratory disorders. For instance, reports from the British literature suggest an array of perplexing conclusions, occasionally contradictory and often inconclusive. As an example, Molyneux and Tombleson[9] state that chronic bronchitis is more prevalent in textile workers with byssinosis complaints, but their figures indicate that male nonsmoking workers in synthetic fiber mills, aged 45–54, have substantially more bronchitis Grade 1 than corresponding workers operating in cotton mills. Fox et al.[10,11] examined textile workers repeatedly, within a 2½-year interval. Although cotton exposed workers appeared to experience a higher loss in spirometry, the authors found no meaningful correlation between dust levels and incidence of bronchitis. In fact, textile workers presented a more favorable trend for frequency of bronchitis than a reference population. Berry

---

* See, for example, Ref. 7, p. 169: "More than half of these persons could not be located," and, further, on pp. 169–170: "We do not know what percentage of the population which met these expanded criteria was actually seen."

et al.[12,13] found that operatives working in cotton mills experience yearly losses of spirometry greater than that manifested by workers operating in synthetic fiber mills. However, these differences existed almost exclusively in comparison with one of the synthetic mills surveyed, whereas workers from the other control mill were not distinguishable from the cotton mill workers. Furthermore, the higher figure of FEV_1 decay per annum (54 ml/year) appears wholly consistent with the similar value observed in British non-mine workers by an earlier survey.[14]

In accordance with these observations, the official Compensation Board in the United Kingdom does not recognize mere chronic bronchitis in cotton exposed textile workers as work related.[15] Indeed, the British Ministry of Pensions stated in 1965 that textile workers have lower prevalence of bronchitis than could be expected on the basis of age and geographic location.[9]

MORTALITY FOR RESPIRATORY DISORDERS

Mortality patterns, for either respiratory or other causes, have been repeatedly studied in the United States and in England. The earliest meaningful record is that published by the Registrar General in 1938 for the United Kingdom and analyzed by Schilling and Goodman.[16]

The picture emerging from these data suggests that the number of deaths from cardiovascular and cerebrovascular causes for certain textile categories (grinders and strippers) exceeds the expected frequency. The correction of these data for respiratory deaths, while reducing somewhat the magnitude of the excess, does not eliminate it. In fact, with the exception of grinders and strippers, the textile population did not appear to experience any excess mortality from respiratory disease, and the simultaneous excess of mortality from other than respiratory disorders strongly suggests a more complex etiology than simply dust exposure.

Berry and Molyneux more recently released data on follow-up studies concerning the mortality of textile workers exposed to cotton.[17] These writers conclude that "The mortality did not show any increase in deaths due to any of the causes that earlier writers had found to be associated with exposure to cotton. . . ." Almost simultaneously with this observation, mortality from a follow-up of hemp workers in Northern Ireland has been published by Elwood et al.[18–20] This follow-up study concludes denying an "*effect on survival of either exposure to dust or byssinosis*."[19]

In the United States, three independent investigators have concluded with results perfectly concurring with the negative data obtained in the hemp and cotton workers in the United Kingdom, namely that work in cotton textile mills does not appear to cause any significant surge in mortality from respiratory disorders.[21–23] Paradoxically, a less frequent rate of mortality at times appears to characterize textile workers exposed to cotton in relation to general populations.[22,23] Even when mortality is examined on the basis of duration of employment, no excess of respiratory deaths could be convincingly identified.[22]

PATHOLOGY

The reports on the morphologic effects of cotton dust exposure are limited. The earlier observations of Gough on the "byssinosis bodies" suggest a finding of occasional occurrence and trivial diagnostic meaning.[24] The selected cluster of autopsy data published by Edwards et al.[25] remains fraught with the limitations of an uncontrolled study. The attempt to update this study by Rooke[26] concludes in a picture suggesting a pathological diagnosis consistent with "asthmatic bronchitis."

The observations by Pratt et al.[27–29] from the United States converge in suggesting the minimal, if existent, effect of cotton exposure in terms of hyperplastic changes of the simple bronchitis variety, a lesion which is not associated with significant obstruction to airflow.

NEGATIVE SURVEYS

On the other hand, although seldom quoted by the current literature, an impressive amount of reports converge to exclude any significant respiratory disablement caused by cotton dust in textile workers in the United States and throughout the world. An extensive review of the textile industry, conducted in the early 1930s by the Public Health Service, denied the occurrence of significant dust injury in workers exposed to cotton dust.[30,31] Smith[32] in New York State, and Ritter and Nussbaum[33] in the Mississippi mills equally minimized or denied the occurrence of significant respiratory diseases of chronic or irreversible nature. Similar studies done in Canada[34] and in England in hemp workers, as well as the studies quoted above[9–13,24,35] have excluded, or, at least seriously questioned, chronic bronchitis as a likely consequence of organic dust exposure. In Australian textile mills, the survey of a stratified random sample comprising 252 employees exposed to cotton dust, demonstrated the classical Monday reversible loss of ventilatory functions, but did not detect any unusual prevalence of chronic bronchitis symptoms, nor could the enhancement of cigarette smoking effect by cotton dust exposure be observed.[36]

In the United States several surveys analyzing, in the aggregate, over 1500 exposed workers, have failed to demonstrate either a significant excess of chronic respiratory disorders or a disproportionate loss in ventilatory function.[37–39] It should be noted that the combined number of exposed subjects studied in the surveys which the OSHA 1978 Cotton Dust uses as evidence for cause and chronic effect is far less, in both quality and quantity, than the sum total of workers examined by these negative reports.

CONCLUSIONS

Published reports throughout world literature consistently recognize the effects of exposure to cotton dust in the acute and self-limited ventilatory response.

This phenomenon is typically reversible within a time interval of minutes or hours. The relationship of this effect to the development of persisting respiratory injuries, frequently observed in a textile population exposed to cotton dust, is undocumented. The popular belief holding that the acute phenomenon evolves into a chronic clinical manifestation such as chronic bronchitis or simply chronic obstructive airflow disorder, is not supported by defensible published studies. Indeed, prospective epidemiologic studies of careful and pertinent design are not available to verify claims of cause and effect between dust exposure and ventilatory response etiologically related to chronic respiratory impairment.

On the contrary, surveys of exposed populations obtained with adequate controls for confounding variables such as sample selection, cigarette smoking, and social factors of airway pathology other than strict occupational exposure, do not suggest a cause and effect association between exposure to textile dust and chronic or irreversible respiratory disorders. In other words, the prevalence of chronic respiratory disorders in the textile population does not appear to differ from the prevalence of the same disorders in groups of workers not exposed to cotton and related organic dust. Conversely, studies purporting the existence of such a relationship are either inadequately controlled or inconclusive.

A host of mortality studies completed recently in the United States, England, and Northern Ireland have further minimized the possibility of any major health effects attributable to cotton and/or hemp dust exposure. The mortality of exposed textile workers, in fact, *does not differ* from that of appropriate reference populations. The analysis of the cotton workers' experience, according to the separate occupational categories of preparation, yarn processing, and weaving, has failed to document any association of mortality with duration of employment and specific exposure.

Obviously, disorders of trivial or limited pathology are not usually reflected in excessive rates of mortality. Although these negative mortality studies cannot be used to deny the occurrence of such disorders, these results discount health effects of major importance, such as factors limiting survival and causing a major disability.

In conclusion, it would be quite appropriate to state that, in the face of these converging data, the frequency and extent of respiratory disorders in the textile worker population does not indicate significant respiratory effects referrable to the specific occupational exposure, other than byssinosis, interpreted as a self-limiting and reversible acute disorder.

SUMMARY

A review of the world literature fails to offer conclusive observations documenting the evolution from an acute specific ventilatory response to a chronic and irreversible effect as an etiologically significant progress. Within a textile population exposed to cotton dust, a barrage of conflicting, and often negative findings, riddle the attempt to document a cause-and-effect connection between cotton dust exposure and significant chronic respiratory effects in textile workers. Chronic symptoms of bronchitis and effort dyspnea do not appear to occur in excessive or unusual frequency in exposed textile populations. Even pulmonary performance cannot be considered more impaired than that observed in relevant control populations.

A range of mortality studies encompassing the experience of textile workers exposed for several decades to cotton dust inhalation in the United States, England, and Northern Ireland does not provide evidence for or suggest trends upholding an irreversible and consistent or injurious effect of cotton dust exposure.

While the converging results of such varied and multiple documentation do not exclude a permanent injurious effect of cotton dust, they certainly make such an effect far less probable than commonly assumed, and certainly limited in extent, if any should exist.

REFERENCES

1. Mareska J, Heyman J: Quoted in Bouhuys A: Byssinosis: Scheduled asthma in the textile industry. Lung 154:3–16, 1976.
2. Collis EL. Quoted in HMSO, Dust in Card Rooms in the Cotton Industry, Report of the Departmental Committee, London, His Majesty Stationery Office, 1932.
3. Bokser YA, Ryabova SD: Pneumoconiosis in cotton mill workers. Quoted in Ref. 6.
4. Prausnitz C: Investigations in respiratory dust disease in operations in the cotton industry. Med Res Counc Spec Rep Ser 212, 1936.
5. Schilling RSF: Byssinosis in the British cotton textile industry. Br Med Bull 7:52–6, 1950.
6. Caminita BH, Baum WF, Neal PA, Schneiter R: A review of the Literature Relating to Afflictions of the Respiratory Tract in Individuals Exposed to Cotton Dust. Pub. Health Bull. #297, US Gvt. Print. Off., Washington, DC, 1947.
7. Bouhuys A, Schoenberg JB, Beck GJ, Schilling RSF: Epidemiology of Chronic Lung Disease in a Cotton Mill Community. Lung 154:167–86, 1977.
8. Gilson JC: Industrial Bronchitis. Proc. Roy. Soc. Med. 63:857–64, 1970.
9. Molineux MKB, Tombleson JBL: An epidemiological study of respiratory symptoms in Lancashire Mills, 1963–1966. Br J Ind Med 27:225–34, 1970.
10. Fox AJ, Tombleson JBL, Watt A, Wilkie AG: A survey of respiratory disease in cotton operatives. Br J Ind Med 30:42–7, 1973.
11. Fox AJ, Tombleson JBL, Watt A, Wilkie AG: A Survey of Symptoms, Dust Estimations, and the Effect of Smoking Habit. Br J Ind Med 30:48–53, 1973.
12. Berry G, McKerrow CB, Molyneux MKB, et al: Br J Ind Med 30:25–36, 1973.
13. Berry G, Molyneux MKB, Tombleson JBL: Relationships between dust level and byssinosis and bronchitis in Lancashire cotton mills. Br J Ind Med 31:18–27, 1974.
14. Higgins ITT, Oldham PD: Ventilatory capacity in miners—A five year follow-up study. Br J Ind Med 19:65–76, 1982.
15. Penumoconiosis and Allied Occupational Chest Diseases, Diagnosis and Procedure for Claiming Industrial Injuries Benefits, 2nd Impressions, London, Her Majesty's Stationery Office, 1975, p 10.

16. Schilling R, Goodman N: Cardiovascular Disease in Cotton Workers: Part I. Br J Ind Med 8:77–87, 1951. Part II, Br J Ind Med 9:146–156, 1952.
17. Berry G, Molyneux MKB: A mortality study of workers in Lancashire cotton mills. Chest 79(Suppl):11S–15S, 1981.
18. Elwood PC, Thomas HF, Elwood JH: Mortality of flax workers. Lancet ii:747–48, 1981.
19. Elwood PC, McAulay IR, Elwood JH: The flax industry in Northern Ireland twenty years on. Lancet i:1112–1114, 1982.
20. Elwood PC, Thomas HF, Sweetam PM, Elwood JH: Mortality of flax workers. Br J Ind Health 39:18–22, 1982.
21. Daum S: Mortality patterns among textile workers. In: *Cotton Dust,* A Symposium, Atlanta, GA, Nov. 12–13, 1974, ACGIH, Cincinnati, OH, 1974.
22. Merchant JA, Ortmeyer C: Mortality of employees of two cotton mills in North Carolina. Chest 79(Suppl):6S–11S, 1981.
23. Henderson VL, Enterline PE: An unusual mortality experience in cotton textile workers. J Occup Med 15:717–19, 1973.
24. Parkes WR: Occupational Lung Disorders, Ind. ed. London, Butterworth, 1982.
25. Edwards C, Macartney J, Rooke G, Ward F: The pathology of the lung in byssinotics. Thorax 30:612–22, 1975.
26. Rooke GB: The pathology of byssinosis. Chest 79(Suppl):67S–71S, 1981.
27. Pratt PC, Vollmer RT, Miller JA: Epidemiology of pulmonary lesions in non-textile and cotton textile workers: A retrospective autopsy analysis. Arch Environ Health 35:133–138, 1980.
28. Pratt PC, Vollmer RT, Miller JA: Prevalence and severity of morphologic emphysema and bronchitis in non-textile and cotton textile workers. Chest 77(Suppl):323–325, 1980.
29. Pratt PC: Comparative prevalence and severity of emphysema and bronchitis at autopsy in cotton mill workers vs. control. Chest 79(Suppl):49S–53S, 1981.
30. Britten RH, Bloomfield JJ, Goddard JC: The Health of Workers in a Textile Plant. US Publ. Health Bull. #207, Washington, DC, 1933.
31. Bloomfield JJ, Dreessen WC: The Health of Workers in Dusty Trades, IV Exposure to Dust in a Textile Plant. US Publ. Health. Bull. #208, Washington, DC, 1933.
32. Smith AR: Report on workers exposed to cotton batting dust. Ind Bull (NY) 21:50, 1942.
33. Ritter WL, Nussbaum MA: Occupational Illnesses in cotton industries. II. Chronic respiratory problems. J Ind Hyg Toxicol 27:47–51, 1945.
34. Roman CL: Some reflections upon the health and mortality of cotton textile workers. Can Med Assoc 55:398–401, 1946.
35. Mair A, Smith OH, Wilson WA, Lochart W: Dust diseases in Dundee textile workers. Br J Ind Med 17:272–8, 1960.
36. Field GB, Ouen P: Respiratory function in an Australian cotton mill. Bull Eur Physiopathol Respir 15:455–68, 1979.
37. Morgan WKC: Statement, OSHA Hearings, April 19, 1977.
38. Bradford JM, Ingram R: Small Airways Disease in Cotton Workers, Terminal Report (Mimeograph). Emory University, Atlanta, GA, Feb. 29, 1979.
39. Weill H: A Report, *Brown Lung,* Special Hearing, Dept. HEW. Washington, DC, US Government Printing Office, 1978.

12 Medical Monitoring of Lung Disease in the Workplace

Brian Boehlecke

Periodic assessment of the respiratory health of workers (medical monitoring) is an important component of a comprehensive surveillance program to control occupational lung disease.[1] It should not be used as a replacement for sound work practices, control technology, or environmental monitoring to reduce worker exposure to hazardous substances to the lowest feasible levels. This chapter presents some basic considerations in the use of medical monitoring to protect the health of workers.

PURPOSES OF MEDICAL MONITORING

Medical monitoring may be used to detect trends in the health status of groups of workers (epidemiologic studies) or to detect individual workers with potentially reversible adverse health effects of exposure (screening for case finding).[2,3] Table 12-1 lists objectives of epidemiologic studies and case finding surveys of workers. Epidemiologic studies may be necessary to recognize an association between illness and a given work environment because that environment results in only a small increase in the incidence of a relatively common disease (e.g., chronic obstructive lung disease); such an association will not be recognized without systematic observation of the respiratory health of a large number of workers. Also, the long latency between certain exposures and effects (e.g., asbestos exposure and bronchogenic carcinoma) may obscure the association. New substances or new combinations of familiar substances may

Table 12-1. Purposes for Medical Monitoring

- I. Epidemiologic Studies
  - A. Determine types of risk to health associated with work environment
    1. Detect a new or previously unrecognized condition
    2. Establish that increased risk of illness is present for a group thought not to be at risk
    3. Demonstrate an increased risk for a common illness associated with a given exposure (i.e., a nonspecific effect of exposure)
  - B. Clarify the relationship between exposure and effect
    1. Quantify the dose–response relationship
    2. Identify interactions between exposures and/or host characteristics that modify the dose–response relationship (including biologic synergism among multiple exposures and host characteristics predisposing to adverse effects due to exposure)
  - C. Evaluate the effectiveness of environmental controls to reduce adverse health consequences
- II. Screening for Case Finding
  - A. Detect and intervene to reverse or minimize adverse health consequences of exposure for affected individuals
  - B. Detect workers with conditions predisposing to future clinical impairment

produce effects not easily predicted from previous experience or analogy. Insight into the relationship between health effects and cumulative dose or rate of exposure to toxic agents can often be gained only through careful medical monitoring in coordination with environmental and biological sampling. Host factors predisposing to illness and interactions among multiple exposures may modify dose–response relationships derived from other worker groups, necessitating continued medical monitoring to evaluate the effectiveness of environmental control programs thought to be adequate to prevent adverse health effects. Focusing more on the individual, screening for case finding seeks to identify workers who have a condition that is either clinically important itself or is predictive of a future impairment. Detection of such conditions is important if intervention, such as removal from further exposure, can prevent, reverse, or minimize impairment.[4] As mentioned above, medical screening should not be used as a replacement for a good environmental control program, but is particularly necessary in evaluating the effectiveness of environmental controls in preventing occupationally related lung disease in the presence of a lack of precise understanding of the relationship between exposure to toxic agents and adverse health effects.

EPIDEMIOLOGIC STUDIES

Important Considerations in Design

Although most industrial medical monitoring programs will be primarily designed for purposes of case finding unless specifically conducted as research projects, physicians involved in monitoring programs should be aware of the principles of epidemiologic studies. These principles, as applied to the occupational setting, have recently been reviewed.[5] When designing a medical monitoring program for epidemiologic investigations, one must clearly establish the magnitude of effect one wishes to be able to detect. The statistical power of a study is the probability that a significant difference between two study groups (e.g., workers with high and low exposure) will be found, given that a true difference of a certain magnitude is present between the populations of interest. Among the factors that determine the power are the number of subjects in the two study groups; if insufficient numbers of workers are studied, a large difference between workers with high and low exposures may go undetected. For example, an average yearly decline in forced expiratory volume in one second (FEV_1), which is 30 ml in excess of that associated with aging alone, might be considered important to detect in a working group with exposure to a respiratory hazard. This excess decrement would result in an average loss of 900 ml in a 30-year working period, a clinically important loss. If the FEV_1 of workers with an average of two years exposure to the hazard were compared to that of a control group, approximately 1090 workers and 1090 controls would be needed to result in an 80% probability (power) of finding a difference between the two groups significant at the 5% level.[6] If a difference of 15 ml per year were considered important, four times as many subjects would be needed to achieve the same power. One should plan a monitoring program with adequate power to detect a difference considered important, or the finding of no significant difference between exposed and control groups may be misleading. Longitudinal (follow-up) studies may be more efficient in detecting effects of exposure than single comparisons (cross-sectional studies) if the average duration of exposure is short. Table 12-2 gives the number of subjects needed to have an 80% power of detecting a significant difference between workers and controls if the workers have a true excess loss of 30 ml per year in FEV_1. The follow-up study is much more efficient if workers have been exposed for an average of four years or less. It is also useful to note that performing measurements of FEV_1 every six months does not improve the efficiency of the longitudinal study much over that of yearly testing. However, serious errors of interpretation of follow-up studies can occur if testing is performed only at the beginning and end of a period of observation, since spurious results at either point may markedly

Table 12-2. Number of Subjects in Each of Two Groups (Workers and Control) Needed to Detect an Increased Annual Loss of FEV_1 of 30 ml per year in the Workers Compared to Controls with Significance level of 0.05 and Power of 0.8[a]

Length of Follow-up or Exposure (Years)	Interval Between Measurements			
	6 Months	1 Year	Beginning and End Only	Single Cross-Sectional Study Only
1	530	530	530	4356
2	128	153	153	1089
4	45	53	59	272
8	30	32	36	68

[a] Adapted from Berry G: Longitudinal observations. Their usefulness and limitations with special reference to the forced expiratory volume. Bull Physiopathol Respir 10:643–655, 1974.

affect the calculated rate of change of the variable under study. Large but unexplained variation in pulmonary function may be observed at certain times in a group of workers being followed closely using standardized equipment and methods.[7]

Interpretation

When interpreting results of epidemiologic studies of workers exposed to potential respiratory hazards, one should bear in mind that statistical significance is not synonymous with clinical significance.[3,8] If large enough sample sizes are studied, very small differences (e.g., in mean FEV_1) between an exposed and a control group may be statistically significant. Calculation of a 95% confidence interval for the difference in means may allow more thoughtful interpretation of whether the largest likely difference between the two groups has any practical significance. On the other hand, lack of an overall effect of exposure does not necessarily mean that some individuals are not adversely affected. Clinically important losses in function in a few subjects may be obscured by nearly normal values for the majority of the group. This has been demonstrated in groups of cigarette smokers.[9] One should consider the distribution of values of the variable of interest, as well as group trends, if important effects are not to be missed.

SCREENING FOR CASE FINDING

The variability of physiologic response among workers in the same environment is one reason why screening for case finding may be needed, even though workplace concentrations of toxic substances are maintained at levels thought to be safe. Table 12-3 lists reasons for variability in health effects among workers. The exposure may vary markedly between individuals despite similar working conditions[10] and the biologic response to the same dose of toxic material may vary due to intrinsic differences either genetically determined[11] or

Table 12-3. Reasons for Variable Responses Among Workers in the Same Workplace Environment

A. Variable Dose of Toxic Agent
   1. Variations in concentration of toxic agent within workplace
   2. Exposures to same agent from nonoccupational sources (e.g., hobbies)
   3. Previous exposures to same agent
   4. Different contact or absorption of agent due to physiologic factors
      a. Variations in work load (e.g., leading to variations in minute ventilation)
      b. Differences in pharmacokinetics of absorption, distribution, metabolism, or excretion
      c. Preexisting pathology which affects the dose absorbed
B. Variable Response to Same Dose
   1. Intrinsic host factors (genetic, immunologic)
   2. Presence of other diseases
   3. Interaction among multiple exposures, including drugs
   4. Sensitization (perhaps from brief exposures to high concentrations)

acquired from previous exposures or illnesses. Even if a generally safe level of a given substance exists, continuous maintenance of workplace concentrations at or below that concentration may not always be possible. Early detection of health effects through medical monitoring may be necessary to adequately protect all workers from occupational lung disease.

Basic Principles

Comprehensive discussions of the rationale and limitations of health screening for case finding in the general population have recently been published.[12,13] The same basic principles apply to screening programs undertaken in the occupational setting. These principles are outlined in Table 12-4. There should be reasonable agreement in the medical community that the condition sought by screening is an important health problem or is predictive of future impairment. Conditions of uncertain significance (or with uncertain relationships to workplace exposures) should be investigated with epidemiologic studies, but not targeted in medical monitoring for early detection of disease.[3] For

Table 12-4. Principles of Screening for Case Finding[a]

A. The condition sought should be suitable for screening.
   1. It should be an important health problem with serious consequences to the individual or society if undetected and untreated.
   2. It should have a preclinical (latent) phase of reasonable duration during which it can be detected by screening methods.
   3. The natural history should be known.
      a. The probability of progression of "early" stages should be known.
      b. There should be an accepted policy on whom to treat.
   4. The prevalence of the condition should be high enough to avoid excessive false positive screening results relative to true cases (a reasonable predictive value of a positive screening test).

B. A suitable screening test should be available.
   1. The test should be acceptable to the population screened (i.e., safe, not overly unpleasant or time consuming).
   2. The test should be practical (simple to administer, rapid, and low cost).
   3. The test should have adequate reproducibility.
   4. The test should have high validity for detecting the condition sought with the "normal range" reasonably well defined.

C. A suitable intervention (treatment) should be available.
   1. It should alter the course and prognosis of the condition and be more effective if given during the latent or early symptomatic phase of the condition.
   2. It should be acceptable to the screened population so that compliance of cases is adequate to result in an improvement in the outcome.

D. A suitable program should be developed.
   1. It should be systematic and continuous, not a single survey or haphazardly periodic.
   2. Adequate facilities for diagnostic follow-up of screen test positives and for treatment of cases should be available.
   3. It should be cost effective relative to the usual methods of detection and treatment of the condition.
   4. It should be evaluated using an adequate measure of outcome.
   5. Any harm caused by false positive and false negative screening results should be outweighed by the beneficial effects of the program.

[a] Adapted from Wilson JMG, Jungner G: Principles of screening for disease. WHO Public Health Papers, #34, 1968.

example, mucus hypersecretion may or may not be associated with functional impairment of lung function and by itself is not a good predictor of future impairment.[14] Although this finding may be an important indicator of occupational lung disease, by itself it would not be a suitable target for screening. The condition sought should also have a latent or preclinical period during which it can be detected by screening tests before overt signs or symptoms are present. The natural history of the condition should be reasonably well understood; if this is not the case, many "early" cases, which would never have progressed to actual clinically important illness, will be detected by screening and unnecessarily subjected to further diagnostic or treatment procedures. The prevalence of the condition in the screened population should be high enough to prevent excessive numbers of false positive screening results relative to true cases. A screening test is not meant to be fully diagnostic, and further evaluation is usually necessary to establish the diagnosis and determine the proper intervention.[15] A screening test will therefore identify some workers as possibly having the condition sought who, on further evaluation, do not have it (false positives) and will miss some workers who actually have the condition (false negatives). The predictive value of a positive screening test is the proportion of those with a positive screening result who actually have the condition sought.[16] This proportion depends on the prevalence of the condition in the screened group and can be surprisingly small, even for a test with a low false positive rate. Table 12-5 shows the predictive value of a positive test for screening, which correctly identifies 95% of those with disease (95% sensitivity) and 95% of those without disease (95% specificity). If the prevalence is 1 in 100 workers, only 16% of those with a positive screening result would be found to actually have the condition. In some instances the cost and morbidity associated with further evaluation of workers with positive results who do not have the condition may outweigh the benefits to those true cases identified.

Screening Tests

The screening test employed must be acceptable to the workers in terms of safety, comfort, and time if adequate participation is to be obtained. It should also be relatively simple to administer, especially if done at the work site, and of reasonable cost. It should be objective, that is, relatively independent of cooperation and personal bias (on the part of the worker or the technician performing the test). The test should not only give reproducible results if repeated, but should have high validity in detecting the condition sought. The

Table 12-5. Predictive Value of a Positive Screening Test with 95% Sensitivity and 95% Specificity

Prevalence of Condition Sought in Screened Population	Predictive Value of Positive Test (%)
50/100	95
1/100	16
1/1000	2

tests most commonly used in medical monitoring for lung disease are questionnaires, chest radiographs, and basic spirometric measures of ventilatory function. These tests satisfy the criteria just described reasonably well. Standardized methods for administering these tests have recently been described.[17–19] Standardized methodology improves the reproducibility and facilitates comparison of results from groups studied by different investigators. Standardized questionnaires with clearly defined guidelines for administration are vital if symptom prevalence in two or more groups are to be compared.[20] Even with standardized techniques the questionnaire remains a subjective instrument, and responses are greatly influenced by the attitude and understanding of the workers interviewed.[21] Answers to standardized questions should not be used as the sole criteria for decisions on intervention for individuals, but may suggest that further diagnostic investigation is warranted. When specific types of responses to workplace exposures are suspected, specialized nonstandardized questions may be used to identify workers who should receive further diagnostic evaluation.[22] Interpretation of chest radiographs is also subjective. Detection and quantification of the severity of pneumoconiosis depends on the technical quality of the radiograph as well as the training and experience of the reader.[23,24] Films used for medical surveillance of workers exposed to substances causing any form of pneumoconiosis should be read independently by two readers and if the interpretations differ importantly, a third independent reading should be obtained and the consensus interpretation accepted. One of the two initial readers should be certified as an expert (NIOSH "B" reader) in interpreting radiographs for pneumoconiosis using the standardized ILO 1980 classification.[17] Among simple tests of pulmonary function, spirometric measurement of the forced vital capacity (FVC) and the FEV_1 provides the most reproducible results.[25] The average intrasubject coefficient of variation (the standard deviation of a series of values divided by the mean value) for the FEV_1 is approximately 3% in healthy persons, but may be higher for those with obstructive lung disease.[26,27] Measurements of respiratory flows at lower lung volumes and measurements derived from the single-breath oxygen test or the helium-oxygen forced expiratory maneuver are less reproducible and have as yet not been shown to be predictive of later clinically significant reduction in ventilatory capacity.[25]

Although reproducibility is a necessary characteristic of a test that is useful in screening, it is not synonymous with validity, which is the ability to correctly identify those with the condition sought. A test may reproducibly measure a variable that is not an important determinant of current or future health status. For many biologic variables there is no absolute separation between values that indicate an important impairment of health and values that do not. Spirometric measures of pulmonary function show a rather large variation among healthy adults of the same race, sex, age, and size. The predicted value for an individual is only an estimate of the average value for healthy persons. Any arbitrary selection of a "range of normal" will result in a certain proportion of healthy persons being classified as "abnormal." For spirometry the lower limit of normal has often been set at 80% of the predicted value derived from studies of nonsmokers with no history of pulmonary disease or current respiratory symptoms. However, the proportion of older healthy adults classified as abnormal by this procedure is greater than the proportion of younger healthy adults misclassified.[28] Approximately 5% of healthy persons under age 39 years will have values of FEV_1 below 80% of the appropriate predicted value, but nearly 12% of healthy persons over the age of 60 years have values below this level. Recently the recommendation has been made that the lower limit of normal for ventilatory function (e.g., FEV_1) be calculated by subtracting a fixed value from the appropriate predicted value.[29] This method, while not absolutely statistically correct, is an improvement over the fixed percentage of predicted method and will reduce the age bias just described. This is important if a larger proportion of older workers are not to be unfairly excluded from certain jobs due to "abnormally low" spirometry. Another factor affecting spirometry that has not been adequately addressed is race. All of the prediction equations for ventilatory function used most commonly in the United States are based on studies of white subjects only. Several studies have indicated that the FEV_1 and FVC of healthy blacks are lower than those of healthy whites of the same age and standing height.[30–32] Although deriving the predicted value for blacks by applying a fixed percentage reduction to the appropriate values for whites is probably not entirely accurate,[33] using 0.85 to 0.90 of the predicted value of FVC and FEV_1 for whites as the predicted value for blacks of the same age and height is a reasonable approximation based on the results of the studies cited. This approximation will at least reduce the proportion of otherwise healthy blacks who will be classified as having "abnormal" spirometry and thus possibly inappropriately excluded from jobs with potential exposures to respiratory hazards.

Periodic Observation of Lung Function

Periodic measurement of lung function provides an estimate of the rate of change of various measures over time. As discussed above, this may provide a more efficient means of detecting an effect of an environmental agent on the pulmonary function of a group of workers than cross-sectional epidemiologic studies. For individuals the rate of loss of function during a period of observation offers the potential of detecting important responses before significant loss of function has occurred. The current Occupational Safety and Health Administration Standard for Occupational Exposure to Cotton Dust requires periodic pulmonary function testing of workers with an assessment at each examination by a physician of whether a significant change has occurred since the previous examination.[34] The examinations must be conducted at least yearly and for workers with acute decrements in FEV_1 of 5% or more during a single workday the examination must be repeated each six months. Presumably, if a decline in function more rapid than "expected" is observed, appropriate diagnostic procedures and/or intervention (e.g., reduction or cessation of dust exposure) will be undertaken. Unfortunately, interpretation of changes in lung function over relatively short periods of time is difficult. Individuals may show marked variability of loss in FEV_1 for no apparent reason.[8] Also measurement errors make estimates of the rate of decline of even a reproducible measurement like the FEV_1 rather inaccurate when based on observations for less than two years.[6] Even if an individual's rate of decline were known accurately, there is a large variation in annual rate of decline in FEV_1 among healthy persons; rather large deviations from the average expected rate of decline are necessary before one can be confident that the observed rate of decline is abnormally rapid. Predicted values for annual rate of decline in FEV_1 have not been as extensively documented as those for the FEV_1 itself and estimates made from cross-sectional studies may be misleading when applied to a cohort of workers being followed for evidence of an adverse effect of workplace exposure.[7,35] At present, the rate of decline of lung function over a relatively short period of time must be considered a screening test that may be helpful in identifying workers who are experiencing an adverse effect from workplace exposure, but additional diagnostic information (such as a complete medical history) and perhaps confirmation of the rate of decline by repeat testing is usually necessary to properly interpret this test for an individual.

Intervention

Since the purpose of medical monitoring for case finding is to detect abnormalities at a stage in which intervention will improve the prognosis, a suitable means of intervention must be available if screening is to be worthwhile. For occupational illnesses in which progression of severity is closely related to cumulative dose of the toxic agent, removal from exposure at an early stage may provide a safe and effective treatment. Coal workers' pneumoconiosis has been shown to have relatively little effect on lung function when detected in its radiographic early stages, but may cause severe impairment and early death if it progresses to the complicated form.[36] Progression to the complicated form from the earlier stages (simple pneumoconiosis) almost never occurs unless the radiograph has reached category 2 on the ILO classification system of 0 to 3.[37] Radiographic category of simple coal workers' pneumoconiosis is closely related to cumulative exposure to coal mine dust and does not progress after dust exposure is terminated.[38] Therefore, medical monitoring using the chest radiograph and removal to less dusty conditions of all miners who have progressed to category I penumoconiosis seems a fully rational and probably effective means of preventing serious impairment of lung function due to coal workers' pneumoconiosis. For other pneumoconioses, the case is less clear. Exposure to asbestos may produce an interstitial fibrosis that progresses even after exposure is terminated, and it has not been clearly established that removal from exposure at an "early" stage judged by the severity of the radiographic abnormality will alter the course of the illness. However, some evidence has been obtained that progression of radiographic abnormalities and excessive loss of ventilatory capacity are related to the cumulative dose of inhaled asbestos fibers.[39] For this reason the recommendation to remove workers with radiographic signs of fibrosis from further exposure to asbestos has been made.[40]

Efforts to limit cumulative dose of asbestos may also be helpful in reducing the risk for later development of a malignancy. Both epidemiologic and pathologic evidence exists that the risk of malignancy increases with increasing cumulative dose of asbestos fibers.[41,42]

The role of medical monitoring in programs to prevent diseases of the airways induced by agents encountered in the workplace is less certain. Improvement toward normal values of certain measures of pulmonary function has been shown to occur in cigarette smokers who stop smoking[43] and an excessive annual rate of decline in FEV_1 may return toward the rate expected for nonsmokers following the cessation of smoking.[9] These results would suggest that airways disease induced by certain workplace exposures might be also reversed or prevented from progressing if detected "early" and further exposure were reduced or eliminated. The acute decrement in FEV_1 over the workshift and the symptoms of chest tightness during work experienced by some workers exposed to cotton dust appear related to the concentration of cotton dust in the workplace.[44,45] These acute effects are reversible with removal from exposure, but the relationship between acute effects and any chronic effects of cotton dust is not clear. It has not been established that an acute response of either type is a good predictor of a propensity for chronic loss of ventilatory function with continued exposure or that the lack of an acute response indicates a low risk for any chronic effects of exposure. In one prospective study workers who continued to experience chest tightness on the first day of the work week (byssinosis) did show an increased annual loss of FEV_1 compared to asymptomatic workers or workers whose symptoms spontaneously remitted during the period of observation.[45] However, in another follow-up study development of byssinotic symptoms was not associated with an increased rate of decline in FEV_1.[44] Neither could the magnitude of acute changes in FEV_1 over the workshift be related to the rate of decline in FEV_1 during the period of observation. Whether removal of workers with acute symptoms or changes in ventilatory function over the workshift as soon as these findings are discovered is useful and necessary in protecting workers exposed to cotton dust from any chronic impairment of lung function remains to be determined by careful epidemiologic studies. The usefulness of early removal from exposure of workers with occupational asthma has been suggested by studies of workers exposed to dust from western red cedar. Symptomatic workers have been shown to have increased airway responsiveness to nonspecific stimuli (the parasympathetic agonist methacholine) and reduced ventilatory function.[46] After removal from exposure only one half of these workers become asymptomatic and had a significant improvement in pulmonary function after three years of follow-up. Those who retained their symptoms were found to have had a longer period of symptoms prior to diagnosis than those who became asymptomatic. This suggests that earlier recognition of specific symptoms and earlier removal from exposure might improve the prognosis. Further follow-up of these workers is underway to investigate this possibility.

Evaluation of a Screening Program

Even if a suitable intervention is available a screening program should be evaluated for its effectiveness in achieving a net beneficial effect in the screened population and its efficiency relative to other means of delivering health services.[47] The measure used to evaluate the beneficial effect of a screening program should be an adequate indicator of outcome such as specific mortality or morbidity, not merely the number of cases (or potential cases) detected by screening. In a recently reported controlled study of multiphasic health checkups including annual chest radiograph, spirometry, and symptom questionnaire, there was no significant difference in mortality or disability rates from respiratory diseases between the control and study group after 11 years of follow-up.[48] This study may reflect a lack of specific and effective intervention for respiratory disease in the general population. Although this limitation might not apply to a workforce with exposure to a specific toxic agent, the need to evaluate outcome and not process is well illustrated.

One must also consider the adverse effects of screening given in Table 12-6 in determining the net effect on the screened population. Not only do false positive screening tests result in unnecessary costs and sometimes morbidity from the follow-up diagnostic procedures employed, but just labeling a worker as diseased can have negative consequences. Days of illness absence increased for workers labeled as hypertensive by a screening program, even among those whose hypertension was judged by their private physician not to require any treatment.[49] A similar effect might also occur among asymptomatic workers labeled as abnormal due to pulmonary function values below the predicted value.

Even an effective screening program should only be undertaken if it represents the best use of available resources. Other aspects of a complete program for prevention and control of occupational lung disease are discussed elsewhere[50] and generally must compete with medical monitoring for limited funds. Medical monitoring can be made more efficient by measures listed in Table 12-7. Specific application of these measures will depend on the type of exposure and the potential health effects.

Table 12-6. Potential Adverse Effects of a Screening Program

1. Consequences of false positive screening tests
   a. Morbidity associated with follow-up diagnostic procedures
   b. Financial burden
   c. Negative psychological impact
   d. Treatment of those who would never have progressed to important clinical impairment without treatment
2. Consequences of false negative screening tests
   a. Loss of confidence in medical care system
   b. False sense of security resulting in important symptoms of disease being ignored
3. Consequences of true positive screening tests
   a. Morbidity associated with the labeling a worker as "diseased"

Table 12-7. Measures to Increase the Efficiency of a Screening Program

A. Target a group at high risk
   1. Define group by exposure or other characteristic associated with the condition sought
   2. Prescreen with simple and safe test (e.g., questionnaire) to identify those potentially at increased risk
B. Increase the specificity of the screening test
   1. Use an intrinsically more specific test
   2. Use multiple tests in series
C. Optimize the frequency of periodic testing
   1. Consider factors which influence the optimum frequency of screening
      a. Duration of the preclinical phase
      b. Lead time gained by screening
      c. Variability of exposure concentrations
      d. Importance of cumulative dose and peak exposures
      e. Relationship between prognosis and stage at which treatment is initiated

MEDICAL MONITORING FOR RESPIRATORY SYSTEM CANCER

Medical monitoring for one important type of occupational lung disease has not yet been discussed. Certain occupational exposures result in an increased risk for development of cancer of the respiratory system.[51] The same basic principles described above apply to screening for cancer, and specific considerations have been described in detail elsewhere.[13,15,52] Uncontrolled trials using chest radiographs with or without sputum cytologic examination for screening have generally shown no net improvement in mortality from lung cancer in the screened group,[53–55] although one study suggested an improved case fatality rate for screen-detected cancers.[56] A large-scale randomized controlled trial in a health maintenance organization showed no difference in mortality from lung cancer after 11 years of follow-up between the study group receiving yearly chest radiographs and the control group receiving standard medical care.[48] The lack of an improved prognosis for lung cancer detected by chest radiograph as an isolated round lesion is consistent with this result.[57] This lack of a demonstrated beneficial effect of screening for nonoccupational lung cancer has led to a questioning of the applicability of medical monitoring for lung cancer in the occupational setting.[58] Currently large controlled trials of screening for lung cancer in high-risk groups (male cigarette smokers over age 45 years) are being conducted at the Mayo Clinic, the Johns Hopkins Hospital, and the Memorial Sloan-Kettering Cancer Center. The Mayo Clinic study group is screened with a chest radiograph, sputum cytologic examination, and questionnaire every four months. Recently published results show no statistically significant difference for mortality from lung cancer between the study and control groups.[59] These studies do show that lung cancer can be detected in asymptomatic subjects by acceptable screening procedures and that a larger proportion of lung cancers detected by screening are in "earlier" stages than those not detected by screening.[60] One must also consider that like all screening programs, those for cancer may have adverse effects. False positive screening tests occur for both chest radiographs and cytologic examinations.[53,61–63] Even with all currently available diagnostic techniques, some patients will be subjected to major surgical procedures for benign conditions.[64] In addition to the potential negative impact on individual workers, screening may well reduce resources used for preventive programs such as worker education and reduction of environmental concentrations of toxic materials. A recent review of the efficacy of screening for lung cancer in workers exposed to asbestos concludes that even for this relatively high-risk group, screening is unlikely to produce significant health benefits.[65] The authors suggest that funds would be better spent on programs to control cigarette smoking. Even in a group of workers with an established increased risk for lung cancer, careful analysis suggests that at present a screening program is unlikely to provide a beneficial effect on the health of workers.

SUMMARY

Medical monitoring for lung disease in the workplace is useful for epidemiologic research into the relationship between exposure and disease and for detecting individuals with adverse consequences from workplace exposures (cases). Different considerations apply to screening programs designed for these two purposes. Not all respiratory conditions are suitable as targets for workplace screening programs designed to detect cases and all screening programs should be evaluated for their effectiveness in providing a net beneficial effect on the health of the workforce. At present, screening for lung cancer appears unwarranted, but use of questionnaires, chest radiographs, and spirometry to detect workers with pneumoconiosis or occupational airways disease may be useful in preventing or minimizing functional impairment. Even a screening program with beneficial effects should only be undertaken if it represents the best use of limited resources for safeguarding and improving the health of workers.

ACKNOWLEDGMENT

This work was supported in part by a Fellowship from the Parker B. Francis Foundation.

REFERENCES

1. ATS Statement (S Brooks, Chmn): Surveillance for respiratory hazards in the occupational setting, Am Rev Respir Dis 126:952–956, 1982.
2. Environmental and health monitoring in occupational health. WHO Tech Rep Ser 535, 1973.

3. Early detection of health impairment in occupational exposure to health hazards. WHO Tech Rep Ser 571, 1975.
4. Wilson JMG, Jungner G: Principles of screening for disease. WHO, Public Health Papers #34, Geneva, 1968.
5. Lebowitz MD: Epidemiological recognition of occupational pulmonary diseases. Clin Chest Med 2(3):305–316, 1981.
6. Berry G: Longitudinal observations. Their usefulness and limitations with special reference to the forced expiratory volume. Bull Physiopathol Respir 10:643–655, 1974.
7. Diem JE, Jones RN, Hendrick DJ, et al: Five-year longitudinal study of workers employment in a new toluene diisocyanate manufacturing plant. Am Rev Respir Dis 126:420–428, 1982.
8. Boehlecke BA, Merchant JA: The use of pulmonary function testing and questionnaires as epidemiologic tools in the study of occupational lung disease. Chest 79(Suppl):114–122, 1981.
9. Fletcher C, Peto R, Tinker C, Speizer F: The Natural History of Chronic Bronchitis and Emphysema. London, Oxford University Press, 1976, pp 83, 129.
10. Zielhuis RL: Biological monitoring. Scand J Work Environ Health 4:1–8, 1978.
11. Menkes HA, Cohen BH, Levy DA, et al: Genetic factors in chronic obstructive lung disease. Bull Eur Physiopathol Respir 16(Suppl):357–364, 1980.
12. Canadian Task Force on the Periodic Health Examination: The periodic health examination. Can Med Assoc J 121:1193–1254, 1979.
13. American Cancer Society guidelines for the cancer-related checkup. Recommendations and rationale. CA 30(4):194–240, 1980.
14. Ref 9, p 149.
15. Commission on Chronic Illness: Chronic Illness in the United States, Vol 1. Cambridge, MA, Harvard University Press, 1957.
16. Vecchio TJ: Predictive value of a single diagnostic test in unselected populations. N Engl J Med 274:1171–73, 1966.
17. Occupational Safety and Health Series No. 22 (Rev), Guidelines for the Use of ILO International Classification of Radiographs of Pneumoconioses, Revised Edition, 1980, International Labor Office, Geneva, Switzerland, 1980.
18. Epidemiology Standardization Project, Benjamin Ferris, Principal Investigator. Am Rev Respir Dis 118(6) Part 2, Dec 1980.
19. Gardner RM, Glindmeyer HW, Hankinson JL: Standardization of lung function measurements: Spirometry and field testing. In: Occupational Lung Diseases: Research Approaches and Methods, eds. Weill H, Turner-Warwick M. New York, Marcel Dekker, 1980.
20. Samet JM: A historical and epidemiologic perspective on respiratory symptom questionnaires. Am J Epidemiol 108:435–446, 1978.
21. Samet J, Speizer F, Gaensler F: Questionnaire reliability and validity in asbestos exposed workers. Bull Physiopathol Respir 14:177–188, 1978.
22. Brooks SM: The evaluation of occupational airways disease in the laboratory and workplace. (Symposium Proceedings on Occupational Immunologic Lung Disease). J Allergy Clin Immunol 70:56–66, 1982.
23. Reger RB, Morgan WKC: On the factors influencing consistency in the radiographic diagnosis of pneumoconiosis. Am Rev Respir Dis 102:905–915, 1970.
24. Reger RB, Smith CA, Kibelstis JA, Morgan WKC: The effect of film quality and other factors on the roentgenographic categorization of coal workers' pneumoconiosis. Am J Roentgenol 115:462–472, 1972.

25. Becklake MR, Permutt S: Evaluation of tests of lung function for "screening" for early detection of chronic obstructive lung disease. In: The Lung in the Transition Between Health and Disease, eds. Macklem PT, Permutt S. New York, Marcel Dekker, 1979.
26. Cochrane GM, Prieto F, Clark TJH: Intrasubject variability of maximal expiratory flow volume curve. Thorax 32:171–176, 1977.
27. Hruby J, Butler J: Variability of routine pulmonary function tests. Thorax 30:548–553, 1975.
28. Miller A, Thornton JC, Smith H Jr, Morris JF: Spirometric "abnormality" in a normal male reference population: Further analysis of the 1971 Oregon survey. Am J Ind Med 1:55–68, 1980.
29. Crapo RO, Morris AH, Gardner RM: Reference spirometric values using techniques and equipment that meet ATS recommendations. Am Rev Respir Dis 123:659–664, 1981.
30. Rossiter CE, Weill H: Ethnic differences in lung function: Evidence for proportional differences. Int J Epidemiol 3:55–61, 1974.
31. Lapp NL, Amandus HE, Hall R, Morgan WKC: Lung volumes and flow rates in black and white subjects. Thorax 29:185–188, 1974.
32. Lanese RR, Keller MD, Foley MF, Underwood EH: Differences in pulmonary function tests among whites, blacks, and American Indians in a textile company. J Occup Med 20:39–44, 1978.
33. Schoenberg JB, Beck GJ, Bouhuys A: Growth and decay of pulmonary function in healthy blacks and whites. Respir Physiol 33:367–393, 1978.
34. Department of Labor, Occupational Safety and Health Administration: Occupational exposure to cotton dust. Final mandatory occupational safety and health standards. Fed Regist 27350–27463, June 23, 1978.
35. Glindmeyer HW, Diem JE, Jones RN, Weill H: Non-comparability of longitudinally and cross-sectionally determined annual change in spirometry. Am Rev Respir Dis 125:544–548, 1982.
36. Morgan WKC, Handelsman L, Kibelslis J, et al: Ventilatory capacity and lung volumes of US coal miners. Am Rev Respir Dis 113:531–559, 1974.
37. McLintock JS, Rae S, Jacobsen M: The attack rate of progressive massive fibrosis in British coal miners. In: Inhaled Particles, III, ed. Walton WH. Surrey, Unwin, 1971, p 933.
38. Jacobsen M: New data on the relationship between simple pneumoconiosis and exposure to coal mine dust. Chest 78(2)(Suppl):408–410, 1980.
39. Jones RM, Diem JE, Gibson JC, et al: Progression of asbestos radiographic abnormalities: Relationships to measures of dust exposure and annual decline in lung function. Am Rev Respir Dis 119(Suppl):224, 1979.
40. Weill H: Basis for clinical decision making. Chest 78(2):382–383, 1980.
41. Selikoff IJ, Lee DHK: Asbestos and Disease. New York, Academic Press, 1978.
42. Whitwell F, Scott J, Grimshaw M: Relationship between Occupations and asbestos-fibre content of the lungs in patients with pleural mesothelionia, lung cancer and other diseases. Thorax 32:377–386, 1977.
43. Cherniak RM, McCarthy DS: Reversibility of abnormalities of pulmonary function. In: The Lung in the Transition Between Health and Disease, eds. Machlem PT, Permutt S. New York, Marcel Dekker, 1979.
44. Berry G, McKerrow CB, Molyneux MKB, et al: A study of the acute and chronic changes in ventilatory capacity of workers in Lancashire cotton mills. Br J Ind Med 30:25–36, 1973.

45. Fox AJ, Tombleson JBL, Watt A, Wilkie AG: A survey of respiratory disease in cotton operatives. Part I. Symptoms and ventilation test results. Br J Ind Med 30:42–47, 1973.
46. Chan-Yeung M, Lam S, Koener S: Clinical features and natural history of occupational asthma due to western red cedar (*Thuja plicata*). Am J Med 72:411–415, 1982.
47. Sackett DL: Evaluation of health services. In: Public Health and Preventive Medicine, 11th ed, ed. Last J. New York, Appleton-Century-Crofts, 1980.
48. Dales LG, Friedman GD, Collen MF: Evaluating periodic multiphasic health checkups: A controlled trial. J Chronic Dis 32(5):385–404, 1979.
49. Haynes RB, Sakett DL, Taylor DW, et al: Increased absenteeism from work after detection and labeling of hypertensive patients. N Engl J Med 299:741–744, 1978.
50. Harber P: Prevention and control of occupational lung disease. Clin Chest Med 2:343–355, 1981.
51. Cole P, Goldman MB: Occupation. In: Persons at High Risk of Cancer: An Approach to Cancer Etiology and Control, ed. Fraumeni J. New York, Academic Press, 1975.
52. Cole P, Morrison AS: Basic issues in population screening for cancer. J Natl Cancer Inst 5:1263–1272, 1980.
53. Lillienfeld A, Archer PG, Barnett CH, et al: An evaluation of radiologic and cytologic screening for the early detection of lung cancer: A cooperative pilot study of the American Cancer Society and the Veterans Administration. Cancer Res 26:2083–2121, 1966.
54. Brett GZ: Earlier diagnosis and survival in lung cancer. Br Med J 4:260–262, 1969.
55. Boucot KR, Weiss W: Is curable lung cancer detected by semiannual screening? JAMA 224:1361–1365, 1973.
56. Nash FA, Morgan JM, Tomkins JG: South London lung cancer study. Br Med J 2:715–721, 1968.
57. Weiss W, Boucot KR: The prognosis of lung cancer originating as a round lesion. Am Rev Respir Dis 116:827–836, 1977.
58. Morgan WKC: Screening for occupational cancer. Chest 74:239–240, 1978.
59. Taylor WF, Fontana RS, Ulenhopp MA, Davis CS: Some results of screening for early lung cancer. Cancer 47:1114–1120, 1981.
60. Melamed MR, Flehinger BJ, Zaman MB, et al: Detection of true pathologic stage 1 lung cancer in a screening program and the effect on survival. Cancer 47:1182–1187, 1981.
61. Gryzbowski S, Coy P: Early diagnosis of carcinoma of the lung: Simultaneous screening with chest X-ray and sputum cytology. Cancer 25:113–120, 1970.
62. Stitik FP, Tockman MS: Radiographic screening in the early detection of lung cancer. Radiol Clin North Am 16:347–366, 1978.
63. Melamed M, Flehinger B, Miller D, et al: Preliminary report of the lung cancer detection program in New York. Cancer 39:369–382, 1977.
64. Baker RR, Tockman MS, Marsh BR, et al: Screening for bronchogenic cancer: The surgical experience. J Thorac Cardiovasc Surg 78:876–882, 1979.
65. McNeil BJ, Eddy DM: The costs and effects of screening for cancer among asbestos-exposed workers. J Chronic Dis 35:351–358, 1982.

13 The "Black Lung" Act: A Pitfall?

Attilio D. Renzetti, Jr.

Coal workers' pneumoconiosis as distinct from silicosis became both a recognized medical entity and a compensable disease in Great Britain in the early 1940s as a result of the comprehensive study of chronic pulmonary diseases in South Wales coal miners by the British Medical Research Council.[1] Coal workers' pneumoconiosis did not become a compensable disease in the United States until the latter half of the 1960s, with the exception of the state of Alabama which passed such legislation in 1952. The reaction to the death of 78 miners in a coal mine explosion at Farmington, West Virginia, on November 20, 1968, and a subsequent strike by most of the 40,000 miners in that state played a vital role in the passage of similar legislation not only by that state and a number of others but also by the Federal Government as the Federal Coal Mine Health and Safety Act of 1969 (Act). The Act defined the term *pneumoconiosis* to mean "a chronic dust disease of the lung and its sequelae, including respiratory and pulmonary impairments, arising out of coal mine employment." By providing the "Black Lung Benefits" the Act revived the term "black lung" which was first used in the medical literature over a hundred years ago to describe the black expectoration and deposition of black matter in the lungs of Scottish coal miners.[2] Its conversion to a legal term by Congress was unfortunate, since its legal definition did not ultimately conform to the medical definition of coal workers' pneumoconiosis, and it has come to be used by coal miners to support their impression that most, if not all, chronic respiratory impairments they might develop were due to coal workers' pneumoconiosis and thereby compensable. To compound the problem from the standpoint of medical science, the United States Congress reinforced the miners conceptions in the 1972 amendment to the Act. Here they expanded the legal definition of "black lung" to include "dust-induced" bronchitis and emphysema and further specified that a negative chest x-ray could not be used as a basis for denying compensation! This trend was carried even further with the enactment of the Black Lung Benefits Reform Act of 1977 in which eligibility for benefits was expanded to include "any respiratory or pulmonary impairment arising out of employment in or around coal mines." However, in fairness it should probably be emphasized at this point that the enormous personal, social, and economic problems created by this legislation stem as much from the rules and regulations written for its implementation as from the language in the Act itself and in its amendments. Before analyzing this legislation with respect to its intent to compensate workers' disability by their exposure to coal mine dust, a brief review of the current state of the relevant medical knowledge is in order.

Coal workers' pneumoconiosis results from the inhalation and deposition in the lung of respirable coal mine dust. The lung tissue reaction to the dust may produce coal macules, coal nodules, or progressive massive fibrosis.[3] Associated with the coal macule, especially in the higher categories of simple coal workers' pneumoconiosis, there occurs a minimally destructive process termed focal emphysema.[4] Since lung biopsy is very rarely indicated in this or other occupational lung disorders, the chest radiograph is ordinarily the only definitive method for diagnosing the presence of coal workers' pneumoconiosis in life.

Given the circumstance of exposure to respirable coal mine dust, what respiratory functional impairment, if any, can be anticipated according to the findings on a properly read and technically satisfactory chest x-ray[5] of a nonsmoking subject without evidence of any respiratory disease other than possible coal workers' pneumoconiosis? The overwhelming evidence is that the presence of the histopathologic lesions of coal workers' pneumoconiosis of insufficient extent to produce radiographic abnormalities does not result in any cardiorespiratory impairment.[6,7] Further, even those nonsmoking miners with simple coal workers' pneumoconiosis (radiographic categories 1, 2, 3), where some sophisticated tests of lung function may be abnormal, significant respiratory functional impairment hardly ever occurs.[7,8] On the other hand, miners with progressive massive fibrosis frequently, although not invariably, do sustain significant cardiorespiratory functional impairment, particularly with categories B and C.[9]

At this juncture the question may legitimately be asked, can coal mine dust damage the respiratory apparatus by mechanisms other than those associated with coal workers' pneumoconiosis? It has now been well established that exposure to coal dust may give rise to a form of chronic bronchitis called "industrial bronchitis."[8] However, this form of bronchitis is not associated with emphysema, and, although it may result in minor decrements of ventilatory capacity, it hardly ever produces clinically significant airflow limitation and is therefore not a cause of significant respiratory impairment.[7,8]

Finally, however brief, no discussion of the current state of knowledge relating coal mine dust exposure to the development of disability can be complete without reference to the single most important confounding variable that permeates this subject, namely, cigarette smoking. The best current perspective on this subject has been recently provided in an extensive review by Elmes,[10] who concluded "that dust exposure contributes little to morbidity or mortality compared with the workers' smoking habits."

From a strictly medical viewpoint the administration of the Act for the determination of eligibility for benefits can be criticized on at least four major counts. First, the diagnosis of coal workers' pneumoconiosis by x-ray was accepted without regard to the qualifications and experience of radiologists in the reading of x-ray abnormalities resulting from dust or other occupational exposures. Rereading of x-rays by experts was essentially disqualified from the determination. It should be noted that as a result of the "Black Lung Benefits Amendments of 1981," effective January 1, 1982, a second reading of x-rays is permissible. Second, the diagnosis of coal workers' pneumoconiosis by histopathology of lung tissue was equated with total disability without regard to the extent of the disease. Thereby, simple coal workers' pneumoconiosis of even category 1 was sufficient to provide eligibility for benefits. Third, respiratory functional impairment of a degree sufficient to meet certain objective criteria was attributed to coal workers' pneumoconiosis in the absence of either radiographic or histopathologic evidence of this disease. The vast majority of such cases undoubtedly had chronic obstructive pulmonary disease as a result of long-term cigarette smoking. Fourth, total disability was adjudged to be present on the basis of the results of ventilatory function tests and measurements of arterial blood gas tensions from tables of values whose validity for this purpose must be seriously questioned. Such obvious and well-known criteria for normality as age, sex, and altitude were neglected in these tables and the levels set as criteria for disability result in some normal older subjects qualifying! In this respect, it must be pointed out that revised ventilatory and arterial blood gas criteria that became effective on March 31, 1981, go a long way toward correcting previous defects.[11] However, even these standards have not met with uniform acceptance by all experts.

From the criticisms enumerated above it would have been predictable that the Act has resulted in the award of monetary benefits to a large number of coal miners who did not have coal workers' pneumoconiosis, or who had the disease without significant respiratory impairment, or who, with or without this disease, had some respiratory impairment, clinically significant or not, as a result of chronic respiratory disease unrelated to coal dust exposure, particularly cigarette smoking-induced chronic obstructive pulmonary disease. In fact, support for this view has now been documented by two studies by the General Accounting Office of the United States Government. A review by the General Accounting Office of random samples, of 200 pre-1973 black lung claims approved by the Social Security Administration and of 205 post-1973 claims approved by the Department of Labor indicated that in 88.6% and 84% of the cases, respectively, "medical evidence was not adequate to establish disability or death from black lung"![12,13]

From an economic standpoint, the cost of the "black lung" benefits program has been staggering. In the eight years from enactment, 1969 through

1977, almost 6 billion dollars were paid to 365,512 claimants who filed claims in the period.[12] The successful claimants represented 65.2% of the living miners and 74.1% of the survivors who had filed claim for benefits.[12] These figures become all the more startling from a medical view when they are compared to the results of prevalence studies of coal workers' pneumoconiosis in United States coal mines for comparable time periods. Medical examinations by the U.S. Public Health Service showed for the period of October 1969 to July 1971 an overall prevalence of almost 30%, of which 2.5% was progressive massive fibrosis in working coal miners, and the 30% figure has been judged too high due to overreading of x-rays.[6,14] Although conceded to be an underestimate, the results of the National Coal Workers Autopsy Study indicate pneumoconiosis as a cause of death in 4% of the first 1299 cases studied to date.[15] It seems obvious then that there is a large discrepancy between the number of miners judged to be disabled by coal workers' pneumoconiosis under the Act and the number that can reasonably be expected to have reliable medical evidence for the disease. Further, according to the Secretary of Labor, the more liberal eligibility criteria introduced by the 1977 amendments will result in an estimated 1.6 billion dollars to be paid in benefits for the fiscal year of 1979.[12] Even more important to consider is the estimate that legal, medical, and administrative costs have amounted to about as much as the benefits. This translates into a total cost of approximately 15 billion dollars for the entire program through 1979!

The provision of financial assistance to disabled workers by a just and equitable system would seem to be a goal with which no one can quarrel. Unfortunately the black lung program as it has operated has also resulted in the disruption of many aspects of society in coal mining communities. The denial of benefits to one miner and the granting of benefits to his neighbor or coworker when there is no substantial difference in their medical conditions leads to personal hostility toward the system and sometimes even between friends. The legal contest between claimants and coal companies serves only to strain relations between workers and management and between unions and industry. Physicians practicing in coal mining communities are put in the awkward position of being expected to help their patients gain black lung benefits when the medical evidence does not warrant such a stance. These are only some personal observations, but I suspect there may be many other adverse social effects of which I am unaware.

I believe I am correct when I say that the great majority of the community of specialists in pulmonary and occupational medicine are of the opinion that the "Black Lung Act" represents an example of how *not* to design legislation that is intended to provide worker's compensation for occupational lung diseases. Apparently, however, we have not succeeded in educating our legislators in this regard, since the past few years have seen repeated new legislation introduced in the U.S. Congress for other single occupational diseases such as asbestosis ("white lung") and byssinosis ("brown lung"). Fundamentally, there is no sound medical reasons for dealing with occupational lung diseases on a piecemeal basis. It would be preferable to design a system incorporating certain fundamental principles applicable to all occupational lung diseases. First among these would be that all disabled workers receive equal treatment under the law. Second, decisions regarding causation of any respiratory impairment should take into account both occupational and nonoccupational hazards (such as smoking, obesity, asthma, cardiovascular disease). In addition, such decisions should utilize all available scientific data, including the results of appropriate epidemiologic studies. Third, respiratory impairment should be determined by highly qualified physicians. Finally, respiratory disability should be determined by highly qualified professionals from the fields of law, economics, and education as well as the health sciences. Systems that incorporate such principles have been demonstrated to operate successfully in the United Kingdom and Quebec, Canada and have recently been recommended by the American Thoracic Society.[16] Further, these principles should be applicable to nonoccupational lung diseases as well. In addition to providing for equality under the law for disabled persons, legislation incorporating such principles should theoretically lead to a marked reduction in the use of both the medical and adversary systems and thereby to a diminution in the costs to society of current disability programs.

REFERENCES

1. Medical Research Council of Great Britain: Chronic pulmonary diseases in South Wales coal miners (1942, 1943). Med Res Counc Spec Rep Ser (Lond) 243, 244, 1943.
2. Thomson W: On black expectoration and deposition of black matter in the lungs. Med Clin Tr, 20:230, 1836.
3. Kleinerman J, Green F, Harley RA, et al: Pathology standards for coal workers' pneumoconiosis. Report of the Pneumoconiosis Committee of the College of American Pathologists to the National Institute for Occupational Safety and Health. Arch Pathol Lab Med 103:375, 1979.
4. Heppleston L: Chronic pulmonary emphysema. Am J Med 31:179, 1961.
5. Guidelines for The Use of ILO International Classification of Radiographs of Pneumoconioses. Revised Edition 1980. Occupational Safety & Health Series No. 22. International Labour Office, Geneva.
6. Morgan WKC, Lapp NL: Respiratory disease in coal miners. State of the art. Am Rev Respir Dis 113:531, 1976.
7. Rom WN, Kanner RE, Renzetti AD, et al: Respiratory disease in Utah coal miners. Am Rev Respir Dis 123:372, 1981.
8. Morgan WKC: Industrial bronchitis. Br J Ind Med 35:285, 1978.
9. Mitchell RS, ed: Physicians' Manual on Coal Workers' Pneumoconiosis and Other Chronic Respiratory Diseases Among Coal Miners. NIOSH, Washington, DC, U.S. Government Printing Office, 1981.
10. Elmes PC: Relative importance of cigarette smoking in occupational lung disease. Br J Ind Med 38:1, 1981.
11. Standards for Determining Coal Miners' Total Disability or Death Due to Pneumoconiosis. Department of Labor, Employment Standards Administration, Part V. Fed Regist 45(42):13,540, Feb 29, 1980.

12. Report to the Congress of the United States by the Comptroller General. Legislation allows black lung benefits to be awarded without adequate evidence of disability. United States General Accounting Office, HRD 80-81, July 28, 1980.
13. Ref 12, HRD-82-86, Jan 19, 1982.
14. Morgan WKC, Burgess DB, Jacobson G, et al: The prevalence of coal workers' pneumoconiosis in U.S. coal miners. Arch Environ Health 27:221, 1973.
15. Green RHY, Laqueur WA: Coal workers' pneumoconiosis. Pathol Annu Pt 2 333, 1980.
16. Disability legislation for occupational lung disease. A statement of an ad hoc committee of the American Thoracic Society. ATS News 7(3):29, Summer 1981.

Index

Page numbers followed by f *indicate figures; page numbers followed by* t *indicate tables.*